About IFPRI

The International Food Policy Research Institute (IFPRI), a research center of CGIAR, provides research-based policy solutions to sustainably reduce poverty and end hunger and malnutrition in low- and middle-income countries. IFPRI was established in 1975 to identify and analyze alternative national and international strategies and policies for meeting the food needs of the developing world, with particular emphasis on low-income countries and on the poorer groups in those countries. Partnerships, communications, capacity strengthening, and data and knowledge management are essential components for translating IFPRI's research to action and impact. The Institute's regional and country programs play a critical role in responding to demand for food policy research and in delivering holistic support to country-led development. IFPRI collaborates with partners around the world.

www.ifpri.org

About CGIAR

CGIAR is a global research partnership for a food-secure future, dedicated to transforming food, land, and water systems in a climate crisis. CGIAR science aims to reduce poverty, enhance food and nutrition security, and improve natural resources and ecosystem services. As the world's largest agricultural innovation network, its research is carried out by 15 CGIAR Centers working around the world in close collaboration with hundreds of partners, including national and regional research institutes, civil society organizations, academia, development organizations, and the private sector.

www.cgiar.org

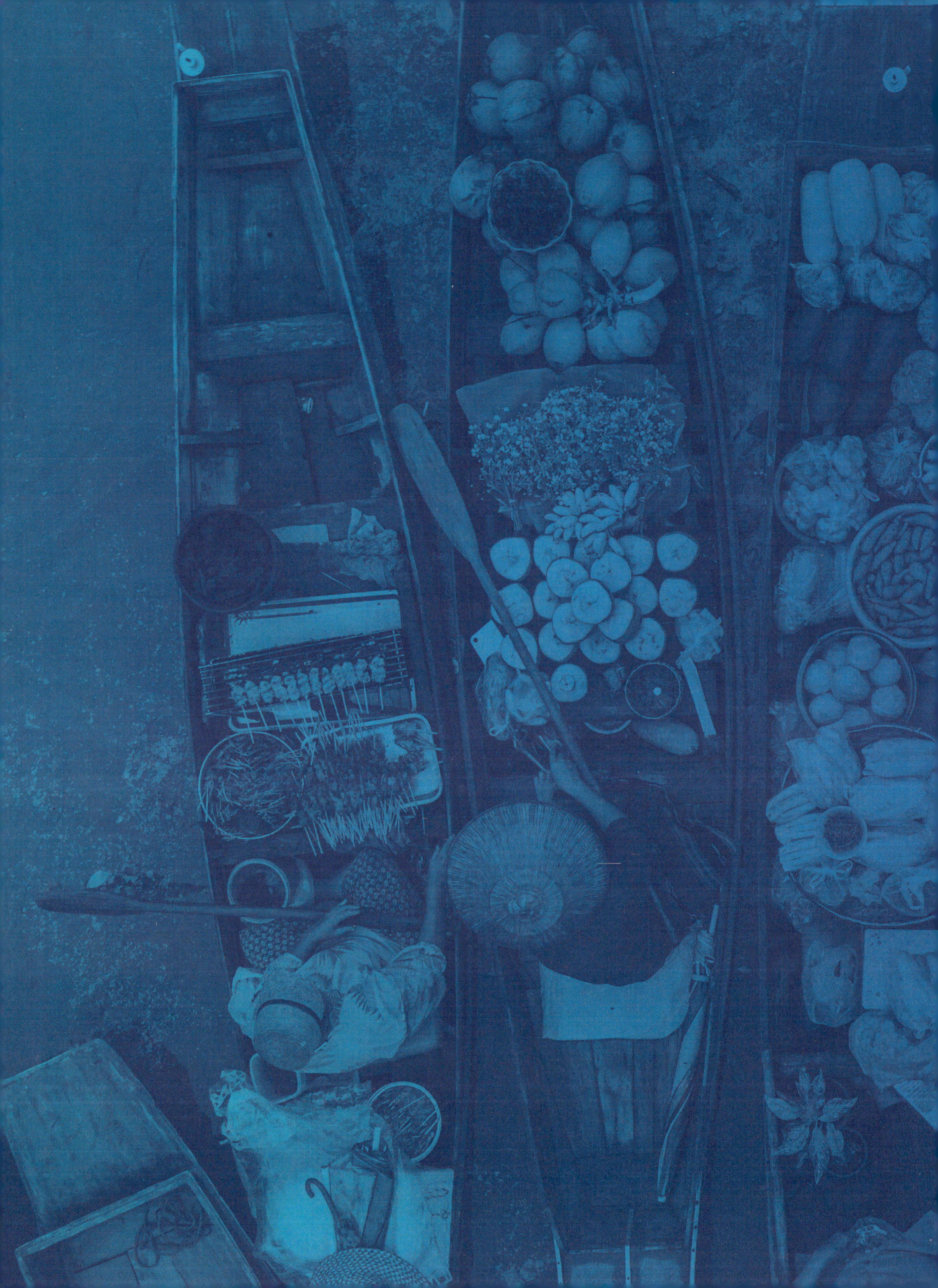

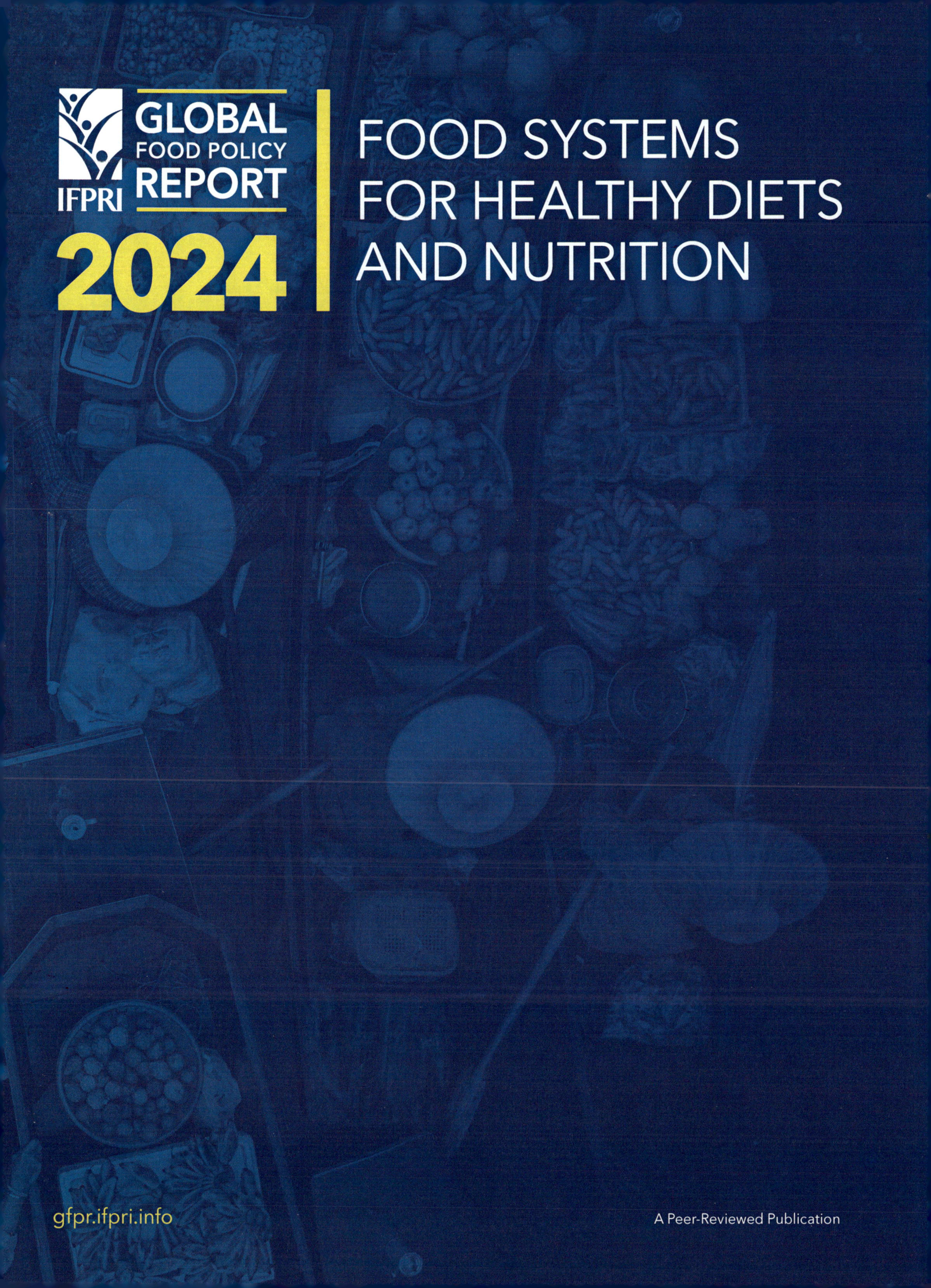

IFPRI

GLOBAL FOOD POLICY REPORT

2024

FOOD SYSTEMS FOR HEALTHY DIETS AND NUTRITION

gfpr.ifpri.info

A Peer-Reviewed Publication

RECOMMENDED CITATION: International Food Policy Research Institute. 2024. *2024 Global Food Policy Report: Food Systems for Healthy Diets and Nutrition*. Washington, DC: International Food Policy Research Institute. https://hdl.handle.net/10568/141760

International Food Policy Research Institute
1201 Eye Street, NW
Washington, DC 20005-3915 USA
www.ifpri.org

ISBN: 978-0-89629-464-6
ISSN: 2329-2873
HANDLE: https://hdl.handle.net/10568/141760
Cataloging-in-Publication Data is available from the Library of Congress.

Photo credits
COVER: Avigator Fortuner / Shutterstock.com.
CHAPTER IMAGES: p. 8 EyeEm / Freepik; p. 18 Sven Torfinn / Panos Pictures; p. 26 POP-THAILAND / Shutterstock.com; p. 36 Luis Overlander / Shutterstock.com; p. 46 Shirlyn / Shutterstock.com; p. 54 Sven Torfinn / Panos Pictures; p. 62 Hariyanto Teng / Shutterstock.com; p. 72 TLF Images / Shutterstock.com; p. 82 Andrzej Kubik / Shutterstock.com.

BOOK LAYOUT: Jason Chow
EDITORIAL MANAGER: Pamela Stedman-Edwards

Contents

Foreword

The world is at a pivotal moment in our understanding of both the imperative to put healthy and sustainable diets within reach of all people and the pathways to reaching this goal. In recent decades, evidence has increasingly shown the critical importance of healthy diets for addressing all forms of malnutrition and improving a wide range of human health and welfare outcomes. Evidence is also growing on the environmental and climate impacts of our food systems and the foods that make up our diets. Global commitment to improving nutrition has risen in recognition of the unique potential of healthy diets to reshape the future for both human and planetary well-being, but there is still a long way to go.

Despite our understanding of the importance of healthy diets and the need for policies, programs, and innovations to improve diet quality, less than half of the world's population consumes diverse diets that include adequate amounts of nutritious foods. Progress in addressing malnutrition has stalled in many places, and the impacts of climate change on food systems are becoming increasingly apparent. We are facing many challenges, but focusing on diets to improve nutrition and well-being can guide our efforts.

Moving forward on food systems transformation for healthier diets will require commitments to prioritize healthy diet goals for diverse population groups, as well as climate change adaptation and mitigation options that support these goals. Countries will need to identify policy choices, instruments, and actions with a focus on "multi-duty" options and "no-regrets" actions that address all forms of malnutrition and generate net benefits for people and the planet. Financial commitments to making healthy diets affordable, accessible, and desirable must be increased. For all of these efforts, governance will need to be strengthened to navigate trade-offs among development goals and powerful interest groups.

To support this critical effort, the *2024 Global Food Policy Report* examines multiple approaches to addressing poor diets and nutrition from the demand and supply sides and through better governance that, when tailored to specific contexts, can promote a shift toward sustainable healthy diets. IFPRI's many years of work on nutrition and food systems are brought together to provide a strong basis for moving forward. Our consistent focus on delivering evidence around policies and interventions, especially those promoting inclusion and equity for women and other vulnerable groups, will continue to support decision-makers and other food system stakeholders as the need to address diets becomes more widely acknowledged. Drawing on research from IFPRI, other CGIAR Centers, and many other colleagues, the report provides evidence-based policy recommendations at both the global and regional levels, and points the way for further research, analysis, and innovation. I would like to thank Purnima Menon and Deanna Olney for their guidance of this report as well as the many contributing authors and IFPRI's Communications and Public Affairs team for this timely piece.

Healthy diets, sustainably sourced, should be a right for all of humanity. To strengthen human and planetary well-being, we need sincere efforts to address the many challenges impeding the achievement of this goal, especially for the most vulnerable people. We hope this report will provide both information and inspiration for all those contributing to the transformation of food systems for sustainable healthy diets.

JOHAN SWINNEN
Director General, IFPRI
Managing Director, Systems Transformation, CGIAR

As IFPRI continues its engagement with partners around the world on sustainable healthy diets, we are pleased to share their views on key research and action priorities for the next decade.

ISMAHANE ELOUAFI
Executive Managing Director, CGIAR

"To meet our ambitious global development goals on diets and nutrition, we need innovative research across the food system that informs and supports large-scale equitable impacts. People and the planet are at the heart of our efforts, and so our priorities for research and action center on understanding how to make sustainable healthy diets aspirational, affordable, and accessible for all. Generating the evidence required and achieving impact on diets and nutrition at scale will require skills, talents, and collaboration from across CGIAR and our wide network of partners globally."

LAWRENCE HADDAD
Executive Director, Global Alliance for Improved Nutrition (GAIN)

"Two main research questions that we at GAIN would like more evidence to draw from are (a) how to reduce the costs of healthier diets? and (b) how to shift preferences toward healthier diets?

These are big questions, but we need less energy now on assessing how costly healthy diets are or what is being eaten, and more on how to make them less expensive and what drives consumption other than price and income."

PIERRE THIAM
Chef, cookbook author, restauranteur, social entrepreneur

"Across the continent of Africa, which has more arable land than anywhere else, there are miracle foods. Some you may have heard of, like sorghum and millet. Others you probably haven't, like fonio or bambara groundnuts... Hundreds of foods grown by smallholder farmers are still ignored by our food system.

These foods are all different, but they share a few things in common: They are healthy and nutritious. They have stood the test of time – growing through seasons of plenty and poverty. And they offer solutions to many challenges – from hunger to sustainability.

What if the future of food could be found in these ancient foods? And what if smallholder farmers in Africa could help feed the world?"

VÍCTOR AGUAYO
Global Director, Child Nutrition and Development, UNICEF

"UNICEF estimates that 181 million children under 5 globally live in severe child food poverty, threatening their survival, growth, and development. Food systems have a major role to play in bringing this injustice to an end by ensuring that families' food environments make nutritious and diverse foods the most affordable and desirable option for feeding young children.

This also means that the practices and products of the food and beverage industry must comply with global standards to protect children from unhealthy foods and beverages. Unethical marketing of breastmilk substitutes, ultra-processed foods, and sugar-sweetened beverages to children and families must stop."

LYNNETTE NEUFELD
Director, Food and Nutrition Division, Food and Agriculture Organization of the United Nations (FAO)

"Robust data on food availability, affordability, consumption, and drivers of choice must be the foundation for the design and implementation of actions, policies, and messaging to address the multiple barriers to achieving healthy diets from sustainable food systems. Important advances have been made on data access (e.g., FAO's Food and Diet Domain), but gaps remain a critical barrier to identifying needed actions and tracking progress.

The centrality of healthy diets for everyone, everywhere must be elevated on the SDG and climate agendas, and existing tools such as food-systems-based dietary guidelines must be leveraged to inform specific agriculture, trade, consumer-facing, and other actions needed in context to enable healthy dietary patterns."

SOUMYA SWAMINATHAN
Chairperson, M S Swaminathan Research Foundation

"An unhealthy diet is the leading risk factor for poor health globally, with over 70 percent of the world's population unable to afford a nutritious diet. A key priority therefore is to ensure food and nutrition security for all people, everywhere. Global warming, degradation of soil and water, and unpredictable weather events are all making farming more challenging, while also impacting the nutritive content of food.

We need global collaboration and multistakeholder partnerships to leverage advances in science and technology (including genomic technologies and artificial intelligence), to help scale them equitably, and to adopt policies – at the global and national levels – that enable farmers to thrive, while at the same time, feeding the world with nutritious and affordable food."

ASMA KHAN
Award-winning chef and restauranteur, World Food Programme Chef Advocate, and *Time* magazine's 100 most influential people in 2024

"A top priority for solving the challenge of healthy diets and malnutrition is addressing gender inequalities across society. Around the world, women bear the primary burden of caring for families and ensuring healthy diets while also balancing workloads outside the home. New solutions to improve diets for all must acknowledge these gender dynamics and find ways to address the deep social inequalities that affect how people, especially the poor, are forced to eat today."

SOPHIE HEALY-THOW
Youth activist, Lead Group Member, Scaling Up Nutrition Movement (SUN), and winner of the 2024 Global Citizen Prize: Food & Nutrition

"When I imagine a world where everyone can have access to sustainable healthy diets and better nutrition, I think first of what young people want their future to look. When 100,000 young people across the world were asked, 'If you had a decision-maker sitting in front of you, what would you want them to do to create a better food future and what can you commit to doing yourself?', these were their top priorities for the next decade: Everyone should be able to afford healthy and nutritious food. Every child should eat a healthy and sustainable meal at school, college, or nursery. And educate everyone about food and its impact on our planet and our health."

Acknowledgments

The *2024 Global Food Policy Report* was prepared under the overall leadership of Johan Swinnen, Purnima Menon, and Deanna Olney, and a core team comprising Charlotte Hebebrand, Pamela Stedman-Edwards, Claire Davis, Sivan Yosef, and Jamed Falik.

Contributions were made by Kibrom A. Abay, Lina Abdelfattah, Kamiljon Akramov, Harold Alderman, Silvia Alonso, Elodie Becquey, Samuel Benin, Christine E. Blake, Erick Boy, Inge D. Brouwer, Kevin Z. Chen, Saskia de Pee, Eugenio Díaz-Bonilla, Jen Foley, Gabriela Fretes, Aulo Gelli, Jody Harris, Derek Headey, Kalle Hirvonen, Sunny S. Kim, Avinash Kishore, Nadia Koyratty, Neha Kumar, Sikandra Kurdi, Isabel Lambrecht, Jef L. Leroy, Quinn Marshall, Wim Marivoet, Phuong Hong Nguyen, Maria-Teresa Nogales, Natalia Palacios, Sarah Pechtl, Valeria Piñeiro, Kalyani Raghunathan, Danielle Resnick, Marie T. Ruel, Mohsen Sarhan, Samuel Scott, and Victor Taleon.

Production of the report was led by Pamela Stedman-Edwards. Jason Chow was responsible for design and layout. Editorial assistance was provided by Claire Davis, Gillian Hollerich, and Cara Aldridge Young.

We would like to thank IFPRI's donors, including those who supported IFPRI's research through their contributions to the CGIAR Fund: https://cgiar.org/funders/

Glossary

Animal-source foods (ASFs) include meat (such as flesh foods and organs), fish (fish, crustaceans, and bivalves), dairy products (milk and foods derived from milk, such as butter, yogurt, and cheese), and eggs.[1]

Diet-related noncommunicable diseases (NCDs) include cardiovascular diseases (such as heart attacks and stroke, which are often linked with high blood pressure), certain cancers, and type 2 diabetes.[2] Unhealthy diets and poor nutrition are among the top risk factors for these diseases globally.

Double burden of malnutrition describes the coexistence of undernutrition with overweight and obesity, or diet-related noncommunicable diseases, within individuals, households, and populations, and across the life course.[3]

Double-duty actions are interventions, programs, and policies that simultaneously prevent or reduce the risk of both nutritional deficiencies leading to underweight, wasting, stunting, and micronutrient deficiencies, and problems of overweight, obesity, and diet-related noncommunicable diseases.[4] The term **multi-duty action** is also used in a way that is synonymous to double-duty action, because some actions or interventions may be designed to address more than two types of malnutrition (such as iron deficiency and stunting in the child, and obesity in the mother) or other food systems outcomes.

Malnutrition refers to all nutritional status disorders, including deficiencies, excesses, or imbalances in a person's intake of energy and/or nutrients.[5] Malnutrition addresses three broad groups of conditions: undernutrition, micronutrient-related malnutrition (including deficiencies or excess of important vitamins and minerals), and overweight, obesity, and diet-related noncommunicable diseases (such as heart disease, stroke, diabetes, and some cancers).

Processed foods are foods that have been modified through simple food processing aimed to increase durability, stability, and make them more enjoyable by modifying or enhancing their sensory qualities. Examples include canned or bottled vegetables or legumes (pulses) preserved in brine; whole fruit preserved in syrup; tinned fish preserved in oil; smoked or canned fish; some other types of processed animal foods such as ham, bacon, and pastrami; cheeses; and freshly made breads.[6]

Sustainable healthy diets are diets that promote all dimensions of an individual's health and well-being and that are accessible, affordable, safe, and equitable while being culturally acceptable and causing low environmental pressure and impact.[7]

Ultra-processed foods (UPFs) are industrially formulated foods that are energy dense and contain added sugars, oils and fats, salt, colors, flavors, emulsifiers, and other additives. These products are hyper-palatable, have a long shelf life (increasing their convenience), and are often heavily marketed by corporations. Examples include sugar-sweetened beverages, sweet or salty packaged snacks, ice cream, sausages, and instant noodles.

CHAPTER 1

Advancing Nutrition
Food System Policies and Actions for Healthy Diets

PURNIMA MENON AND DEANNA OLNEY

Purnima Menon is senior director, Food and Nutrition Policy, International Food Policy Research Institute (IFPRI). **Deanna Olney** is director, Nutrition, Diets, and Health Unit, IFPRI.

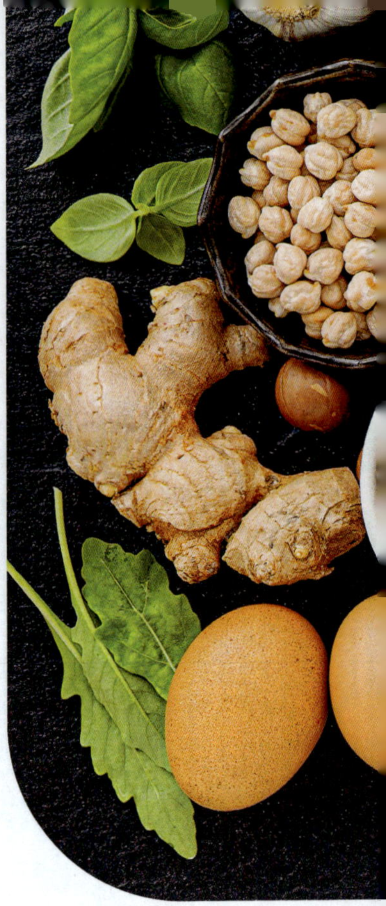

Hunger, food insecurity, and unhealthy diets underpin many critical public health challenges, including all forms of malnutrition and diet-related noncommunicable diseases (NCDs). These health outcomes, in turn, have short- and long-term impacts on the well-being and productivity of human populations worldwide. A recent slowdown in progress in reducing hunger and undernutrition in low- and middle-income countries (LMICs) and a rapid increase in overweight and obesity worldwide, together with the challenges that climate change is imposing on food systems, have brought global attention to the urgent need to transform our food systems in ways that ensure sustainable healthy diets are achievable for everyone. Many countries now face a double burden of malnutrition – meaning that undernutrition and micronutrient deficiencies coexist with overweight and obesity, or diet-related NCDs, within individuals, households, and communities, and across the life course (Box 1).

Healthy diets provide the nutrients needed for an active, healthy life. They include a diversity of foods – fruits, vegetables, legumes, nuts, whole grains, and varying amounts of animal-source foods (ASFs). Healthy diets limit consumption of foods high in sugar, salt, and fat, and provide high concentrations of nutrients, fiber, and other protective elements. The foods that make up a healthy diet vary according to local food availability, cultural context, and individual preferences. Individual physiological characteristics, including age, physical activity, and conditions such as pregnancy or lactation, also determine nutrient requirements.

Today, less than half of the world's population consumes diverse diets that include enough fruits, vegetables, and other nutritious foods.[1] For many people, these nutrient-dense foods are unaffordable, not readily available, or not preferred for a variety of reasons. In LMICs, diets are rapidly evolving to include higher consumption of ultra-processed foods (UPFs), a shift that has resulted from changing livelihoods and lifestyles, as well as the increased availability and marketing of these less expensive foods. Overconsumption of ASFs also continues to grow in some regions of the world, though many vulnerable populations who could benefit from nutrient-dense ASFs cannot access or afford sufficient quantities of these foods.

Food systems are also recognized to have significant environmental and climate-related impacts. Agriculture and other food systems-related activities are estimated to contribute around one-third of global greenhouse gas emissions,[2]

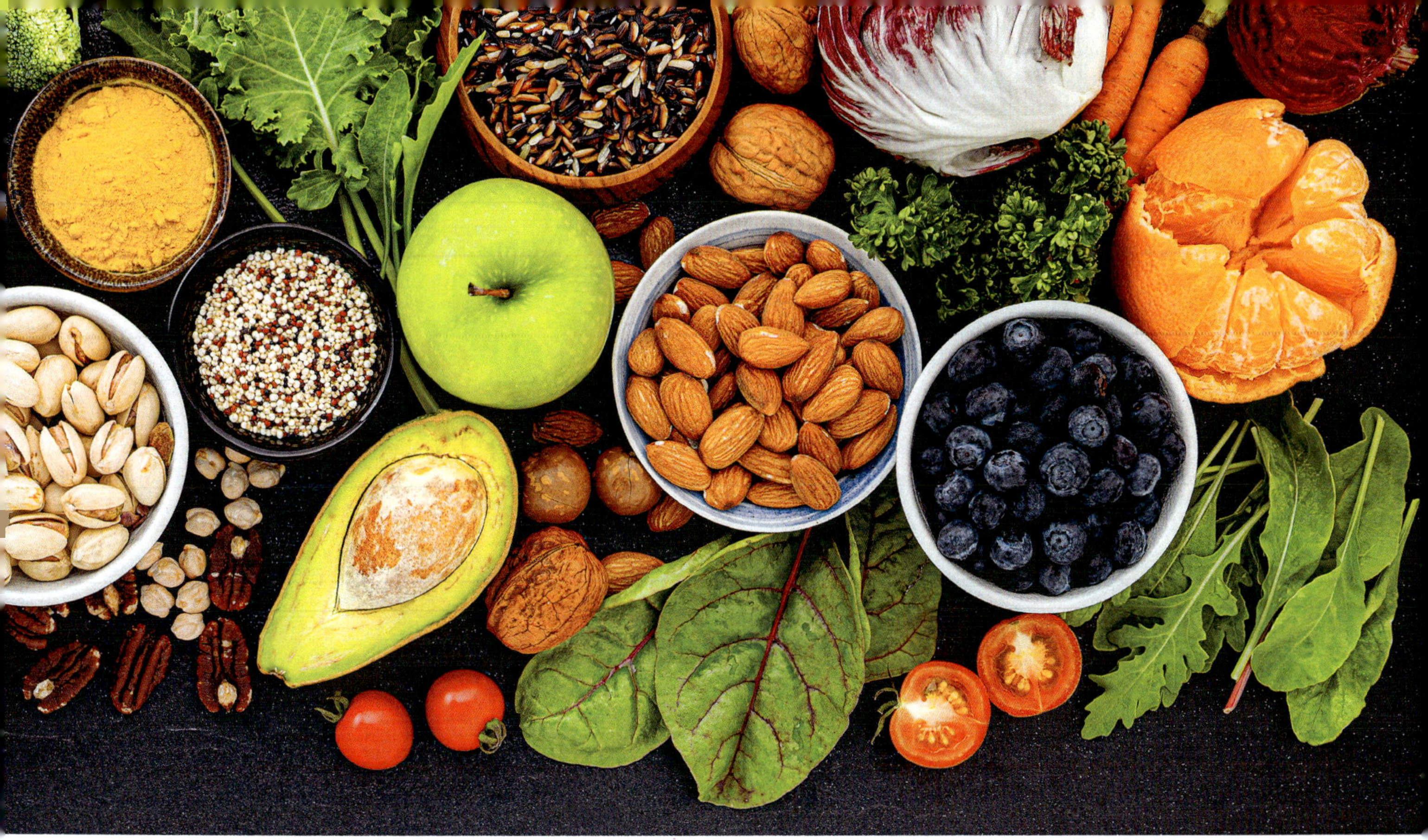

BOX 1 MALNUTRITION AND DIET-RELATED NONCOMMUNICABLE DISEASES

Over the last several years, progress in addressing hunger and malnutrition has slowed as a result of compounding crises, including the COVID-19 pandemic, rising food prices, natural disasters, and ongoing conflicts around the world. Globally, the share of people facing hunger rose from 7.7 percent in 2014 to more than 9 percent in 2022, affecting between 691 and 783 million people.[a] Micronutrient deficiencies, often called "hidden hunger," affect more than half of children under five years old and two-thirds of adult women.[b] Millions of children under five remain affected by stunting (148.1 million) and wasting (45 million).[c]

At the same time, overweight and obesity and associated noncommunicable diseases (NCDs) are on the rise globally. As of 2022, 43 percent of adults were overweight, and 16 percent were living with obesity, more than double the rate 30 years ago.[d] Unhealthy diets are the leading risk factor for NCDs,[e] which are responsible for more than 73 percent of deaths globally.[f] The prevalence of diet-related NCDs, including cardiovascular disease, certain cancers, and type 2 diabetes, is increasing in many countries. Dietary improvements such as increasing fruit and vegetable intake can reduce NCD-related deaths by 20 percent.[g]

and they often negatively affect land quality, water use, and biodiversity. Thus, the environmental footprint of food production and dietary choices requires greater consideration. At the same time, climate change and natural resource degradation will impact our food supply and the nutritional content of crops, requiring greater attention to the development of agricultural technologies and infrastructure that can ensure the availability of nutritious foods necessary for healthy diets.

Amid these complex, interconnected challenges, the global focus on how to leverage food systems for nutrition has shifted toward sustainable healthy diets that promote well-being for both people and the planet. *Sustainable healthy diets* promote all dimensions of an individual's health and well-being, and are accessible, affordable, safe, and equitable while being culturally acceptable and causing low environmental pressure and impact.[3] Ensuring all of these characteristics is only possible if diets are considered within the wider context of the whole food system, from the farm to the consumer, and its links with numerous other sectors, from education to infrastructure.

A CONSUMER-FOCUSED FOOD SYSTEMS FRAMEWORK FOR SUSTAINABLE HEALTHY DIETS

The High Level Panel of Experts on Food Security and Nutrition[4] (HLPE), the science-policy interface of the United Nations Committee on World Food Security, has developed a food systems framework to provide a holistic, multisectoral understanding of food systems that places healthy diets as one of the key goals of food systems transformation, along with economic growth, social equity, and environmental sustainability. In an adaptation of the HLPE framework (Figure 1), we highlight the centrality of consumers, their behaviors, and their food environments, as well as food supply chains, in determining diets, and show that the quality, quantity, diversity, safety, and adequacy of diets are key drivers of nutrition and health outcomes.

By prioritizing diets as a critical entry point for tackling all forms of malnutrition and diet-related NCDs, this framework allows us to consider the wide range of possible policies and actions to meet realistic, measurable goals for food systems transformation (Chapter 2). It also highlights the need for food systems actors to coordinate with other systems to address many of the underlying determinants of malnutrition, such as health, social protection, education, and women's empowerment. Multiple solutions have the

FIGURE 1 A consumer-focused food systems framework for sustainable healthy diets

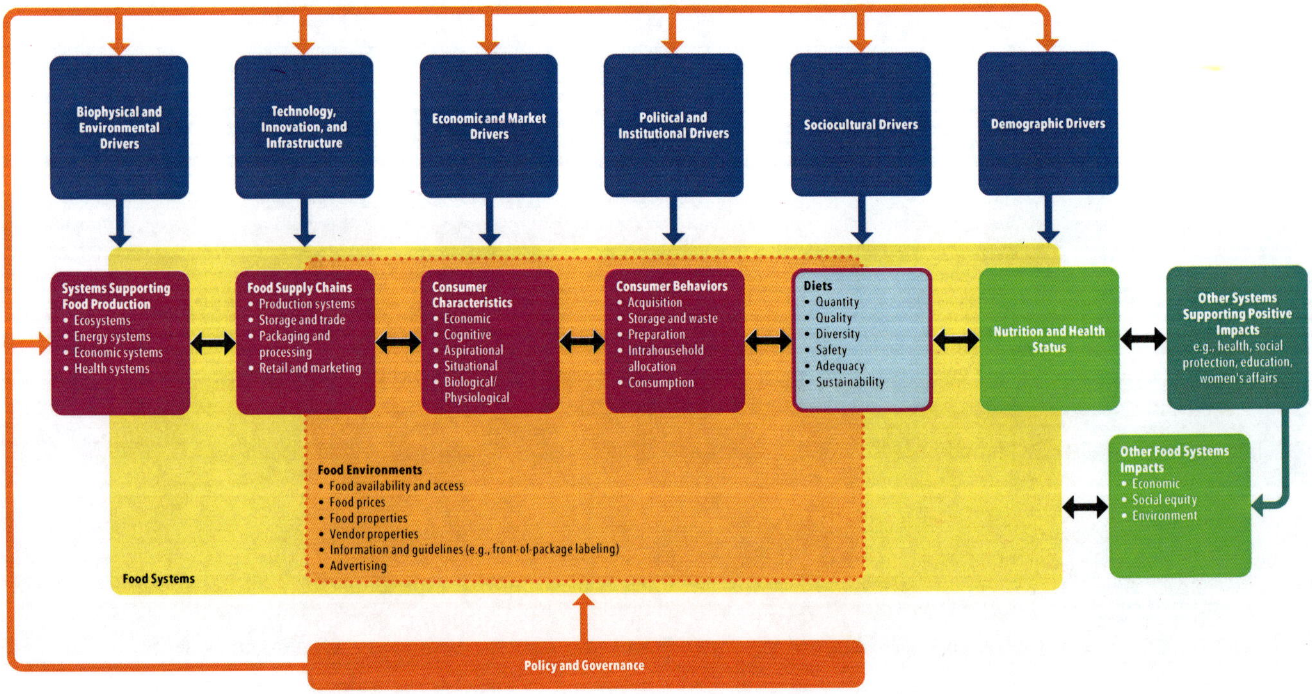

Source: Adapted from High Level Panel of Experts on Food Security and Nutrition of the Committee on World Food Security, *Food Security and Nutrition: Building a Global Narrative Towards 2030* (Rome: 2020).

potential to propel a shift toward sustainable healthy diets, including demand-side approaches that promote changes in consumer behavior; measures to make healthy diets more affordable; fiscal policies that promote healthy foods over less healthy options; and other changes in food environments, such as marketing and retail strategies. On the supply side, increasing the availability and lowering the costs of foods that contribute to healthy diets is essential.

In the thematic chapters and regional sections of this report, IFPRI researchers and colleagues review what we know about approaches across the food system to address desirability, affordability, accessibility, and availability constraints to achieving sustainable healthy diets and the challenges and opportunities we will face going forward. No single intervention can accomplish the change we need: to achieve sustainable healthy diets, meaningful actions must be interlinked and supported by good governance.

ADDRESSING DEMAND, AFFORDABILITY, AND FOOD ENVIRONMENTS

Shifting demand toward healthier diets will require consumer-level changes in preferences and improved understanding of healthy diets, access to affordable nutritious foods, and improvements in food environments. Efforts to address these challenges must start with better assessment of the drivers of food choice, including consumer preferences, affordability, intrahousehold dynamics, market conditions, and entry points for government policies. In turn, increasing demand for healthier foods can potentially increase production and lower costs for these foods, but these systemic impacts of population-wide dietary shifts remain to be studied.

SUPPORTING HEALTHIER FOOD CHOICES

Individual food choices and consumer behavior directly shape diets, even in low-income settings where choices are limited by poverty, high prices, and constraints to availability (Chapter 3). Creating demand for healthy diets requires shifting both personal and collective preferences toward nutritious foods.[5] Actions designed to strengthen demand for healthy and sustainable diets must be context specific. They should build on relevant patterns and trends in cultural, social, economic, and food environments and consider the supply-side constraints to healthy choices.

Several approaches are promising. National food-based dietary guidelines offer practical guidance on specific food groups, nutrients, and diets appropriate to a specific country-level context. These guidelines can help consumers make healthy food choices, and provide the basis for public education, labeling and advertising policies, and food production priorities. To date, more than 100 countries have developed these guidelines,[6] but many do not meet all the requirements of a healthy diet, and some LMICs still have no national guidelines.

Social and behavior change (SBC) interventions use technical, social, and information platforms to provide education and behavioral models that support healthier diets.[7] As stand-alone interventions, SBC efforts have had mixed results, and evidence is limited on SBC efforts to reduce the consumption of unhealthy foods in LMICs. However, adding SBC as a complement to other nutrition and diet-related programs is essential to increase the effectiveness of various multisectoral interventions that aim to generate demand for healthy diets by addressing supply constraints that limit food choice, such as availability and affordability.[8] These include nutrition-sensitive agriculture programs, such as home gardening programs,[9] and social protection programs that provide in-kind or cash transfers, which can improve dietary diversity and intake of micronutrient-rich foods, especially among women and children.[10]

The design and targeting of SBC must take gender into consideration, as empowering women and increasing household access to nutritious food can also improve the diets of young children, who are especially vulnerable to malnutrition and poor development outcomes (Box 2).

BOX 2 GENDER AND DIETS

For healthy diets to provide lifelong benefits, they must become a part of individual and household eating patterns over the life course. Nutrition plays a critical role in ensuring optimal development during the first 1,000 days of a child's life – from conception to the second birthday – and beyond. Adolescent girls and women face special nutritional needs related to their growth and development, reproductive status, and health. Women's diets and nutrition matter not only to their own health and well-being, but also to that of their children.

Yet women and their children suffer the greatest burden of malnutrition, with millions affected by micronutrient deficiencies and undernutrition.[a] The causes of malnutrition are multifactorial, but include suboptimal diets, food insecurity, health status, social and gender relations, and education, among others. Social norms, gender dynamics, and roles within households can limit access to healthy diets, although their influence varies across contexts. Even as women around the world have entered the workforce and spend more time outside the home, they continue to bear a tremendous care burden, including daily meal preparation for their families.

Empowering women can contribute to restructuring the social environment so that they have the resources to better care for themselves and their families, including being able to demand healthier foods. Nutrition-sensitive agriculture programs, social protection, and biofortified or fortified foods have also proven effective in improving dietary diversity and consumption of micronutrient-rich foods, as well as nutrition outcomes, among women and children.[b] Moving forward, understanding the combined impacts of women's time and workload constraints and intrafamilial dynamics around food will be essential to identifying practical solutions to ensure healthy diets for families around the world.

ADDRESSING THE HIGH COSTS OF HEALTHY DIETS

Affordability is a major constraint to healthy diets in LMICs (Chapter 4). The cost of a healthy diet is a relatively new metric that involves measuring people's access to a range of safe and nutritious foods. This cost is defined as the least expensive combination of locally available items, including fruits, vegetables, and other nutrient-dense foods that align with food-based dietary guidelines. Several such metrics exist to determine diet costs, but they all indicate that healthy diets are unaffordable for at least 2 billion and perhaps more than 3 billion people, many of them in South Asia and Africa.[11] Better understanding of the scale and scope of the affordability problem will require national and subnational monitoring of healthy diet affordability, including of food prices and wages.

Unaffordability is the combined result of poverty and the relatively high cost of nutrient-dense foods, as compared to calorie-dense staple foods. The cost of a healthy diet far exceeds the income of many of the world's poor, with more than 84 percent of the population in low-income countries and almost 68 percent in lower-middle-income countries considered "diet poor."[12] Existing social protection measures in these countries barely begin to meet this tremendous need.[13] Poor infrastructure and logistics make storage and transport of perishable products difficult, and agricultural policies and consumer subsidies that support staple crops have kept prices for those foods relatively low. Given the scale of the problem, it would cost at least $1.3 trillion per year to provide the world's diet poor with enough cash to afford healthy diets. Solving the problem thus demands multiple investments.

Healthy diets can be made more affordable by accelerating pro-poor economic growth to catalyze more equitable growth and increase incomes. Across countries, there is also evidence that well-targeted social protection programs can reduce diet poverty;[14] projections show that a 2 percent increase in spending on these programs in LMICs could reduce the number of diet poor by almost 100 million. In addition, realigning agricultural policies toward nutrient-dense foods and scaling up investment in transport, infrastructure, and logistics could reduce the relative price of these foods and increase their availability. However, addressing the

BOX 3 ULTRA-PROCESSED FOODS

Ultra-processed foods (UPFs) are industrially formulated products that are energy dense and contain added sugars, oils and fats, salt, colors, flavors, emulsifiers, and other additives. Examples include sugar-sweetened beverages, ice cream, sausages, instant noodles, and packaged snacks.

Availability and consumption of UPFs have expanded rapidly everywhere, in wealthy and poor areas, and rural and urban areas alike.[a] These products are easy to prepare and convenient to eat away from home, have a long shelf life, and are hyperpalatable.

These foods contribute to diet-related noncommunicable diseases by leading to overconsumption of energy, saturated fats, sugar, and salt, and by replacing more nutritious foods. In some settings, the displacement of nutrients by these foods may contribute to children's poor diets and undernutrition. Emerging evidence suggests that the food industry's pervasive marketing of these products, often targeted to children and adolescents, and the pressure food and beverage companies apply to limit regulation, labeling, and standards contribute substantially to consumer preferences for these products and their growing share in diets.

problems of incomes and relative costs may not be sufficient to improve diets because of dietary preferences for more calorie-dense and nutrient-poor foods. Nutrition-sensitive social protection and nutrition education, as well as changes in food environments, will need to be scaled up to increase demand for healthy foods.

IMPROVING FOOD ENVIRONMENTS

The food environment is the context in which people choose what to eat, where to buy those foods, and where, when, and how to eat (Chapter 5). In LMICs, these dynamic environments are undergoing dramatic changes due to urbanization, rural transformation, and associated shifts in consumer preferences. Unfortunately, food environments increasingly cater to, and even fuel, the growing preference for UPFs (Box 3). These foods are now available from all types of food vendors, including informal and online vendors as well as traditional retailers. In LMICs, the availability and affordability of fresh foods is affected by long supply chains, seasonal variability, and limited infrastructure. These factors, along with food handling practices that can reduce food safety, all affect demand.

Food marketing – across all settings and forms of media – primarily promotes less healthy food options, and is often targeted to children and adolescents. While evidence on the impact of advertising to these age groups is limited for LMICs, studies from high-income countries suggest that exposure to traditional and digital promotional material shapes young people's food preferences, choices, and diets.

Policy interventions to make food environments more conducive to healthy eating include providing information and incentives to consumers, such as labeling foods high in fat, salt, and sugar, and fiscal measures to nudge consumers toward healthier diets, such as taxes on sugar-sweetened beverages. Mandatory labeling and taxes on unhealthy products have had positive results in the Americas, providing a model that could be expanded to other regions. Other interventions, such as limiting the promotion of UPFs to children, show promise, but industry pushback has been strong, and implementation has been slow. More study is also needed on interventions that aim to change what products are offered or how they are positioned in retail settings. In addition, new approaches must address the emerging threats and opportunities created by the growing digital food environment. Further study of policy and actions to promote access to and demand for nutrient-dense foods will be essential to promoting a shift toward healthy diets.

IMPROVING THE AVAILABILITY OF HEALTHY AND SUSTAINABLE FOODS

There are multiple pathways to improving the availability of healthy and sustainable foods that can contribute to making them affordable, accessible, and desirable for consumers. These include leveraging food crops for better nutrition, ensuring the availability of sustainably produced ASFs, and strengthening value chains and markets (Box 4), as well as promoting food safety for nutritious foods.

LEVERAGING FOOD CROPS FOR BETTER NUTRITION

In combination with interventions to increase desirability, accessibility, and affordability, increasing the year-round availability of nutritious plant-based foods will be essential to making sustainable healthy diets attainable (Chapter 6). Crops that deliver energy and high concentrations of vitamins, minerals, phytochemicals, and dietary fiber – fruits, vegetables, and whole grain and nutrient-enriched staples – are among the principal components of healthy diets.[15] Yet consumption and access to these foods is inadequate among many poor and at-risk populations, and global availability is too low to support adequate consumption. Moreover, the nutritional quality and availability of foods eaten in LMICs are projected to deteriorate because of climate change and unsustainable resource use.[16]

Several strategies can increase the availability of nutritious plant-based foods. Investments in crop diversity, such as introducing new species or intercropping, can increase the year-round availability of diverse foods. In addition, "orphan crops" – locally produced crops that have been neglected in breeding programs or underused – can be promoted to fill nutritional gaps.[17] Whole grains can also be promoted, instead of more processed grains, to increase nutrient intake. Yet, the ultimate impact on diets will depend on the interplay with food environments and consumer demand.

Food fortification and biofortification of staple crops are also well-established strategies for addressing micronutrient deficiencies. They can offer an equitable and affordable means of delivering nutrients, especially to vulnerable populations. In many households, women and children consume staple foods every day but have little access to more nutritious foods, so fortification can be critical in providing essential nutrients for these populations.[18] Biofortification enhances the micronutrient density of widely consumed staple crops and can be readily integrated into existing cropping systems to address deficiencies. In addition, large-scale fortification of staple foods during postharvest processing, especially when mandated by law, can reduce micronutrient deficiencies and has been implemented in many countries, with particularly positive results for adults.[19]

THE ROLE OF ANIMAL-SOURCE FOODS

Small quantities of ASFs – meat, fish, dairy, and eggs – can contribute substantially to diet quality and health (Chapter 7).[20] While global ASF consumption has been rising sharply in recent decades, this increase masks major differences across regions and even within countries. While consumption in high-income countries is often excessive,[21] other populations would benefit from greater consumption of ASFs. These foods play a particularly important role in meeting higher nutritional needs in early childhood, adolescence, pregnancy and lactation, and old age. For these groups especially, ASFs are an excellent source of high-quality protein and bioavailable micronutrients that can be difficult or impossible to obtain from plant-based foods.[22] However, ASFs are unaffordable for many of the populations who would most benefit from consuming them.

Incorporation of ASFs into sustainable healthy diets requires consideration of their substantial environmental impacts, including greenhouse gas emissions, land and water use, and biodiversity loss. However, environmental impacts vary greatly among ASF products and production systems. In mixed crop-livestock systems, which are common among smallholders, there can be productive synergies between crop and livestock production, such as use of manure as fertilizer.[23]

BOX 4 TRADE AND MARKET SYSTEMS LINK FOOD AVAILABILITY AND CONSUMPTION

In today's world, major commodities move around the world in diverse ways and forms, often traveling long distances from point of production to point of consumption. Global, regional, and local trade play a strong role in shaping the availability and prices of food all around the world, with important implications for diets and nutrition. Globally, there is greater incentive to trade agricultural commodities and food products that have a longer shelf life and stability over long distances, such as ultra-processed foods (UPFs). Fruits and vegetables and other perishable products are also traded across borders and are often sourced from developing countries, but higher transport costs put these out of reach of poor consumers. Prices for perishable healthy foods are also determined at a more local level, as these commodities often cannot be cost-effectively transported within countries, due to infrastructure and other value chain constraints, such as insufficient cold storage. Improving the affordability and accessibility of perishable nutrient-dense foods will require scaling up investments in transportation, infrastructure, and logistics for domestic and international trade, as well as diversifying and increasing the supply of these foods through technologies for agricultural production, processing, and marketing (see Chapters 4 and 6).

IFPRI research has focused on the impacts of trade shocks as well as other types of shocks at the national or local level, which can drive up the price of all foods and make healthier food choices even more unaffordable.[a] While export restrictions are not addressed in this report, IFPRI has pointed in particular to the damaging impact of these restrictions on agricultural products. To date, these restrictions are not being disciplined by the World Trade Organization's rules in a meaningful way, driving up the price of food.[b]

More broadly, evidence is increasingly showing that the food that is consumed, even by the rural poor, is often sourced primarily from markets.[c] This is true especially in the Americas, most of South Asia, and Southeast Asia. The functioning of market systems, including the value chains that bring produce and animal-source foods to the food environments of consumers, has profound impacts on the availability, accessibility, and affordability of these nutrient-dense perishable foods. Most notably, lack of infrastructure for transport, storage, and marketing of food and for food safety reduces access to and affordability of these foods. Market systems also influence the largely unregulated availability of UPFs around the world (see Chapter 5). Strengthening the ability of market systems to support better diets and nutrition by offering sustainable, healthy, and convenient foods must be a major priority.

In many LMICs, ASF consumption will need to increase, particularly in infants and young children. With so many people unable to afford a healthy diet, improving consumption will require a combination of greater farm productivity and market efficiency to reduce prices, as well as an increase in household incomes. Food safety for these perishable products will also need to be addressed, especially in the informal markets that serve many LMIC consumers.[24] In other regions, excess ASF consumption will need to decrease to reduce both diet-related NCDs and environmental impacts. Together, these shifts could benefit human health and lead to a more equitable distribution of ASFs produced within sustainable limits.

GOVERNANCE FOR BETTER DIETS AND NUTRITION

Enabling environments for better diets and nutrition must include attention to leadership, governance, and political economy, including the interplay of diverse actors with an interest in shaping food systems outcomes for the future. Sound governance is essential for implementing the broad range of policy interventions required to improve diet quality and nutrition (Chapter 8).[25] Bundling these different policy options is often the most effective approach, but is not always feasible when state capacity is low. A state's capacity includes its administrative capacity, namely its ability to develop policy, impose regulations, and deliver public services, all of which depend on sufficient technical staff, current data, coordination mechanisms, reach, and impartiality.[26] Capacity also includes the state's ability to raise taxes and mobilize funds for food system investments.[27]

Substantial state capacity and positive political incentives are critical to meeting administrative needs for policy implementation and managing trade-offs across nutrition goals and other objectives. Government engagement with food companies and other interest groups, which may either oppose or support government goals, is likewise shaped by state capacity and political incentives. Where powerful actors lack incentives to support policy implementation, policies are more likely to be contested. Along with the government and private sector, citizen engagement and grassroots movements can also play a transformative role in improving diets and nutrition. This engagement is most likely to flourish when governments are committed to ensuring civic space for such movements.[28]

Governance can be strengthened in multiple ways. To ensure that policies for diets and nutrition are sustainable and scalable, policy analysis can be expanded to include an assessment of governance capacity. Governance constraints that limit capacity and ability to navigate industry influence should be identified and addressed. In addition, governments should provide an enabling environment for citizen agency through policy transparency and government accountability, and for growth of successful grassroots movements that can support better diets and nutrition. In complex and ever-moving governance conditions, it is clear that leadership for better diets and nutrition must coexist in diverse sectors and be effectively deployed toward diverse positive outcomes.

CHALLENGES AND OPPORTUNITIES

A food systems approach for sustainable healthy diets offers many promising opportunities, but also entails a set of difficult challenges (Chapter 2). Success will require a truly multisectoral approach that tackles the need for sustainable healthy diets from multiple directions and with "multi-duty" tools that address different forms of malnutrition and consider the wide range of factors that shape diets and their contributions to nutrition and health outcomes.

Achieving optimal consumption of diverse food groups to support healthy diets in various contexts and populations will also require a range of context-specific policies and initiatives that focus on demand, food environments, and supply. While fruits and vegetables are universally recognized as essential to healthy diets, low consumption of these healthy foods is a global problem. The relatively high prices of nutritious plant-based foods, as well as ASFs, must be addressed to improve diets for low- and middle-income households. In addition, at all income levels, consumer knowledge, intrahousehold dynamics, and tastes and preferences must be addressed to build demand for healthy food options.

A critical challenge lies in managing the actions of diverse stakeholders and inherent conflicts of interest. Numerous trade-offs will need to be identified and negotiated, not only between interest groups, but also across critical development goals for well-being and sustainability. Although healthy diets are generally perceived to be more environmentally sustainable than unhealthy diets, the footprint of food systems is large,[29] and there are likely to be trade-offs between optimal diets and sustainability goals.

Finally, despite emerging efforts to improve data on food systems, publicly available information remains sorely lacking on what populations eat, where food is sourced from, drivers of people's consumption choices, characteristics of food environments and markets, and composition of food supplies. Well-tested methods, tools, and indicators as well as increased data collection are needed to analyze and monitor complex food systems and their different components, including their environmental impacts. Improving the available evidence base can support LMICs in diagnosing diet and nutrition challenges and drivers, testing and scaling solutions, and monitoring progress. Urgent efforts are needed to support governments and other actors at all levels – from global to local – in using data and evidence to guide national nutrition plans, identify effective entry points for improving diets, set goals for their own food systems transformation efforts, and navigate trade-offs and conflicts of interest along the way.

Achieving sustainable healthy diets will require substantial investments in high-impact food systems actions, with a keen focus on addressing dietary gaps and enabling populations to build healthy dietary patterns sustainably and equitably. Global commitments to nutrition are strong, but the world is not moving fast enough to deploy effective strategies and financing, or to establish financing and accountability mechanisms to meet Sustainable Development Goal 2, which targets malnutrition.[30] Meeting this goal will be no small feat, but evidence is emerging from numerous creative efforts.[31] In our dynamic world, it is crucial that we continue to build the evidence base needed to strengthen these ongoing efforts. We must identify successes, but we must also identify failures – fast – because there is little time to lose, especially for those who are most vulnerable to the combined impacts of climate change and social inequalities. In the chapters that follow, we explore the recent evidence on what works and what does not, the challenges we face, and opportunities for transforming food systems to ensure sustainable healthy diets for everyone.

CHAPTER 2

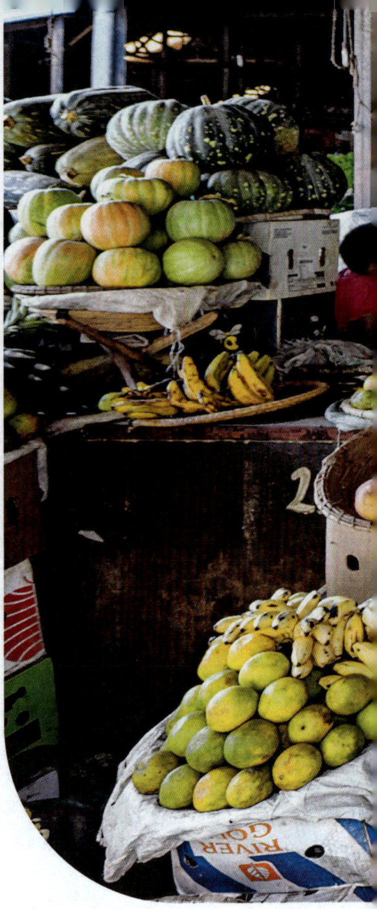

Diets and Nutrition
The Potential of a Food Systems Approach

MARIE T. RUEL AND INGE D. BROUWER

Marie T. Ruel and **Inge D. Brouwer** are senior research fellows, Nutrition, Diets, and Health Unit, International Food Policy Research Institute.

KEY MESSAGES

- Priorities in nutrition research and practice have evolved over many years as new evidence has become available on preventing and addressing different forms of malnutrition.
- Experiences with nutrition-sensitive agriculture highlight the importance of holistic, multisectoral frameworks for addressing malnutrition.
- Adopting the "food systems for sustainable healthy diets" framework helps position consumers and their food environments in the global food systems transformation agenda.
- Anchoring sustainable healthy diets as one of the key outcomes of food systems transformation helps prioritize diets as a critical entry point to tackle all forms of malnutrition.
- The focus on diets, rather than on nutrition and health outcomes, helps set feasible goals for food systems transformation.

A number of investments are needed to make food systems work for diets and nutrition:

- For sustainable healthy diets to translate into optimal nutrition and health, food systems will need to coordinate with other systems that address the underlying determinants of malnutrition – such as health, social protection, education, and women's empowerment – and will require greater coordination among food systems actors.
- Methods, tools, and indicators for measuring consumer behavior and food environments are urgently needed to evaluate and monitor food system solutions for sustainable healthy diets.
- For policymakers, using the food systems paradigm creates new opportunities to revamp national food-based dietary guidelines to incorporate health and environmental considerations. Using this paradigm also provides an opportunity to address all forms of malnutrition and incorporate multi-duty actions in national nutrition plans and other relevant sectoral strategies.

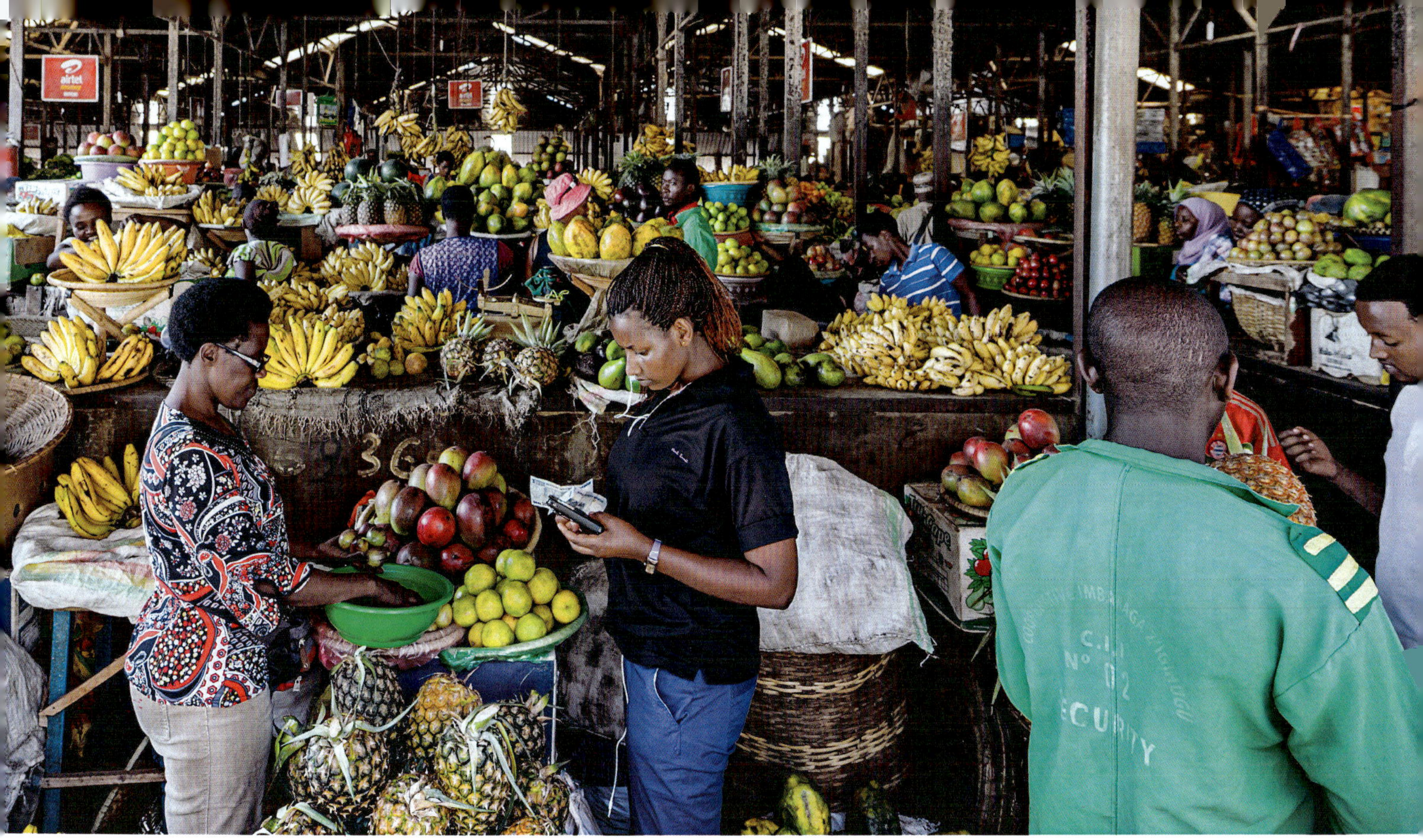

Over the last century, priorities in nutrition research and practice have evolved as new evidence on the prevention and treatment of different forms of malnutrition has become available. A succession of paradigms have shaped the narrative on nutrition challenges and their solutions, with important implications for investments.[1] As food systems have increasingly become the organizing principle for work on nutrition and diets, "food systems for sustainable healthy diets" has emerged as the latest paradigm in nutrition.

The 2021 United Nations Food Systems Summit (UNFSS)[2] has been instrumental in shaping this new paradigm by positioning nutrition and diets in global discussions and national plans on food systems transformation. Until recently, large agrifood systems investments focused primarily on producing more food, especially staple crops, to address global food insecurity and availability constraints. The UNFSS, however, proposed a new framework to shift the global dialogue on hunger and undernutrition to a more holistic approach that positions healthy diets (to address all forms of malnutrition) as one of the ultimate goals of food systems transformation, along with economic growth, social equity, and environmental sustainability.[3] The UNFSS also led to the creation of the Coalition of Action on Healthy Diets from Sustainable Food Systems for Children and All,[4] which aims to foster coordinated multi-duty actions (see Glossary) to tackle all forms of malnutrition. Although there is broad consensus on the importance and urgency of food systems transformation for sustainable healthy diets, there is much less clarity on how to address the new complexities and trade-offs among outcomes and how to bring about the needed transformation.

In this chapter, we first summarize how learning from decades of work on the linkages between agriculture and nutrition paved the way to adopting the new food systems for sustainable healthy diets framework (see Figure 1, Chapter 1). We then reflect on the emerging challenges and opportunities that arise for the nutrition community as we navigate this new global agenda. This discussion sets the stage for the following chapters in the report, which present the inherent complexities of defining and operationalizing food systems transformation to achieve sustainable healthy diets for all.

NUTRITION-SENSITIVE AGRICULTURE: WHAT HAVE WE LEARNED?

Nutrition-sensitive agriculture (NSA) programs incorporate specific nutrition goals and interventions and address some of the underlying determinants of child nutrition: adequate income, access to food in sufficient quantity and quality, optimal caregiving resources and practices, and access to health services and a safe and hygienic environment. The early years of the 21st century saw rising interest and research on the role of agriculture in accelerating progress to improve child nutrition, especially during the first 1,000 days of a child's life (from conception to the second birthday). A first breakthrough came with HarvestPlus,[5] the pioneering work on breeding for nutrition. This work showed that biofortified staple crops with higher concentrations of micronutrients could improve micronutrient intake and status as well as diet quality (see Chapter 6).[6] At the time, evidence on the linkages between agriculture and nutrition showed little or no impact of agricultural interventions on child anthropometric indicators or complementary feeding practices.[7] After sharpening objectives, design, and targeting of nutrition intervention packages as well as strengthening evaluations, subsequent studies showed more consistent positive impacts on household food security, consumption of nutritious foods, and dietary diversity among mothers and children. Some studies also observed positive impacts on child health indicators and on maternal knowledge, well-being, and empowerment.[8] Greater benefits were achieved by incorporating robust health and nutrition behavior change communication and women's empowerment activities in these programs. Impacts on child stunting, wasting, and micronutrient status, however, remained limited. These impacts were found only in programs that added water, sanitation, and hygiene (WASH) interventions to prevent or reduce infections and/or distributed micronutrient supplements to complement poor diets in areas with limited access to nutrient-rich foods.[9]

This evidence suggests that although NSA can effectively improve food security and diet quality, improving anthropometric or nutritional status outcomes requires significant additional inputs from other key sectors that contribute to nutrition (including nutrition counseling, access to and use of health and WASH services, and women's empowerment interventions). The resulting programs may be overly complex, expensive, and operationally challenging. Thus, evidence from more recent NSA evaluations supports the use of *diets*, as opposed to child anthropometry, as the main goal of NSA programs, because improving diets is a much more achievable and reasonable goal for community-based (largely rural) agriculture and food production-focused programs. This key insight is also critical for incorporating nutrition into food systems – focusing on diets, rather than nutrition and health outcomes, helps set realistic goals for food systems transformation.

FOOD SYSTEMS FOR SUSTAINABLE HEALTHY DIETS: NEW OPPORTUNITIES AND CHALLENGES

NEW OPPORTUNITIES

In the context of the 2021 UNFSS, the interest in NSA expanded to the broader food systems that host agriculture and to the challenges of leveraging food systems to improve diets and tackle all forms of malnutrition. While NSA mainly addresses undernutrition in young children and their mothers in rural contexts, persistent undernutrition now coexists with overweight, obesity, and diet-related noncommunicable diseases (NCDs, see Glossary) due to poor-quality diets and other changes in lifestyles that affect both urban and rural populations and individuals at all stages of life.[10] As consumers shift from traditional to more modern lifestyles, and more women work away from home and earn income, the need for convenience and the modernization of the food supply have led to greater reliance on prepared, ready-to-eat foods and meals, and excessive consumption of cheap processed and ultra-processed foods (UPFs, see Glossary).[11] These diets lead to overconsumption of energy, saturated fats, sugar, and salt, and are associated with overweight and obesity and a range of NCDs.[12]

NSA programs alone are not well suited to tackling the complex dynamics of modernizing food systems, urbanization, and rapidly changing diets and related nutrition and health challenges. While these programs continue to be important as a form of social protection for poor rural households, they are only a small component of the much broader food systems that produce, process, distribute, and market foods that are made available to consumers through the food environments where they procure food.

Thus, using a food systems for sustainable healthy diets framework to position diets and nutrition in the global food system discourse is beneficial for several reasons. This approach helps bring consumers, food environments, and sustainable healthy diets into the global development agenda, and it fosters linkages between food, diets, and the environment, compelling a rethinking of the definition of healthy diets to include environmental concerns.[13] It also places a focus on households and on the importance of intra-household dynamics in achieving nutrition and health outcomes. In addition, the food systems framework brings together different sectors by fostering engagement and coordination among all actors and sectors essential to improving nutrition and diet outcomes.

NEW CHALLENGES

Despite the benefits outlined above of taking a food systems approach to sustainable healthy diets, such a shift inevitably comes with challenges. We briefly describe four main challenges, as examples of the complexity of this new framework.

TRADE-OFFS WITHIN SUSTAINABLE HEALTHY DIETS. The definition of healthy diets has changed over time, as research has continued to evolve on diets, foods, and food groups (and their optimal range of intake) that help prevent all forms of malnutrition and protect from diet-related NCDs. Adding sustainability to the healthy diet definition requires considering the environmental footprint of diets as another key outcome. Healthy diets are generally perceived to be more environmentally sustainable than unhealthy diets because they include an abundance of plant-based foods, moderate to no animal-source foods (ASFs, see Glossary), and no UPFs. But adding sustainability to the definition of healthy diets may create significant trade-offs between healthiness goals and diets' environmental footprint (see Chapters 6 and 7).

The role of ASFs, especially meat and fish, in sustainable healthy diets highlights the complexity of these trade-offs. In Viet Nam, for example, modeling showed that adding a sustainability criterion to the design of a standard healthy diet required reducing the amount of ASFs in the diet, which disproportionately reduced the ability of women of reproductive age to meet their micronutrient needs compared with men.[14] In Viet Nam and many other low- and middle-income countries where large-scale fortification of staple foods or micronutrient supplementation may be out of reach, especially for marginalized populations, a minimum amount of ASFs is required for women of reproductive age, infants and young children, and adolescent girls to meet all their nutrient needs (see Chapter 7).[15]

ACHIEVING OPTIMAL CONSUMPTION OF A DIVERSITY OF HEALTHY FOOD GROUPS AND AVOIDING UNHEALTHY FOODS TO SUPPORT HEALTHY DIETS IN VARIOUS CONTEXTS AND POPULATIONS. Fruits and vegetables (F&V) are universally recognized as a cornerstone of healthy diets for all contexts and populations. Higher consumption of F&V has a well-documented protective effect against diet-related NCDs,[16] and there is no known upper limit where consumption becomes unhealthy. Low consumption of F&V, however, is a global problem that affects all countries.[17] Availability, affordability, and seasonality of F&V may limit consumption in some areas, but a study conducted in four countries of sub-Saharan Africa found that F&V had low income and price elasticities.[18] An analysis of 164 countries also found small and insignificant price and income elasticities for vegetables (and fruits, to some extent) in the six world regions studied, and for both men and women across age groups.[19] These findings imply that economic incentives, including increasing F&V affordability through lower prices or higher incomes, may not be sufficient (in many contexts) to boost consumption. Approaches that create demand are essential if the health and nutrition benefits of

F&V consumption are to be reaped globally (see Chapter 3). Consumption of other nutritious food groups, including whole grains, legumes, and nuts, also needs to increase dramatically in all regions of the world to achieve optimal levels. Increasing demand for these foods would also require tackling constraints related to availability, desirability, access, and affordability.[20]

UPFs have been receiving close attention, with the consensus being that these foods have no role in sustainable healthy diets. Evidence shows that a higher percentage of total energy consumed from UPFs is associated with poorer diet quality and various health issues, including higher risks of obesity, diabetes, cardiovascular diseases, cancer, common mental disorder outcomes, anxiety, and mortality.[21] Despite overwhelming evidence on the negative health impacts of UPFs, nuanced questions remain about the definition of UPFs, their role in sustainable healthy diets, and the mechanisms causing their harmful effects. Moreover, the current definition of UPFs may inadvertently include some foods and food products that are crucial for healthy diets. These include industrially fortified foods, reduced-fat milk products, and specially formulated nutrient-dense and high-energy foods or nutrient supplements to treat or prevent wasting in young children.[22] Additionally, it is unclear whether the processing of UPFs or their energy-dense/nutrient-poor concentration (or the combination of both) plays a greater role in contributing to adverse health outcomes. Some food companies have started to reformulate select UPFs, but if the processing itself is responsible for the health risks, a radical shift away from UPFs would be more beneficial. For the time being, several national food-based dietary guidelines include specific recommendations to limit the consumption of UPFs.[23]

CLIMATE CHANGE AND ITS IMPACTS ON FOOD PRODUCTION AND THE NUTRIENT CONTENT OF CROPS. Climate change affects diets, nutrition, and health through its impacts on food production, which include reductions in the quantity, quality, nutrient content, diversity, safety, and affordability of foods.[24] For food producers and processors, additional impacts come from losses in income and livelihoods as extreme weather events limit crop yields, destroy livestock, and disrupt food production and transportation.[25] Box 1 summarizes results from analyses of the effects of elevated carbon dioxide on the nutrient content of major staple crops and highlights predicted reductions in the global availability of iron, zinc, and protein by 2050, with low- and middle-income countries being most affected. While these findings are disconcerting, it is important to recognize that staples and other cereal crops are not the best sources of bioavailable iron, zinc, and high-quality proteins, and that small amounts of ASFs could easily fill the gap for these nutrients (see Chapter 7). Renewed efforts are needed to leverage food environments and shift consumer demand toward sustainable healthy diets that incorporate an optimal balance of ASFs (small amounts, especially for vulnerable individuals) and plant foods (abundant) to meet all essential nutrient needs (see Chapter 3), while mitigating impacts on planetary health. Efforts to bring biofortification and large-scale food fortification to nutritionally vulnerable populations or subgroups could also help meet essential micronutrient needs for the general population (see Chapter 6). For individuals with higher nutrient needs or in environments where (bio)fortification is not available or accessible, nutrient supplements may be needed.

SCARCITY OF METHODS, TOOLS, AND INDICATORS TO ANALYZE AND MONITOR COMPLEX SYSTEMS AND THEIR DIFFERENT COMPONENTS. Significant investments have been made recently to develop simpler methods and tools to assess dietary intake and to develop and validate indicators to characterize the quality, healthiness,[26] and environmental impact of diets.[27] Recognizing the lack of consensus on indicators that best capture different components of healthy diets, the UN's Food and Agriculture Organization (FAO), World Health Organization (WHO), and UNICEF established the Healthy Diets Monitoring Initiative[28] in 2022 to develop standardized metrics tailored for distinct purposes, in collaboration with national and global stakeholders, and to advocate for the widespread adoption of these measures. Collections of dietary data sets have also been compiled, such as the FAO/WHO Global Individual Food Consumption Data Tool (GIFT),[29] and several low- and middle-income countries have received technical assistance to conduct nationally

BOX 1 IMPACTS OF CO_2 ON GLOBAL MICRONUTRIENT AVAILABILITY

Estimates of the impact of rising carbon dioxide (CO_2) levels on the nutrient content of crops vary, but all point to a decline in the concentration of critical nutrients. A 2017 study projects that, by 2050, the effects of elevated CO_2 levels will reduce the nutrient content of major staple crops by 3-11 percent for iron, zinc, and protein.[a] A more recent analysis finds that increased CO_2 (measured by carbon nutrient penalty, that is, the loss in mineral concentration in plants due to higher atmospheric concentrations of CO_2) would result in losses in global availability of 3-4 percent for protein and iron, and 2-3 percent for zinc.[b] Modeling of atmospheric CO_2 changes that also include CO_2 fertilization and climate effects on productivity indicates much larger losses in the global availability of nutrients (close to 20 percent for protein, 14 percent for iron, and 15 percent for zinc) compared with a scenario that includes expected technological and market development gains by 2050. However, a recent review of the impact of climate change on the micronutrient-rich food supply concludes that yield declines will have greater impacts on the global availability of these nutrients than changes in crop nutrient content or quality.[c] These estimated impacts are expected to disproportionately affect low- and middle-income countries, where large proportions of the population rely mostly on staple crops and other plant sources to meet their protein and micronutrient needs.[d]

representative or other large dietary assessment surveys (for example, through the Intake project[30]). Few countries have established data collection and monitoring systems to track trends in diets and nutrient gaps over time, or to guide the development of national nutrition plans or food-based dietary guidelines. Fortunately, genuine efforts are underway to correct this situation.

Initiatives like the Food Systems Dashboard[31] and the Food Systems Countdown[32] provide new opportunities to track and monitor progress in food systems transformation processes at the global, national, and, in select countries, subnational levels. However, there is a dramatic gap in methods, tools, and indicators to analyze interactions between elements of food systems (for example, in food production, value chains, food environments, consumers, or food system drivers) or assess impacts of interventions at different stages of these systems on diets and other outcomes. Modeling and projections play a critical role in analyzing complex systems, predicting the impacts of different policy scenarios on a range of outcomes, and addressing trade-offs.[33] However, quantitative tools are needed to answer context-specific questions such as how do food environments affect household consumption and individual diets, what are the key drivers of dietary choices,[34] or what are the impacts of food environment- or consumer-targeted interventions on dietary changes. To address these questions and undertake microeconomic research, primary data collection methods and standardized tools and indicators are needed.

LOOKING AHEAD

Adopting the food systems for sustainable healthy diets framework presents a unique opportunity to improve diets and nutrition at one of the most critical times in history, marked by a series of food, economic, climatic, and conflict crises that threaten human and planetary health. Anchoring sustainable healthy diets as one of the key outcomes of food systems transformation helps prioritize diets as a critical entry point to tackle all forms of malnutrition and achieve positive health outcomes. With healthy diets as an additional outcome of food systems transformation, however, greater coordination among food system actors from all disciplines is needed to address increasing complexities in trade-offs and priority setting for key development outcomes.[35] To ensure that sustainable healthy diets translate into optimal nutrition and health, food systems also need to coordinate with other systems that address the underlying determinants of all forms of malnutrition, such as health, social protection, education, and women's affairs.

The focus on food systems for sustainable healthy diets also helps position consumers and their food environments in the global food systems transformation agenda. For this new paradigm to endure and generate positive change, a deeper commitment is required from nutritionists, along with economists, environmental, agricultural, and development scientists, and all food systems actors. Focused efforts are needed to develop, test, and scale up solutions to turn the tide toward sustainable healthy diets without interfering with other critical outcomes of food systems transformation, including economic growth, social equity, and environmental sustainability. For policymakers, using the food systems paradigm creates new opportunities to revamp national food-based dietary guidelines to incorporate health and environmental sustainability considerations. This approach provides an opportunity to address all forms of malnutrition and incorporate multi-duty actions in national nutrition plans and in health, agriculture and food security, social protection, and women's empowerment strategies and policies.

"Focused efforts are needed to develop, test, and scale up solutions to turn the tide toward sustainable healthy diets – without interfering with other critical outcomes of food systems transformation."

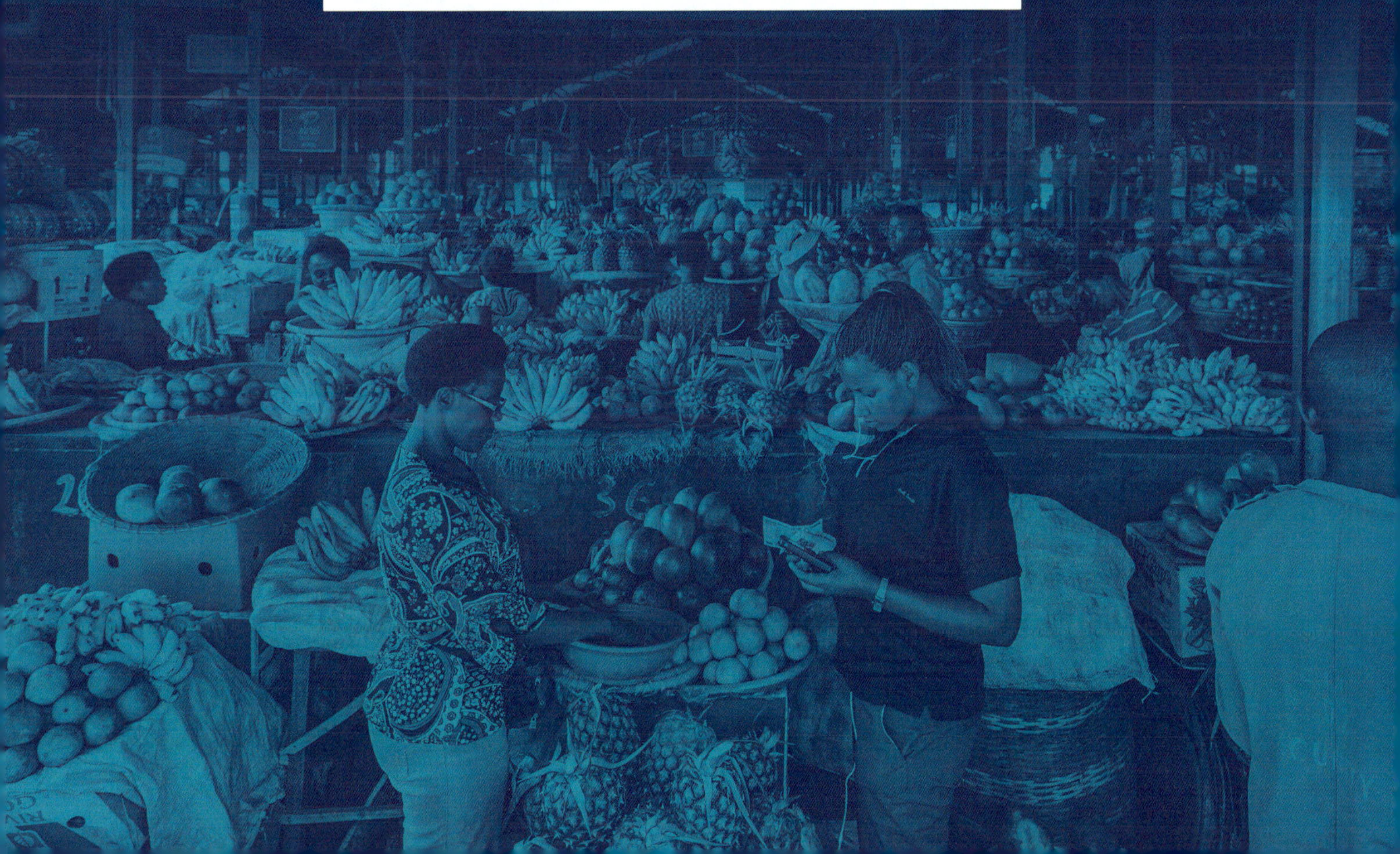

CHAPTER 3

Demand-Side Approaches
Supporting Healthier Food Choices

SUNNY S. KIM, NADIA KOYRATTY, CHRISTINE E. BLAKE, AND NEHA KUMAR

Sunny S. Kim and **Neha Kumar** are senior research fellows, and **Nadia Koyratty** is an associate research fellow, Nutrition, Diets, and Health Unit, International Food Policy Research Institute. **Christine E. Blake** is an associate professor, Health Promotion, Education, and Behavior, Arnold School of Public Health, University of South Carolina.

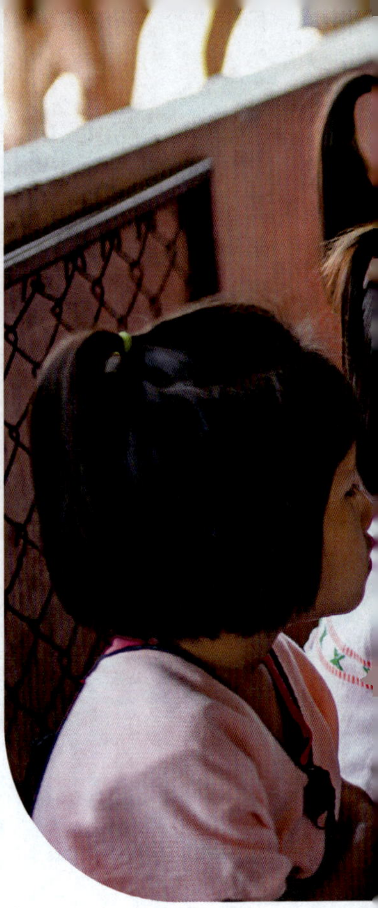

KEY MESSAGES

- Globally, consumption of most foods has increased, but less than half of adults consume diverse diets, and rising consumption of ultra-processed foods is a concerning trend. Efforts to increase the healthfulness and sustainability of diets must focus on quality – not just quantity – of food production or consumption to achieve optimal nutritional status across diverse populations.
- Understanding the drivers of individual food choices, consumer behavior, and food demand is essential to reshape food systems to achieve broad nutrition and sustainability goals. Although many initiatives to transform food systems and promote healthier diets focus on supply-side changes, actions must also focus on the demand-side drivers of food choices.
- Creating demand for sustainable healthy diets requires shifting personal and collective food choice behaviors. Demand-side actions can incentivize sustainable production of healthy foods and improve the enabling environment for healthy diets by influencing consumer preferences and increasing purchasing power.
- Key actions to shift demand include developing national food-based dietary guidelines that define context-specific diets, and promoting behavior change through consumer empowerment and food and nutrition education.
- Nutrition-sensitive agriculture programs, social protection programs, and school meals and school-based nutrition programs are also proven to improve diets and nutrition outcomes when selected and designed based on the intended objectives and context.

To generate and support demand for sustainable healthy diets, it is important to:

- Build understanding of the drivers of food choices, especially the perceptions and values of consumers.
- Develop food-based dietary guidelines to help consumers navigate their food environments and make healthy food choices.
- Strengthen social and behavior change communication to reach a wide audience and build practical skills that nurture an informed consumer base.
- Integrate multisectoral approaches, including agriculture, education, health, and economic policy, within the context of local food systems to help create an enabling environment for healthy food choices.

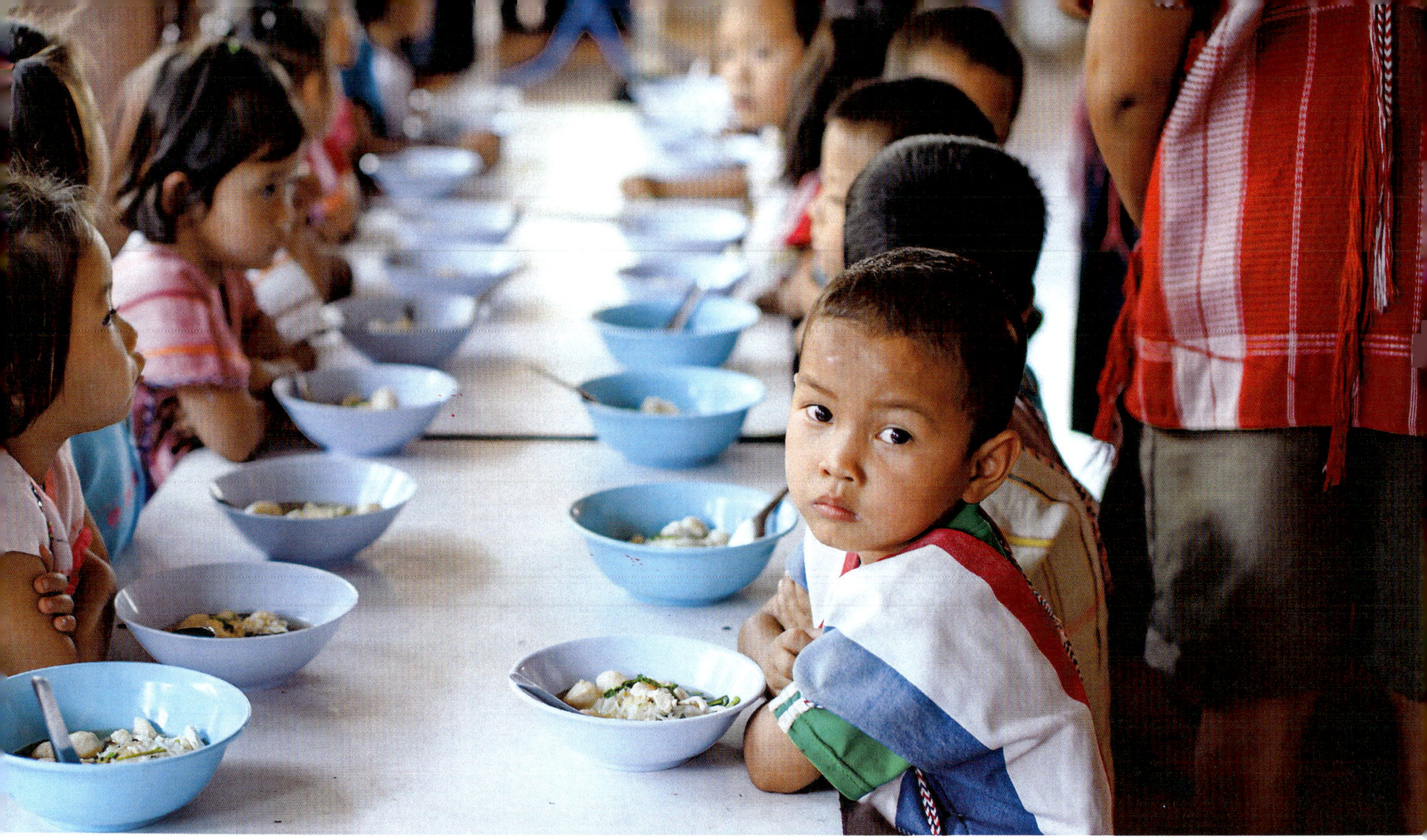

As with most of the world, low- and middle-income countries (LMICs) are grappling with questions of how to support and promote sustainable healthy diets[1] that prevent malnutrition in all its forms while reducing the food system's environmental impacts.[2] Global nutrition and health communities are increasingly coalescing around broad principles for transforming food systems to achieve sustainable healthy diets that promote all dimensions of individuals' health and well-being; exert low environmental pressure; are accessible, affordable, safe, and equitable; and are culturally acceptable.[3] However, health and nutrition challenges remain huge, with one in three individuals globally affected by at least one form of malnutrition, such as hunger, stunting, wasting, micronutrient deficiencies, or overweight and/or obesity, and rising prevalence of diet-related noncommunicable diseases (NCDs).[4]

Current global patterns show increased per capita consumption of most foods, including both animal- and plant-source foods, but less than half of adults worldwide consume diverse diets, and there are concerning increases in consumption of ultra-processed high-fat, high-sugar foods.[5] In countries across most income classifications (lower middle to high income), the share of people consuming salty packaged snacks, instant noodles, and other fast food and sugar-sweetened beverages (SSBs) (as reported in the previous 24 hours) nearly reaches the prevalence of those consuming all five food groups (that is, at least one type of vegetable; fruit; pulse, nut, or seed; animal-source food; and starchy staple) (Figure 1).[6] Efforts to increase the healthfulness of diets must focus on quality, not just on increased food production or greater consumption, to achieve optimal nutritional status across diverse populations.[7] This goal requires understanding of supply, food environment, and demand-related drivers of dietary intake.

Many initiatives to transform food systems and promote healthier diets focus on improvements in food supply (see Chapters 6 and 7) and in food environments (see Chapter 5), addressing availability, accessibility, and affordability of healthy foods in the marketplace. Actions must also focus on demand-side drivers of food choices to achieve sustainable healthy diets.[8] Understanding individual food choices and their net aggregate – which constitutes demand – is essential for any effort to reshape food systems to achieve

FIGURE 1 Consumption of all five food groups, ultra-processed foods, and sugar-sweetened beverages

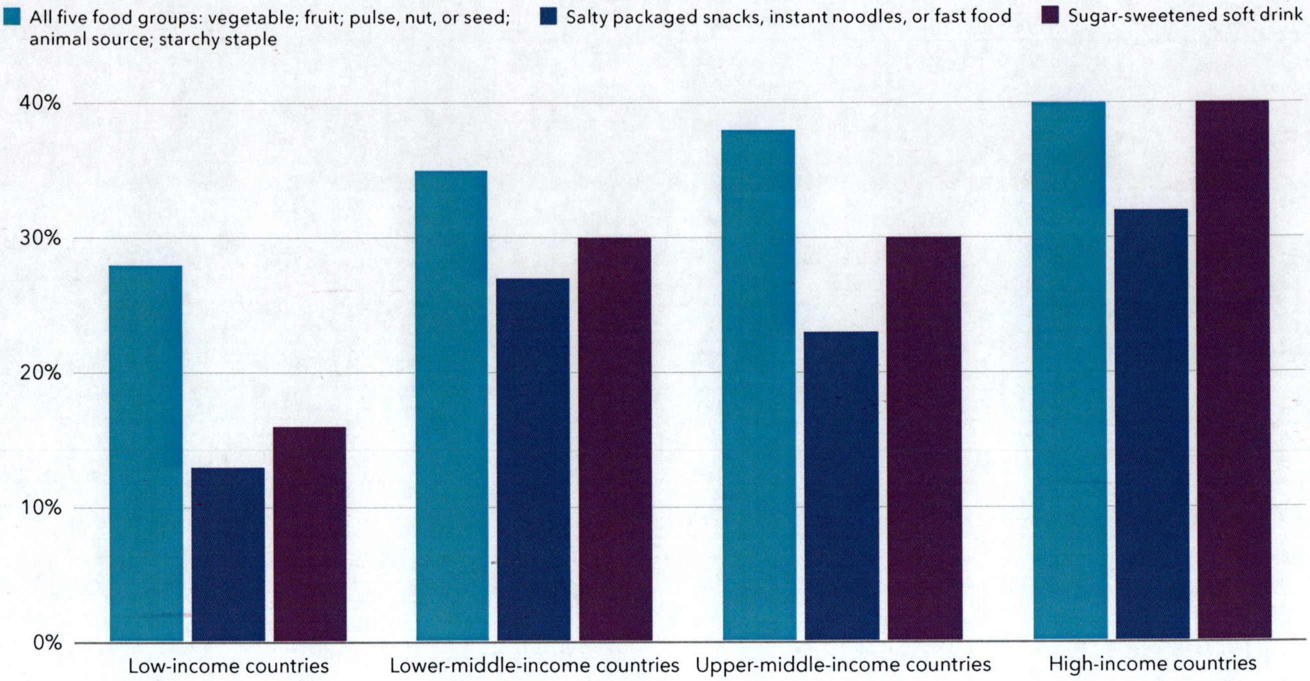

Source: Data from Food Systems Dashboard, www.foodsystemsdashboard.org

Note: Based on 24-hour recall among adults ages 15 years and older. Data from 2021.

broad nutrition and sustainability goals. This chapter presents an overview of food choice and consumer food demand in complex food systems, provides a summary of evidence for demand-side approaches to improve the healthfulness of diets, and identifies key areas where demand-side approaches can foster healthier food choices to achieve optimal health and nutrition.

WHAT ARE DEMAND-SIDE FACTORS, AND WHY DO THEY MATTER?

Food choice and food demand are two related but distinct concepts (Box 1).[9] A common misconception is that people living in LMICs have limited choice. However, even in resource-constrained settings, most

BOX 1 DEFINITIONS

CONSUMER BEHAVIOR: The activities through which individuals engage with markets and how they purchase, use, and dispose of goods and services. In food markets, this includes behaviors related to acquisition, storage and waste, preparation, intrahousehold allocation, and consumption of foods.

FOOD CHOICE: The processes by which people consider what and how to acquire, prepare, store, distribute, and consume foods and beverages.[a]

FOOD DEMAND: The quantity, amount, and type of food that consumers want to buy at a given price, which is determined by the interaction of consumer preferences with market conditions.[b]

FIGURE 2 A consumer-focused food systems framework for sustainable healthy diets

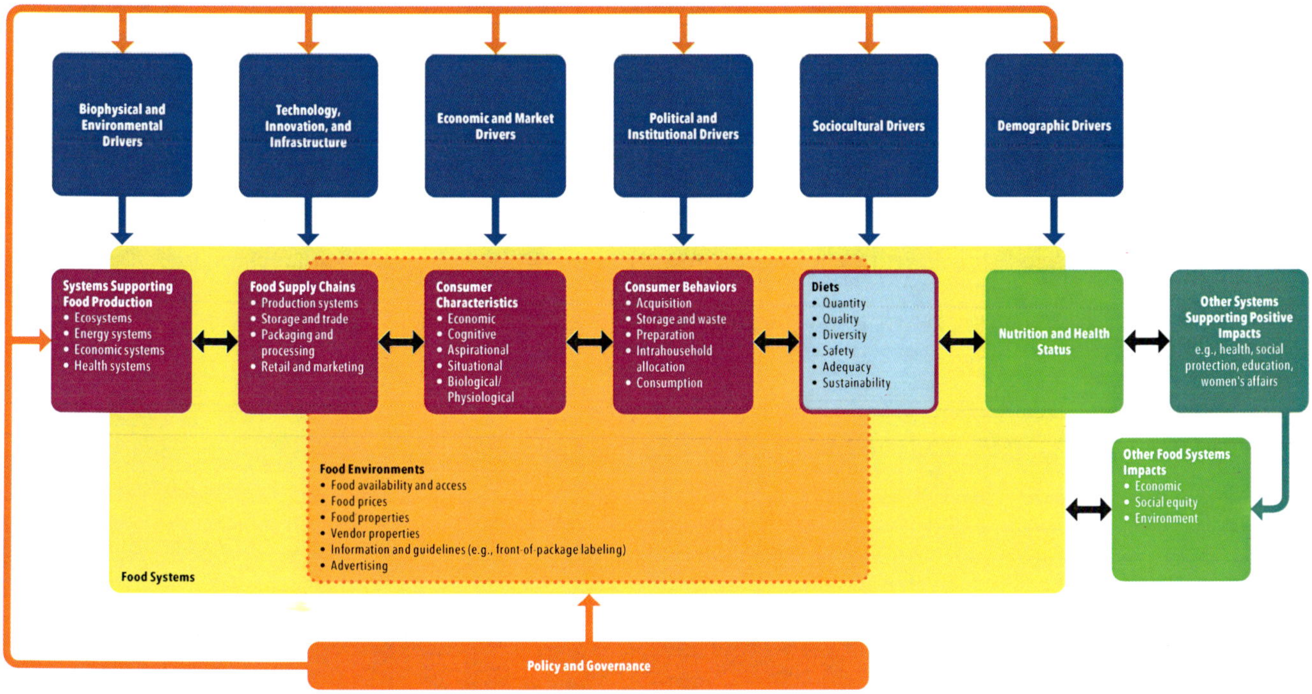

Source: Adapted from High Level Panel of Experts on Food Security and Nutrition of the Committee on World Food Security, *Food Security and Nutrition: Building a Global Narrative Towards 2030* (Rome: 2020).

people have some choice of what foods to prepare, serve, and consume, and when, where, with whom, and how to do so.[10] There are many drivers of these food choice processes that contribute to consumer behavior. Assessment of food demand provides insight into relationships between consumer characteristics (their tastes and preferences) and market conditions that shape consumer behavior, including prices, income levels, availability of substitutes and complements, consumer expectations, and government policies.[11] Understanding food choice processes, consumer behavior, and food demand in the context of dynamic food systems is essential for the development, implementation, and evaluation of demand-side approaches to foster sustainable healthy diets.

In the food systems framework developed by the High Level Panel of Experts on Food Security and Nutrition,[12] consumer behaviors are depicted at the center of the food system. We have expanded this framework to include key consumer characteristics and behaviors (Figure 2). A clearer understanding of the drivers of food choice and consumer behaviors provides an important foundation for developing innovative programs and policies for sustainable healthy diets.[13] For example, knowledge is needed about how consumers think (such as consumer perspectives on food safety),[14] shifting aspirational values and priorities,[15] changes in situational food access and time use due to shifting livelihoods,[16] and individual economic interactions with formal and informal food markets.[17]

Any intervention designed to change demand for certain foods or ways of eating must take into account the particular context, including relevant trends in the cultural, social, economic, and food environments. Further, policies meant to support healthy eating can also have impacts on demand for foods that affect dietary and sustainability outcomes, specifically through the varied trade-offs, priorities, constraints, and facilitators inherent in these policy actions. For example, many communities in LMICs are undergoing dramatic shifts in livelihoods due to broad technological, geopolitical, and environmental changes that affect the reliability of income and reduce time available for food purchase and production. In this context, any intervention that aims to increase demand for healthy foods must account for the complex trade-offs consumers make across income, time, energy, and other considerations. For example, healthy foods that require consistent access to food preparation equipment or substantial preparation time are unlikely to be adopted.

Aligning priorities and efforts across supply- and demand-side sectors is also a major challenge for the successful development and scaling of evidence-based programs and policies for sustainable healthy diets. Ideally, alignment across sectors would ensure the development of food environments that offer access to foods of adequate quality and diversity (supply side), facilitate acquisition of necessary knowledge and skills to increase demand for healthy foods (demand side), and instill the demand for and motivation to apply resources, knowledge, and skills to procure foods and beverages for optimal diets of all household members (demand side). The following sections provide an overview of demand-side approaches for increasing healthfulness of diets, with examples of successful interventions.

WHAT WORKS TO SHIFT FOOD CHOICES AND CONSUMER DEMAND?

Creating demand for sustainable healthy diets[18] requires shifting personal and collective food choice behaviors. The FAO and WHO guiding principles for sustainable healthy diets[19] identify two key demand-side actions: (1) developing **national food-based dietary guidelines** that define context-specific diets; and (2) promoting **behavior change**, including consumer empowerment and food and nutrition education. These demand-side actions can also incentivize sustainable production of healthy foods and improve the enabling environment for production by influencing consumer preferences and increasing purchasing power. Other important interventions to shift diets include **multisectoral approaches**, most notably nutrition-sensitive agriculture, social protection programs, and school meals and school-based nutrition programs. When designed to promote sustainable healthy diets, these programs are often leveraged to generate demand.

NATIONAL FOOD-BASED DIETARY GUIDELINES

Food-based dietary guidelines (FBDGs) encourage healthier and increasingly more sustainable food choices and create environments conducive to better health and nutrition by offering practical guidance on specific food groups, nutrients, and dietary patterns. FBDGs provide context-specific advice and principles for healthy diets and lifestyles based on evidence, and respond to a country's public health and nutrition priorities, food production and consumption patterns, sociocultural influences, food composition data, and accessibility.[20] FBDGs are shifting toward a more comprehensive approach to diets, with countries now incorporating advice into their guidelines on meal combinations, eating habits, food safety, lifestyle, and sustainability. These guidelines provide a framework for public education, healthcare guidance, food production priorities, nutrition programs, and policies on food labeling and advertising. In Sri Lanka, for example, national FBDGs have led to the development of a "model food plate."[21] This educational tool, representative of a balanced diet, was tailored to align with the cultural palate, locally sourced foods, and nutritional requirements of the Sri Lankan populace. The tool has been integrated into school curricula and used by public health midwives for community-based education.

More than 100 countries have developed tailored national FBDGs, often complemented by visual food guides for consumer education,[22] but not all are implemented, and many LMICs do not yet have national FBDGs. Among the countries with FBDGs, none of the guidelines fully meet all the global recommendations for both encouraged food groups (fruits and vegetables; legumes, nuts, and seeds; whole grains; fish) and discouraged ones (sugar, red meat, processed meat).[23] Even so, a recent analysis of 85 national FBDGs found that their adoption by the population would lead to a 15 percent reduction on average in premature mortality from NCDs and a reduction of 13 percent in greenhouse gas emissions.[24] This decrease in mortality reflects dietary shifts recommended by the FBDGs, such as increased consumption of whole grains

(+19 percent), vegetables (+11 percent), fruits (+10 percent), legumes (+5 percent), fish (+3 percent), and nuts and seeds (+1 percent), and decreased intake of processed and red meats (−4 percent and −3 percent, respectively).[25] The potential effectiveness of FBDGs, if everyone follows the guidelines, varies widely by region, from a 6 percent mortality decrease in Africa – where communicable diseases still pose a significant health risk – to as much as 19 percent in North America, attributed to notable declines in obesity rates. Indeed, the health advantages of adopting FBDGs could equal 10-25 percent of a country's GDP, highlighting the significant value of these dietary guidelines.

While FBDGs are an important starting point for encouraging the uptake and demand for sustainable healthy diets at a population level, adoption of their recommendations remains a major challenge. Clear and consistent policy actions and investments are needed to support fulfilment of the recommendations of FBDGs.

SOCIAL AND BEHAVIOR CHANGE INTERVENTIONS

Social and behavior change (SBC) interventions aim to change individual and collective behaviors by addressing their drivers. SBC interventions leverage informational, technological, and social platforms (for example, counseling or education, mobile phones or wireless technology, mass media, social groups, or gatherings) to apply common behavior change techniques,[26] including:

- providing instructions on how to perform a behavior (such as brochures or recipe cards),
- demonstrating a behavior (such as cooking or feeding sessions),
- providing information on benefits or consequences (such as posters or tv/radio spots),
- using a credible or influential source (such as campaigns with respected leaders or celebrities),
- adding objects to the environment or substituting with alternatives (such as food supplements or kitchen products), or
- restructuring the physical or social environment (such as modifying physical spaces to make behavior easier, engaging groups that are not typically included, or mobilizing communities).

SBC interventions have been successful in influencing consumer behaviors related to consumption of healthy foods, such as fruits, vegetables, whole grains, and some animal-source foods, and in improving dietary diversity. However, SBC interventions have had mixed results in changing consumption of unhealthy foods, including ultra-processed foods and beverages,[27] which is perhaps unsurprising given their intense appeal and commercial force.

Interventions to improve diets often start with awareness and educational efforts. Nutrition education interventions, for instance, assume that consumer knowledge is a key driver of food demand, and evidence shows that diets can be improved by increasing awareness of the health benefits of a diverse diet or the dangers of unhealthy foods. For example, increasing caregiver knowledge and skills about complementary feeding for infants and young children (that is, feeding solid, semi-solid, and liquid foods along with breast milk)[28] have led to significant improvements in children's diets (Box 2).[29] To reduce intake of SSBs such as carbonated sodas and fruit juices, most studies have tested the impact of providing information on the consequences of high sugar intake, but the intervention that has proved most effective among children is modeling or demonstrating appropriate behavior (for example, choosing or preparing less-sweetened alternatives) by parents or other adults.[30]

SBC interventions need to be high quality, equitable, and scalable and to allow for the maintenance of positive food choice behaviors if they are to be successful in achieving sustainable healthy diets and changing the contextual norms underpinning those behaviors. Furthermore, evidence shows that approaches that

BOX 2 NUTRITION EDUCATION FOR PARENTS IMPROVES CHILDREN'S DIETS

In Nigeria, only 22 percent of children achieve minimum dietary diversity, meaning that they consume the minimum recommended number of food groups per day.[a] Fathers are key influencers of children's diets but are not well-informed about which types of foods help children develop. The Alive & Thrive initiative implemented an intensive multichannel social and behavior change (SBC) campaign aimed at educating caregivers on complementary feeding and increasing paternal support for child nutrition. The campaign engaged caregivers by distributing communication materials such as pamphlets, sharing posters at community meetings, delivering information during religious services, offering counseling sessions during home visits from community health workers, disseminating information to fathers via mobile text messages, and using mass media outlets such as television and radio for broader reach. These efforts led to increases in caregivers' nutrition knowledge and in children's consumption of fish and eggs.[b]

Similar successes were observed in Bangladesh, where education on complementary feeding delivered through mass media, interpersonal communication, and community efforts led to improved dietary diversity.[c] In Ghana, a series of drama programs targeted to both mothers and the wider family were broadcast on the radio. These programs aimed to not only educate caregivers on child feeding, but also encourage support from other household members. This campaign led to an increase in health and nutrition knowledge among caregivers and improvements in dietary diversity among young children.[d] These approaches considered the cultural and social norms in these countries, recognizing the role that other family members and society play in influencing children's diets.

The development of practical skills, such as cooking and food preparation, also improves dietary diversity and nutrition outcomes. In Ethiopia, an SBC intervention provided education about adequate feeding practices and cooking demonstrations with the goal of improving complementary feeding and enhancing caregivers' self-efficacy in preparing food and feeding their children.[e] The intervention led to increased consumption of fruits, vegetables, and animal-source foods (including eggs and dairy). In Malawi, a nutrition education intervention targeting pregnant women included a cooking demonstration and food processing activity focused on following the national dietary guidelines.[f] At the end of the intervention, the participants reported improved nutrition knowledge and greater dietary diversity.

Most of the studies described above measured outcomes on diet quality or food groups using a dietary diversity survey module based on maternal reports, which are subject to reporting bias; a few but not all of the studies attempted to measure and account for social desirability bias.

combine interventions to address multiple drivers and multiple socioecological levels (individual, interpersonal, organizational, community, general public) may be more effective than stand-alone interventions.[31]

Unfortunately, development activities or actions such as humanitarian aid can unintentionally increase demand for ultra-processed foods and beverages (Box 3).[32] Such experiences provide cautionary tales that should be considered when designing or implementing food-related interventions.

With or without SBC interventions, integrated multisectoral approaches have been shown to be effective in generating demand for sustainable healthy diets in low-income settings, particularly in addressing barriers by improving access to and affordability of sustainable healthy foods. In the following sections, we highlight three such multisectoral strategies or platforms: nutrition-sensitive agriculture, social protection, and school meal and school-based nutrition programs.

NUTRITION-SENSITIVE AGRICULTURE PROGRAMS

Agriculture programs have potential to improve global food availability and access and to enhance household food security, diet quality, income, and women's empowerment. As part of a broader food systems approach, agriculture programs that integrate nutrition interventions (known as nutrition-sensitive

BOX 3 UNINTENDED CONSEQUENCES: HUMANITARIAN ASSISTANCE IN POST-EARTHQUAKE NEPAL

Nepal has made progress in reducing malnutrition, although childhood stunting and wasting remain significant challenges. In Kathmandu Valley, children under two years of age obtain one-quarter of their calories from unhealthy snack foods and beverages,[a] and only 1.1 percent of Nepalese adults (over 15 years of age) consume at least the recommended 400 grams of fruits and vegetables daily.[b]

A study in a low-income setting in the country revealed substantial changes in food behaviors over the past decade, with increased consumption of rice, meat, and highly processed snack foods.[c] After the devastating earthquake in 2015, Nepal's nutrition transition accelerated, stimulated by the inflow of cash for reconstruction efforts and increased availability of packaged snack foods. The emergency food aid provided after the earthquake included packaged foods like instant noodles.[d] This inadvertently increased demand for unhealthy foods, as people became accustomed to eating these foods.

interventions) and are gender focused can increase agricultural productivity, boost women's agency, and promote nutritious crops that can be consumed by women and children or sold for income. One approach to addressing the challenges of affordability and accessibility of healthy foods – such as fruits and vegetables, which tend to be the most expensive food groups in LMICs (see Chapter 4)[33] – is through home gardening, which can provide direct access to homegrown fresh produce. In rural Bangladesh, major improvements were observed in household-level fruit and vegetable consumption and dietary diversity when agricultural training was combined with nutrition education.[34] In Cambodia, complementary interventions spanning production enhancement, processing or preserving techniques, and nutrition education led women farmers to significantly increase both their yields and personal levels of vegetable consumption.[35]

By increasing household access to nutritious foods, nutrition-sensitive agriculture programs can lead to improvements in the diets of young children, who are especially vulnerable to malnutrition and poor development due to low-quality diets.[36] A recent meta-analysis of studies in several African countries and Cambodia showed that children under five years of age are 64 percent more likely to achieve minimum dietary diversity when exposed to such interventions.[37] In India, children under two years of age were more likely to achieve minimum dietary diversity if their caregivers viewed videos about nutrition and agriculture, compared with those who did not.[38] Similar interventions that combined agriculture programs with nutrition messaging in Ghana, Malawi, and Nepal also showed positive impacts on children's diets.[39]

SOCIAL PROTECTION PROGRAMS

Social protection encompasses public actions intended to support poor and vulnerable individuals and households, including social assistance programs that provide food and cash transfers. These programs function in both urban and rural settings in many LMICs, and evidence shows that they improve food security and reduce chronic poverty at the household level.[40] At the individual level, evidence suggests that social assistance programs are effective in improving dietary diversity and intake of micronutrient-rich foods among women and children.[41] These programs also improve nutrition outcomes such as anthropometric indicators, hemoglobin, and anemia, though they are more effective for women than children.[42] Evaluation of these interventions also provides important lessons on the transfer modality (such as cash or food) and effective design components. For example, in-kind transfers (which often include fortified foods) have been found more likely to improve women's and children's nutritional status, compared with cash transfers.[43] Delivering behavior change communication alongside the transfers has been linked to program effectiveness, and increasing the size of transfers has been linked to improvements in dietary diversity and

BOX 4 WOMEN'S GROUP-BASED PROGRAMS LEAD TO NUTRITION CHANGE IN SOUTH ASIA

Women's groups serve as important social and financial institutions, particularly in South Asia.[a] Originally formed as savings and credit groups, these organizations are now providing platforms to deliver health and nutrition interventions.[b] Studies on the impact of nutrition interventions delivered through women's groups in South Asia suggest that information provision can modify behaviors but does not change nutritional status among women and children. This work also draws attention to important aspects of delivery and design:

1. To have traction, outcomes selected must resonate with and be relevant for the members of the group. The intervention should not only focus on information delivery but also mobilize the community and build their capabilities.
2. Interventions must be intentional (having components with a nutrition focus) and consider the pathways to impact, and they must ensure that the inputs being delivered are adequate for achieving the desired outcomes, are targeting (and reaching) the right group, and are delivered with an intensity and for the duration that is needed to have the desired impact.
3. Nutrition outcomes often depend on factors such as the healthcare system or availability of nutritious foods and/or are constrained by resources available to households. To identify such constraints and address them in design and delivery, interventions must take a holistic view.

consumption of animal-source foods (for more on the role of these foods in healthy diets, see Chapter 7).[44] Success in improving nutrition outcomes varies significantly by the type of social assistance program and its design (for example, target populations, inclusion of fortified foods, and behavior change communication), meaning that programs should be selected and designed based on the intended objectives and the particular context.[45]

Empowering women by enhancing their agency in decision-making, protecting against intimate partner violence, and providing access to education also contributes to restructuring the social environment in ways that better engage women in food systems and generate demand for healthier diets. Women's groups, for example, can play an important role in enhancing the objective of social assistance programs (Box 4).

SCHOOL MEAL PROGRAMS AND SCHOOL-BASED NUTRITION PROGRAMS

School-based initiatives can lay foundational pillars for the development of food preferences, nutritional literacy, and agricultural understanding, fostering demand for healthy foods that are safe, nutritious, sustainable, and affordable from early childhood into adulthood. The Global Survey of School Meal Programs underlines the pivotal role of school meal initiatives as investments in human capital, ensuring that children's fundamental nutritional requirements are met so they can thrive.[46] These programs, such as India's Mid-Day Meal Scheme, demonstrate that providing free meals in primary schools can yield intergenerational nutritional advantages, evidenced by improved growth metrics in the children of beneficiaries.[47]

School meal programs go beyond simply feeding children to also promote awareness of healthy dietary habits and steer food preferences toward nutritious choices. WHO recommends strategies for school-based nutrition programs that include (1) targeting the school curriculum to include nutrition education for children and teaching professionals; (2) restructuring the school food environment through placement or convenience of foods, marketing or promotion, variety or portion sizes of foods, school menu reformulations, and canteen policies; and (3) forming partnerships with students, families, staff, and community members to encourage healthy food purchases and adequate allocation to household members.[48]

Together and individually, these strategies have shown positive impacts on dietary behaviors, notably enhancing fruit and vegetable consumption and reducing fat intake.[49] These interventions can lay the groundwork for lifelong healthy eating habits, not just addressing undernutrition but also preventing obesity and NCDs by fostering more nutritious diets. However, further evidence is needed on the effectiveness of some strategies, underscoring the need for research to inform evolving objectives.[50]

CHANGING COURSE: PRIORITIES FOR GENERATING DEMAND FOR SUSTAINABLE HEALTHY DIETS

Generating and supporting demand for sustainable healthy diets requires an understanding of the drivers of food choices, especially the perceptions and values of consumers. Drawing on the evidence and insights presented in this chapter, we outline the following priorities for fostering this pivotal shift in consumer demand.

DEVELOPING FOOD-BASED DIETARY GUIDELINES. Developing FBDGs tailored to local contexts can empower consumers and help them navigate their food environments to make healthy food choices. These guidelines must not only communicate the nutritional benefits of diverse diets but also emphasize the environmental sustainability of food choices.

STRENGTHENING SOCIAL AND BEHAVIOR CHANGE COMMUNICATION. Robust SBC interventions are essential to effectively shift consumer preferences and habits. These interventions should use a variety of platforms – from traditional media to digital channels – to reach wide audiences. SBC should build practical skills that enable consumers to incorporate diverse, nutritious foods into their daily lives and nurture an informed consumer base that can drive food demand. Engaging influential change agents and using culturally relevant content can enhance the effectiveness of these campaigns.

INTEGRATING MULTISECTORAL APPROACHES. Increasing demand for sustainable healthy diets requires a concerted effort across multiple sectors. This includes agriculture, education, health, and economic policies that collectively create an enabling environment for healthy food choices. These programs should be designed with a deep understanding of local food systems and consumer behaviors to ensure they meet the needs and preferences of the target populations.

By prioritizing these actions, we can generate the demand necessary to drive the transition toward sustainable healthy diets. However, achieving widespread adoption of better diets will also require overcoming socioeconomic and affordability, accessibility, and availability constraints that can make it difficult for households and individuals to act on knowledge gained from interventions. For example, public-private partnerships can play a crucial role in aligning the food industry's incentives with public health and sustainability goals by supporting the development of healthier food products, promoting responsible marketing practices, and increasing the availability and affordability of nutritious food options (see Chapters 4, 5, 6, and 7) that are in the best interest of public health and environmental stewardship. In addition, interventions must be sensitive to the barriers faced by different population groups. This includes ensuring that healthy food options are not only available but also affordable and accessible to all segments of society. Policies and programs should be designed to address the specific needs and constraints of vulnerable groups and reduce inequities in food access and nutrition outcomes. The chapters that follow explore the role of these constraints, including food affordability, the food environment, and supply-side constraints, which must be addressed to increase demand for healthy diets.

CHAPTER 4

Diet Affordability
Understanding the High Cost of Healthy Diets

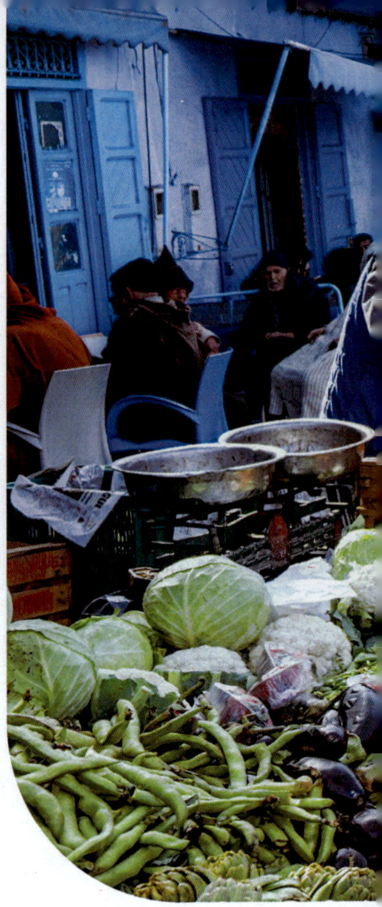

DEREK HEADEY, KALLE HIRVONEN, HAROLD ALDERMAN, SASKIA DE PEE, AND KALYANI RAGHUNATHAN

Derek Headey and **Kalle Hirvonen** are senior research fellows, Development Strategies and Governance Unit, International Food Policy Research Institute (IFPRI). **Harold Alderman** is a senior research fellow, Poverty, Gender, and Inclusion Unit, IFPRI. **Saskia de Pee** is chief of Analytics and Science for Food and Nutrition, United Nations World Food Programme. **Kalyani Raghunathan** is a research fellow, Poverty, Gender, and Inclusion Unit, IFPRI.

KEY MESSAGES

- Healthy diets that provide a range of safe and nutritious foods are not yet affordable for much of the world's population, especially in South Asia and Africa. The cost of a healthy diet is defined as the least expensive combination of locally available items that meet a food-based dietary guideline. This metric, which is relatively new, indicates that between 2 and 3 billion people cannot afford a healthy diet.
- Poverty is a primary factor limiting diets. There is a huge gap between the current food budgets of the world's poor and the spending needed for a healthy diet. Current social protection transfers in Asia and Africa barely begin to fill the healthy diet affordability gap.
- High prices of nutritious foods also limit access to healthy diets. Nutrient-dense foods – especially fruits, vegetables, and animal-source foods – are relatively expensive compared with calorie-dense foods, in part because agricultural policies and consumer subsidies have long favored production of staple crops.
- Provisional evidence suggests healthy diet costs are much higher in countries with poor transport, storage, and logistics infrastructure and services.

To shift actual diets toward healthy diets, we need to:

- Improve national and subnational monitoring of healthy diet affordability, including food prices, expenditures, and wages, in order to strengthen knowledge and provide a strong platform for nutrition interventions.
- Accelerate pro-poor economic growth in low- and middle-income countries (LMICs) through reforms to catalyze more equitable and inclusive growth.
- Increase availability and reduce prices of nutritious foods by repurposing agricultural policies toward nutritious foods and increasing investment in transport, infrastructure, and logistics.
- Scale up nutrition-sensitive social protection in LMICs, including appropriate targeting of vulnerable groups, delivering transfers that come closer to bridging the healthy diet affordability gap, and linking social protection with nutrition education interventions that increase demand for healthy foods and decrease demand for unhealthy foods.

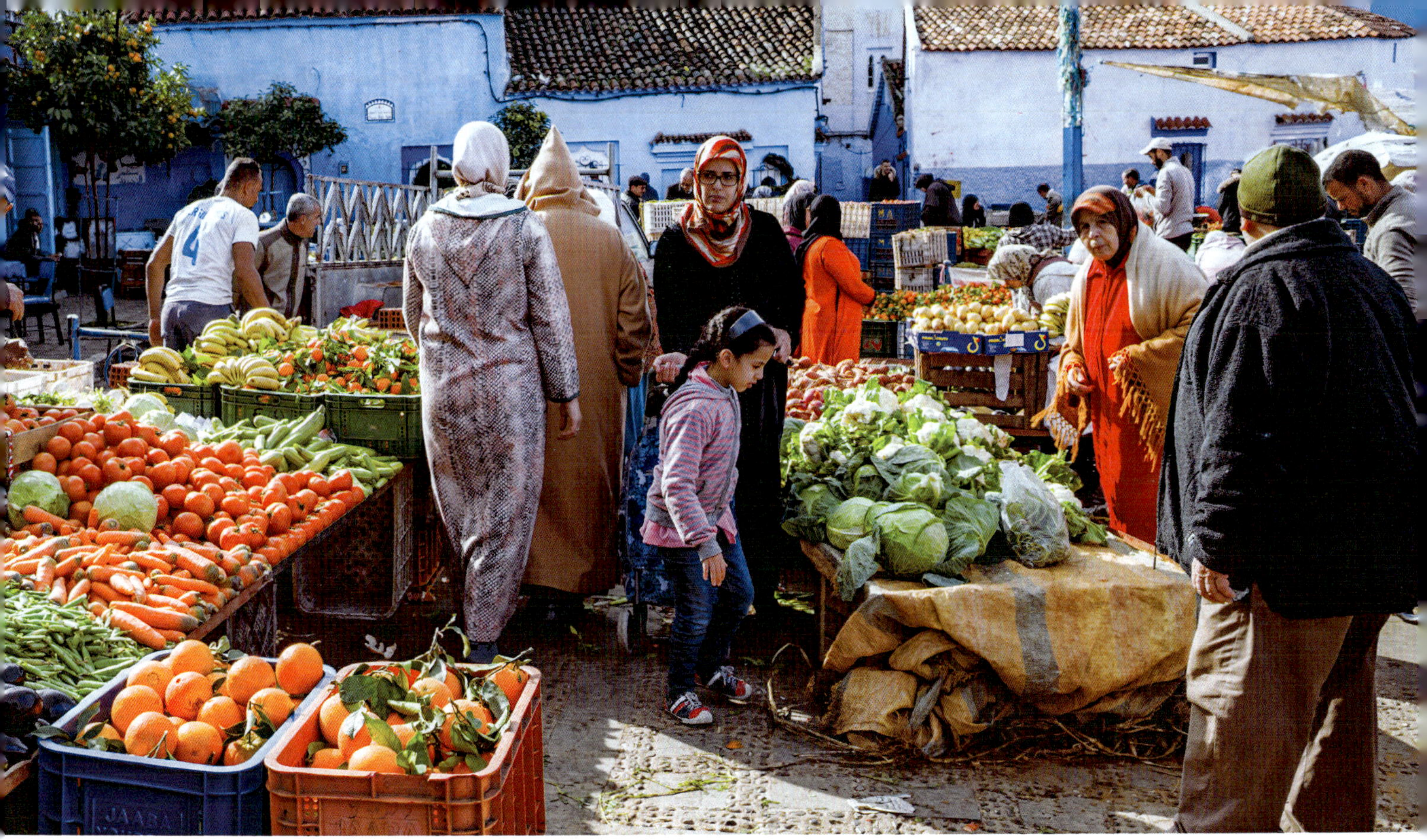

The 1996 World Food Summit defined food security as existing "when all people, at all times, have physical and economic access to sufficient safe and nutritious food that meets their dietary needs and food preferences for an active and healthy life." For many decades, however, food security measurement and policy were chiefly focused on ensuring adequate supplies of calories or calorie-dense staple foods, rather than year-round universal affordability of a wider range of safe and nutritious foods. In the past five years, new metrics of healthy diet affordability have been developed to address this (see Box 1), first in Asian case studies[1] and then in the global context of costing the EAT-Lancet diet[2] and a global healthy diet adopted in the State of Food Security and Nutrition (SOFI) reports.[3] Depending on the methods used and the definition of a healthy diet,[4] it is estimated that between 2 and 3 billion people worldwide – mostly in low- and middle-income countries (LMICs) – cannot afford a healthy diet.

The implications for human nutrition are striking: affordability is a binding constraint to achieving a healthy diet in the world's poorest countries, and it would require truly heroic efforts to improve universal economic access to healthy foods. But what are those heroic efforts? To initiate strategic thinking on this question, this chapter poses several questions.

First, how large are the scale and scope of the affordability problem? How many billions of people cannot afford a healthy diet? In which regions are the "diet poor" concentrated? How large is the gap between their current food budgets and the food spending required to support a healthy diet?

Second, why are healthy diets so unaffordable for so many? Is poverty simply too deep and pervasive? Or do poor people also live in food environments (see Chapter 5) where healthy foods are expensive? If we address affordability constraints, could we really achieve a rapid improvement in diets, or would people's preferences also stand in the way?

Third, what actions are required to not only address the healthy diet affordability problem, but also achieve a shift toward healthy diets by simultaneously addressing behavioral barriers to choosing healthy foods?

BOX 1 MEASURING THE COST AND AFFORDABILITY OF HEALTHY DIETS

The cost of a healthy diet is defined as the least expensive combination of locally available items that meet a food-based dietary guideline (FBDG). This "cost and affordability of a healthy diet" metric (CoAHD) is relatively new, having first been developed in Asian contexts using national FBDGs, and then in global studies on cost and affordability of the EAT-Lancet global reference diet and an alternative global healthy diet now used in the State of Food Security and Nutrition reports. Cost of healthy diet metrics are different from the cost of nutrient-adequate diets designed to meet all essential nutrient requirements. Many organizations (including the World Food Programme) use nutrient-adequacy diet costing for analysis of specific target groups, social protection transfer requirements, and food fortification interventions, which is especially useful in settings where unaffordability of healthy, nutritious diets is widespread and deep. However, a healthy diet consists of more than just nutrients, since healthy foods can help to prevent disease just as unhealthy foods can increase the risk of disease. Moreover, the EAT-Lancet healthy reference diet also has environmental sustainability objectives.

There are four key steps for measuring the cost of a healthy diet:

1. Quantify a hypothetical reference diet consisting of consumption targets for essential food groups that are consistent with FBDGs.

2. Convert food group recommendations into number of servings or grams into calories.

3. Assign food items to the guideline's food group classifications.

4. Convert retail prices of food items into standardized costs per edible calorie.

5. Select the cheapest food items that the reference diet's food group targets.

These healthy diet costs can be expressed in different currencies and in nominal or real terms, but only really assume significance when used to measure the affordability of the least-cost healthy diet or when monitored. The key challenge here is to estimate a realistic food budget for an individual or household. Some studies compare the cost of a healthy diet to a household's actual food expenditures, while others estimate a share of total expenditure or income that might be spent on food. Unfortunately, income/expenditure surveys are infrequently implemented in LMICs (often only every five years, a far lower frequency than the general availability of administrative or other data on prices). In contrast, a recent IFPRI study argues that affordability of healthy diets can instead be monitored at high frequency by comparing healthy diet costs to wage rates for different kinds of low-skilled activities or occupations. The authors show that monthly price and wage data can be used to track the impacts of major economic shocks on healthy diet affordability in crisis-affected countries like Sri Lanka, Myanmar, and Ethiopia, as well as periods of long-term progress in improving affordability of healthy diets.

CoAHD measures can be sensitive to choice of methods and data sources, yet the conclusion that several billion people around the world cannot afford a healthy diet is robust, and the value of CoAHD metrics in capturing key affordability constraints to improving diets is clear. There is, moreover, huge potential scope to expand CoAHD measurement at the national and subnational levels using existing government data.

Source: Tufts Friedman School of Nutrition Science and Policy, "Food Prices for Nutrition" (https://sites.tufts.edu/foodpricesfornutrition/methods/); D. Headey, F. Bachewe, Q. Marshall, K. Raghunathan, and K. Mahrt, "Food Prices and the Wages of the Poor: A Cost-effective Addition to High-frequency Food Security Monitoring," *Food Policy* 125 (2024): 102630; D. Headey, K. Hirvonen, and H. Alderman, "Estimating the Cost and Affordability of Healthy Diets: How Much Do Methods Matter?," IFPRI Discussion Paper 2179, IFPRI, Washington, DC, 2023.

In the remainder of this chapter, we will attempt to answer these questions. We conclude the chapter with a summary of six sets of actions that are instrumental for rapidly achieving a convergence of actual diets in LMICs toward healthy diets.

HOW BIG IS THE PROBLEM?

To illustrate the healthy diet affordability problem at a global level, we report results from an updated empirical analysis of the cost of the EAT-Lancet global reference diet (hereafter ELD).[5] We use the ELD caloric intake recommendations for nine food groups to estimate each food group's minimum cost and the aggregate least-cost ELD for 107 LMICs.

A first key finding is that the sample average for the least-cost ELD diet is $2.98 per person per day in 2017 purchasing power parity (PPP) terms.[6] While this sounds inexpensive for a typical consumer in a high-income country, it is quite costly for consumers in LMICs. The median per capita income in a country like Tanzania is just $2.33 per day, which also needs to cover an individual's non-food expenditure requirements, implying that the ELD is highly unaffordable for a typical Tanzanian.

Why are healthy diets relatively expensive? Figure 1 shows the calorie shares of the ELD as well as its average cost shares. When a food group has a cost share that is smaller than its calorie share, it is a relatively cheap source of calories: generally starchy staples, oils and fats, and sugars. Conversely, when a food group has a cost share that exceeds its calorie share, it is a relatively expensive source of calories even if it delivers micronutrients or high-quality protein relatively cheaply. Fruits, vegetables, and animal-source foods (meat, fish, dairy, and eggs) all have relatively high cost shares and collectively account for 57 percent of the average ELD cost, compared with just 20 percent of calorie shares.

Data from household expenditure surveys allow us to estimate the number of people whose food expenditure is below that country's ELD cost. Table 1 reports cost and affordability of a healthy diet (CoAHD) statistics stratified by World Bank income groups and regions. Column (1) reports the absolute number of people who cannot afford a healthy diet ("diet poor" for short), while column (2) reports each group's share of the global diet-poor, and column (3) reports the prevalence of people unable to afford a healthy diet. This table also reports the difference between an average individual's estimated food expenditure and the healthy diet cost (column 4), which reflects the daily cash transfer that would be required to make a healthy diet affordable to the average person in each region or income group, assuming (optimistically) that the transfer is entirely spent on food. Aggregating this measure for all diet-poor individuals yields the total amount of money that would have to be transferred per day to eliminate diet poverty in a given income or regional group, as reported in column (5).[7]

Table 1 suggests that 2.66 billion people in 128 countries could not afford the ELD in 2017,[8] with around 50 percent of these residing in South

FIGURE 1 The EAT-Lancet reference diet's recommended calorie intake shares versus its cost shares in 107 LMICs

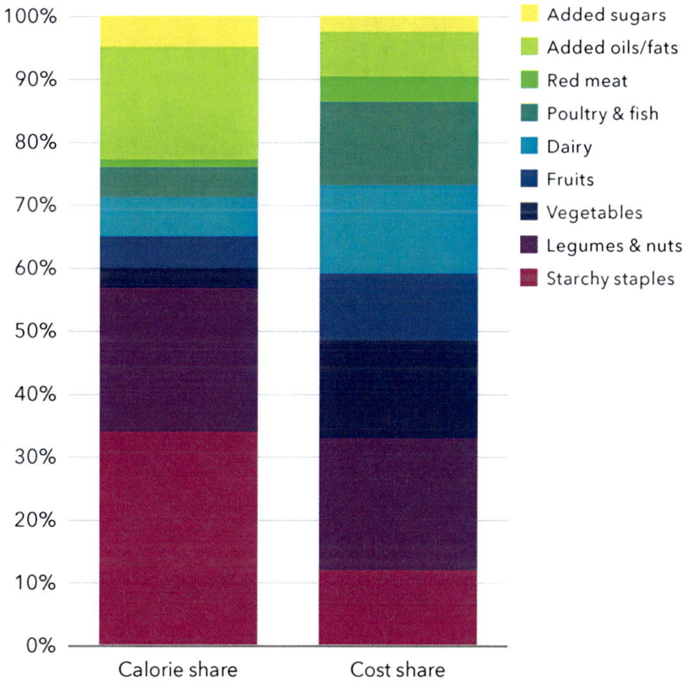

Source: Authors' estimates based on methods described in K. Hirvonen, Y. Bai, D. Headey, and W.A. Masters, "Affordability of the EAT-Lancet Reference Diet: A Global Analysis," *Lancet Global Health* 8, 1 (2020): e59–e66.

TABLE 1 Metrics on "diet poverty" for the EAT-Lancet reference diet, by World Bank income groups and geographic regions, 2017

Income levels and geographic regions	Number of countries	(1) Absolute number (millions)	(2) Share of "global" diet-poor population	(3) Prevalence of unaffordable diet	(4) Daily cost of making healthy diets affordable for an average diet-poor consumer (PPP $) (poverty gap measure)	(5) Aggregate daily cost of making healthy diets affordable for all diet-poor consumers (PPP $ billions)
Income level						
High income	39	11.0	0.4%	1.0%	$0.05	$0.00
Upper-middle income	34	362.2	13.6%	15.0%	$0.44	$0.16
Lower-middle income	35	1913.0	71.7%	67.6%	$1.39	$2.66
Low income	20	382.9	14.3%	84.4%	$1.95	$0.75
Geographic region						
South Asia	6	1315.3	49.3%	76.4%	$1.43	$1.88
Sub-Saharan Africa	38	725.4	27.2%	78.2%	$1.82	$1.32
East Asia and Pacific	13	412.7	15.5%	18.6%	$0.42	$0.17
Middle East and North Africa	9	101.5	3.8%	42.3%	$1.22	$0.12
Latin America and Caribbean	18	93.1	3.5%	17.7%	$0.65	$0.06
Europe and Central Asia	42	16.8	0.6%	2.1%	$0.11	$0.00
North America	2	4.2	0.2%	1.2%	$0.04	$0.00
Global	128	2669.0	100.0%	39.3%	$1.34	$3.56
Global with alternative method	128	2006.7		29.5%	$0.58	$1.17

Note: The main method follows Hirvonen et al. (2020) with a 37 percent fixed non-food cost component, as used in SOFI 2020. The alternative method in the last row of Table 1 adjusts for cross-country differences in demographics, non-food expenditure requirements, and price survey characteristics, as per Headey et al. (2023). PPP $ = purchasing power parity dollars in 2017 terms. See K. Hirvonen, Y. Bai, D.D. Headey, and W.A. Masters, "Affordability of the EAT-Lancet Reference Diet: A Global Analysis," *Lancet Global Health* 8, 1 (2020): e59-e66; and D.D. Headey, K. Hirvonen, and H. Alderman, "Estimating the Cost and Affordability of Healthy Diets: How Much Do Methods Matter?," IFPRI Discussion Paper 2179, IFPRI, Washington, DC, 2023.

Asia, almost 30 percent in sub-Saharan Africa, and just over 15 percent in East and Southeast Asia (see Regional Developments section of this report). In terms of prevalence, three in four people in South Asia and sub-Saharan Africa are estimated to have been unable to afford the ELD in 2017.

These global estimates for 2017, as well as the SOFI reports' estimates, should be treated with some caution for several reasons. First, there are certainly limitations to the underlying data used in global calculations. Price data are for 2017 only, and income/expenditure survey data are often out of date, most notably for India, where the last expenditure survey was implemented in 2011-2012.[9] The number of diet poor in India has almost certainly decreased in the past 12 years. Conversely, economic and other crises in many LMICs since COVID-19 have likely led to increasing numbers of diet poor. For example, military misrule in Myanmar led to a 56 percent increase in the cost of a healthy diet in 2022 and a 14 percentage point increase in the share of people who could not afford that diet (Figure 2).[10] Second, estimation methods matter in global calculations. Drawing on a recent IFPRI study,[11] the bottom row of Table 1 gives alternative estimates that adjust for cross-country differences in demographic structures, non-food expenditure requirements, and price survey characteristics. Strikingly, these adjustments reduce the estimated total number of people who cannot afford the ELD from 2.66 billion to just over 2 billion.

All these considerations suggest an urgent need for updated data and analysis on the cost and affordability of healthy diets at global, regional, national, and subnational levels. Yet, from a practical standpoint, all existing national and global estimates present daunting numbers that highlight the scale of the affordability problem. That problem is immense, and we need to understand why it exists and what to do about it.

WHY ARE HEALTHY DIETS SO UNAFFORDABLE FOR SO MANY? AND WHAT ARE THE SOLUTIONS?

Poverty, price, and preferences represent three barriers to achieving a sustainable shift to healthy diets. The combination of low incomes and relatively high prices for nutritious foods constitutes the key economic barrier to shifting toward healthier diets, but we also need to acknowledge the possibility that economic solutions are necessary but not sufficient. People may not choose to eat healthier diets even when they can afford to do so, or their food environment may have limited availability of healthy foods.

FIGURE 2 Prevalence of households in Myanmar that could not afford a healthy diet, 2022 and 2023

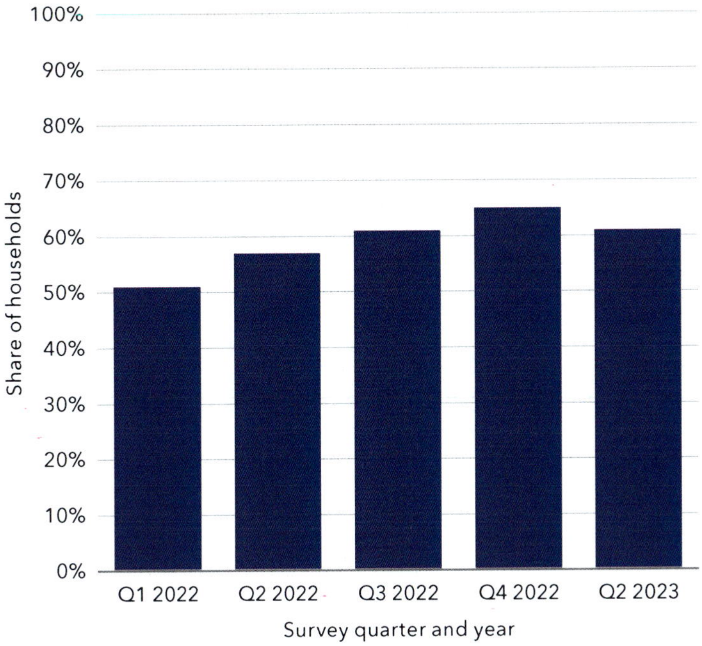

Source: Authors' calculations from IFPRI's Myanmar Household Welfare Survey.

Note: These data reflect the prevalence of households that could not afford a healthy diet during a rapid increase in the cost of living in 2022 and early 2023.

THE POVERTY PROBLEM

ECONOMIC GROWTH. Too many people in the world simply do not earn enough to purchase the recommended quantities of healthy foods in their food environments. How quickly could economic growth improve the affordability of healthy diets in LMICs? To explore this question, we use cross-country regressions to estimate the responsiveness of healthy diet affordability to economic growth. We estimate that a 1 percent increase in per capita GDP is associated with a 1.3 percent reduction in the number of people who cannot afford the minimum cost of the ELD (on average). These results imply that faster economic growth can indeed be expected to help address the affordability problem. However, it is important to know that population growth works in the other direction, by increasing the absolute number of people who cannot afford a healthy diet; a 1 percent increase in population is associated with a 1.8 percent increase in the number of diet poor. Hence economic growth needs to substantially outpace population growth rates, which remain high in sub-Saharan Africa especially (2.5 percent annually as of 2020).

SOCIAL PROTECTION. While economic growth is a critical long-term driver of improved affordability of healthy diets, nutrition-sensitive social protection programs could offer a more immediate means to bridge affordability gaps. However, the current social protection gap – the difference between actual social protection transfers and the level needed to make healthy diets affordable – is enormous. The unadjusted affordability estimates in Table 1 show that the average diet-poor person in a low-income country would require a transfer of \$1.95 per day to afford a healthy diet, which falls to \$1.39 per day in lower-middle-income countries. Those transfers, however, are unrealistic compared to actual transfers. During the extraordinary circumstances of COVID-19, for example, poorer households in lower-middle-income countries in Asia typically received around \$0.50 per day (in cash or in kind). For a household of five, that amounts to \$0.10 per individual, which is woefully insufficient compared with the

$1.39 required to close the gap. It follows that such a modest transfer would also have only a very limited impact on diet quality.[12]

Even so, social protection can still play a role in improving healthy diet affordability. First, in upper-middle-income countries, the affordability challenge is less fiscally overwhelming (Table 1), suggesting that nutrition-sensitive social protection programs in these countries have a realistic prospect of promoting a shift toward achieving affordability of healthy diets. Second, in poorer countries, social protection programs could aim to target the most nutritionally vulnerable groups, such as through maternal and child cash transfers[13] or specially formulated fortified foods for pregnant and breastfeeding women and young children, rather than giving very small transfers to a larger swathe of the population.[14] Third, there is surely scope to scale up social protection in LMICs through internal reallocation of LMIC government expenditures and more generous development assistance to social protection programs. Globally, 1.5 billion people are assisted by social safety nets,[15] with LMICs spending an average of only 1.5 percent of GDP on these programs.[16] Across countries, there is a statistically significant association between social protection spending and decreases in diet poverty. We use that association to project that if LMICs spent 2 percent or more on social safety nets, they could reduce the number of individuals unable to afford the ELD by 95.5 million in 2030.[17]

THE PRICE PROBLEM

Previously, we noted that the average price of the ELD in LMICs is a costly $2.98 per day in 2017 dollars, and that many healthy foods are quite costly for consumers. There are many ways to reduce prices of healthy foods, but for all of them, important trade-offs exist in terms of fiscal costs, the speed at which prices might change, and financial sustainability.

AGRICULTURAL SUPPORT. In the short run, agricultural support through producer subsidies, price subsidies, or border protection measures (such as tariffs) can either increase or decrease consumer prices. The 2022 SOFI report[18] finds that support to agricultural production in richer countries generally focuses on staple foods, dairy, other protein-rich foods, and sugar. In LMICs, rice, wheat, and sugar are often subsidized, while fruits and vegetables are supported much less or even taxed. Consumer price subsidies – which have potential to support healthier diets – are rare in LMICs because of their fiscal cost. They are also likely to be regressive because better-off households consume more nutrient-dense foods than poorer households.

In many Asian countries, rice and wheat are subsidized both for producers (through input subsidies and price supports) and for consumers (as through India's Public Distribution Scheme; see South Asia regional section). The subsidies to farmers almost certainly inhibit diversification into healthy food production, but offering consumers cheaper grains frees up room in household food budgets for spending on non-staple foods, potentially allowing for greater dietary diversification.

However, diversifying agricultural production could have significant effects on relative prices. Healthy foods that are highly perishable would experience the largest price reductions from a given productivity gain, because these commodities cannot be cost-effectively imported or exported except through regional cross-border trade. In other words, prices for perishable healthy foods are set at a more local level, so an increase in supply of a perishable food from an improved production, processing, or marketing technology could result in a sizable sustained reduction in its price, benefiting consumers, but also potentially benefiting producers if productivity gains offset declining prices. Some of these perishable foods may also be attractive investments for other reasons, including for the private sector, especially if strong consumer demand creates scope for sustained expansion of production and domestic marketing. Moreover, from an R&D perspective, fruits, vegetables, and many livestock or aquatic foods are often historically neglected, meaning that additional investments are likely to have notable impacts on productivity, whereas crops like rice, maize, and wheat that benefited from the Green Revolution now face diminishing returns on investment.[19] An additional criterion relevant for selecting high potential commodities for new agricultural R&D

investments is their potential to influence poverty reduction, important in its own right, but also instrumental to achieving a shift toward healthy diets through income effects.

These may seem to be logical assertions, and they are also testable in simulation tools such as IFPRI's RIAPA model,[20] but is there historical evidence that productivity gains in perishable healthy foods translate into reduced real prices? A clear example comes from eggs, which are highly perishable and not easily traded, but are characterized by such steep economies of scale that the transition of small backyard production systems to commercial farms results in massive productivity gains. Unsurprisingly, there is a very strong cross-country correlation between greater commercialization in a country's poultry sector and lower egg prices.[21] We also observe declining egg prices in poultry success stories, such as India in the 1990s and Myanmar in the 2000s. In Myanmar, commercialization from 2008 to 2017 resulted in a 35 percent reduction in the real price of eggs and a 30 percent reduction in the price of poultry meat.[22] Whether the same types of real price reductions are feasible for fruits, vegetables, and legumes or for other animal-source foods is less certain, but this is an important area for future research.

INFRASTRUCTURE AND LOGISTICS. The efficiency of infrastructure and transport logistics can also be expected to affect the costs of a healthy diet, because transport and storage are important for enabling both domestic and international trade as well as for reducing food loss and waste. To explore this, we use the World Bank's transport and infrastructure logistics quality index, which ranks countries from 1 (low quality) to 5 (high quality). Figure 3 shows much higher ELD costs in countries with poorly developed transport and infrastructure logistics, while ELD costs fall quite sharply as countries' logistics scores improve. For countries with the worst scores (less than 2.5 out of 5), predicted ELD costs are around $3.00 per capita, but this steadily falls to less than $2.50 per capita for countries with the best transport, storage, and infrastructure logistics scores.[23] Assuming this relationship holds true for future infrastructure investments and reforms, we simulate the impacts of improving transport and infrastructure logistics in LMICs by raising each country's score by a full point, capped at a maximum index score of 3.75 (China's current score).[24] A regression-based prediction suggests that the average healthy diet cost in LMICs would fall by 11 percent, and that the baseline number of people unable to afford a healthy diet globally would fall by 143 million, from 2.66 billion to 2.52 billion.

Of course, improving transport and infrastructure logistics isn't easy or cheap. From 2007 to 2022, World Bank data suggest that LMICs improved their ratings by 0.3 points, but there were also dramatic and diverse individual success stories on this front, notably Rwanda (+1.37 points), Egypt (+1 point), Philippines (+0.94 points), Armenia (+0.82 points), China (+0.8 points), and Viet Nam (+0.7 points). Hence, there does seem to be considerable scope for countries to drive down diet costs – and improve value chain efficiency and economic growth more generally – through ambitious but smart investments in infrastructure, and logistics.

FIGURE 3 EAT-Lancet diet costs by country transport and infrastructure logistics ratings (scaled 0–5)

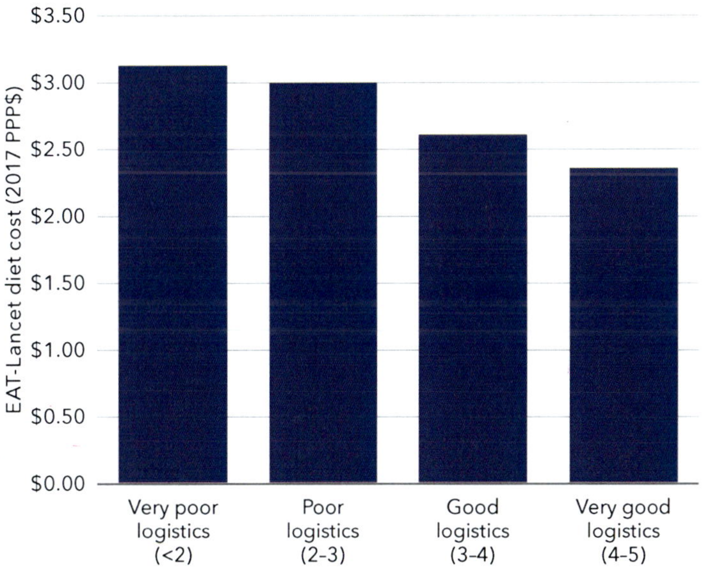

Source: Authors' estimates from the World Bank's 2017 International Comparison Program food price data in 2017 purchasing power parity (PPP) dollars, and World Bank logistics rankings for 128 countries, including high-income countries as well as LMICs.

Note: The World Bank index ranks countries from 1 to 5 which we present as ranging from low quality to high quality

FIGURE 4 Consumption availability relative to the EAT-Lancet reference intake levels, by GDP quartile, 2021

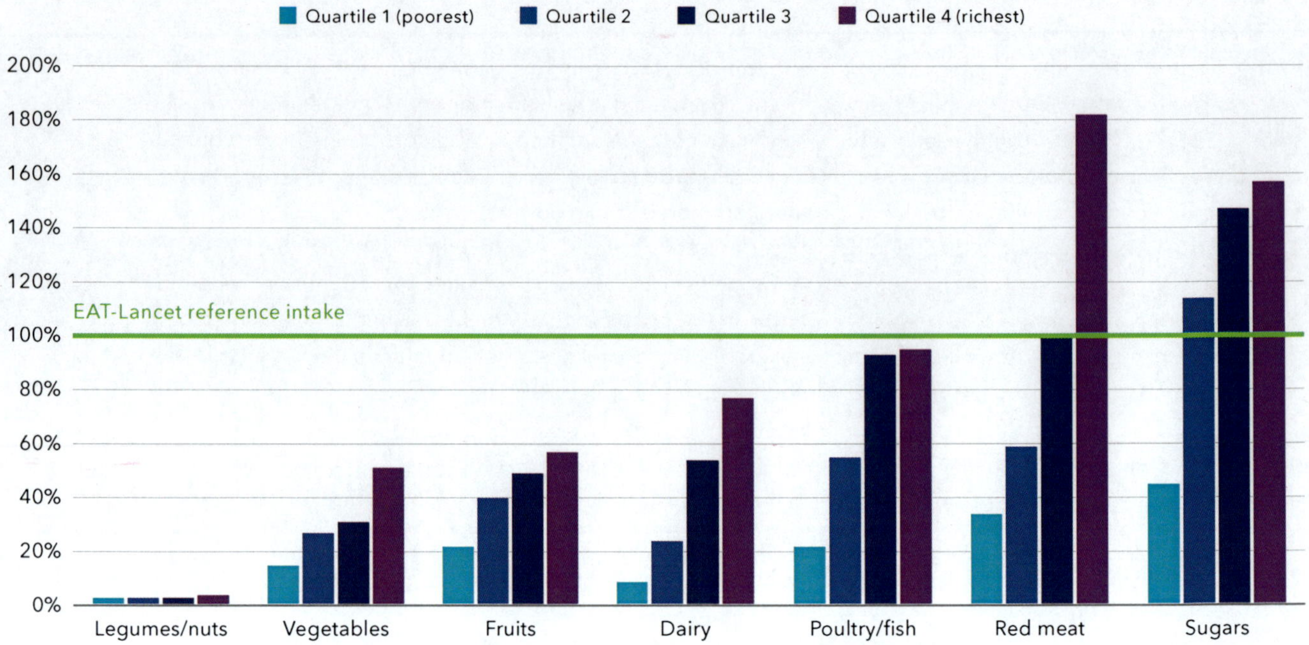

Source: Authors' estimates from FAO Food Balance Sheets for 186 countries for 2021.

Note: Quartiles disaggregate GDP per capita from the poorest group (0 to 25th percentile) to the richest (75th to 100th percentile).

THE PREFERENCE PROBLEM

If, tomorrow, all poor people in the world were given the $1.3 trillion required to afford a healthy diet (Table 1), would they actually choose to consume that diet? Or would tastes, convenience, culture, and poor nutritional knowledge – loosely called "preferences" here – prevent a shift to healthy diets? A simple means of exploring this question is by looking at how diets typically evolve as per capita incomes increase, and whether consumption levels of specific foods converge to global recommendations at high income levels. We do this by reporting average per capita food supplies from the FAO's Food Balance Sheets[25] relative to the reference intakes of the ELD, organized by quartiles of GDP per capita (Figure 4). In brief, it appears that latent demand for sugar and animal-source foods is strong (unhealthily so for red meat), but that consumer preferences for vegetables and fruits are relatively weak, while legume and nut consumption is only a fraction of the recommended ELD intake and does not notably increase with GDP. Thus, GDP growth in LMICs would likely lead to only a partial shift to healthy diets (meeting goals for animal-source food consumption), with the underconsumption of legumes and nuts, fruits, and vegetables persisting even with significant economic growth.

Can policies and programs shift food preferences at scale through demand-side or food environment interventions? That is the subject of ongoing research in CGIAR and elsewhere (see Chapters 3 and 5), and much of the existing evidence is limited to quite specific types of interventions, such as programs targeted at mothers of young children, rather than the general population or other groups of interest, such as adolescents. Arguably, one example of success at scale is the promotion of dairy products in Thailand, a country with no tradition of dairy consumption. To support dairy farmers and promote nutrition, the Thai government launched a national school milk program and dairy promotion campaign in the late 1980s.[26] Such was the success of the program that dairy products are now closely associated with improved child nutrition in Thailand, to the point where there are concerns about excess dairy consumption among middle-class children.[27]

POLICY ACTIONS TO ACHIEVE A SHIFT TO HEALTHIER DIETS

We estimated that more than 2 billion people in 128 countries cannot afford the EAT-Lancet diet, and it would cost at least $1.3 trillion per year to provide them enough cash to afford such a diet. The scale of the healthy diet problem is therefore immense, and solving it will require a range of revolutionary actions, rather than any single "silver bullet." We propose six such sets of actions:

IMPROVE THE NATIONAL AND SUBNATIONAL MONITORING OF HEALTHY DIET AFFORDABILITY. This includes actions to improve not only food price data collection and analysis, but also wage monitoring[28] and the wider use of high-frequency welfare surveys, including phone surveys.[29] Such actions will (1) strengthen the economic and nutritional dimensions of early warning systems; (2) improve research, evidence, and knowledge; and (3) provide a stronger platform for nutritional advocacy at the national level.

ACCELERATE MORE RAPID AND PRO-POOR ECONOMIC GROWTH IN LMICS. While LMIC growth rates are partly determined by external forces, there are many reforms that countries can implement to catalyze faster and more equitable growth.

REALIGN AGRICULTURAL POLICIES AND INVESTMENTS TOWARD NUTRITIOUS FOODS (including fortified foods and other processed foods) to make healthier, nutritious diets more affordable, through either price or income mechanisms. Repurposing agricultural policies to support healthier diets is one critical component; another involves strategically reforming the composition of agricultural investments toward high-return non-staple foods, especially perishable nutritious foods that offer potential to reduce retail prices for consumers. Economic modeling tools can be used to assess synergies and trade-offs between nutrition objectives (dietary changes) and economic and environmental objectives.

SCALE UP INVESTMENT AND REGULATION OF INVESTMENTS IN TRANSPORTATION, INFRASTRUCTURE, AND LOGISTICS SYSTEMS relevant to domestic *and* international trade in food and agriculture. This entails not just hard infrastructure investments, but also a focus on developing efficient businesses in the "hidden middle" of the food system, namely transport, logistics, storage, processing, and other wholesale trading functions.

SCALE UP NUTRITION-SENSITIVE SOCIAL PROTECTION IN LMICS in terms of coverage, size, nutritional adequacy, and comprehensiveness of transfer packages and the intensity of nutrition education interventions. We know that nutrition-sensitive cash and food transfers can be particularly efficacious for mothers and children; we need to know more about the effects of nutrition-sensitive social protection on other demographic groups.

SCALE UP "DOUBLE DUTY" INTERVENTIONS TO INCREASE DEMAND FOR HEALTHY FOODS AND DECREASE DEMAND FOR UNHEALTHY FOODS. Evidence on large-scale efforts to shift consumer preferences is admittedly limited (see Chapters 3 and 5), although there are indications that school-feeding programs have helped sustain healthy preferences into adulthood, such as dairy programs in Thailand and other Asian countries. More evidence and experimental programming are needed.

In the context of a nascent scientific literature, we do not claim that there is exhaustive evidence to quantify the impact of these actions individually or together: more systematic research on these questions is greatly needed. Nevertheless, it seems clear that any single set of actions could not solve the problem within a desirable timeframe. Achieving convergence toward healthier diets in LMICs requires a combination of aggressive actions on multiple fronts – it requires a revolution in the way we think about food policy's fundamental role in providing healthy diets, for all people, at all times.

CHAPTER 5

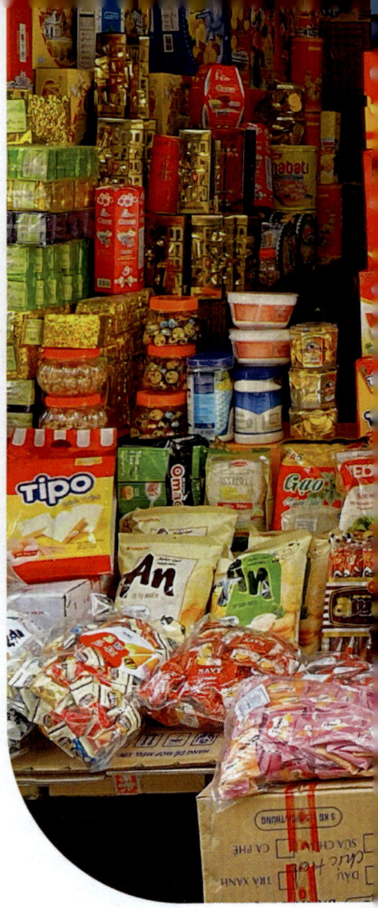

Food Environments
Improving Their Healthfulness

GABRIELA FRETES, QUINN MARSHALL, AND JEF L. LEROY

Gabriela Fretes and **Quinn Marshall** are associate research fellows and **Jef L. Leroy** is a senior research fellow, Nutrition, Diets, and Health Unit, International Food Policy Research Institute.

KEY MESSAGES

- Food environments in low- and middle-income countries (LMICs) are undergoing dramatic changes. Their important role warrants attention from researchers to better understand how they are impacting diets, and from decision-makers to develop policies and actions for food environments that promote sustainable healthy diets for all.
- Ultra-processed foods are now ubiquitous and heavily consumed in both urban and rural areas. These cater to increasing demand for convenience from busy consumers and are heavily marketed, especially to children and adolescents.
- Fruits, vegetables, and other nutrient-dense fresh foods are often available from informal vendors in LMICs, but food safety remains a serious challenge, and availability is subject to high postharvest losses, deterioration in quality, and seasonal fluctuations.
- Online grocery and food delivery services are changing how consumers engage with food environments, while social media is opening up new avenues for marketing and advertising of (primarily unhealthy) foods that are difficult to monitor and regulate.

A variety of policies and actions can improve food environments to promote sustainable healthy diets:

- Mandatory front-of-package labeling systems and taxes have reduced consumption of unhealthy foods and beverages in LMICs, particularly in the Americas, and could be expanded to other regions.
- Restrictions on marketing of unhealthy products, especially to children and adolescents, hold promise for reducing consumption of ultra-processed foods but require further evaluation.
- To address new threats created by the digital food environment, valid metrics for monitoring and research are urgently needed to assess the impact on dietary habits and to inform effective, enforceable regulation of marketing.
- Policies and actions designed to promote access to healthy foods, including fresh produce and animal-source foods, require further research in LMICs. Studies examining subsidies for healthy foods and retail-level interventions such as product placement have been limited to high-income countries, and those for retail-level interventions are still inconclusive.

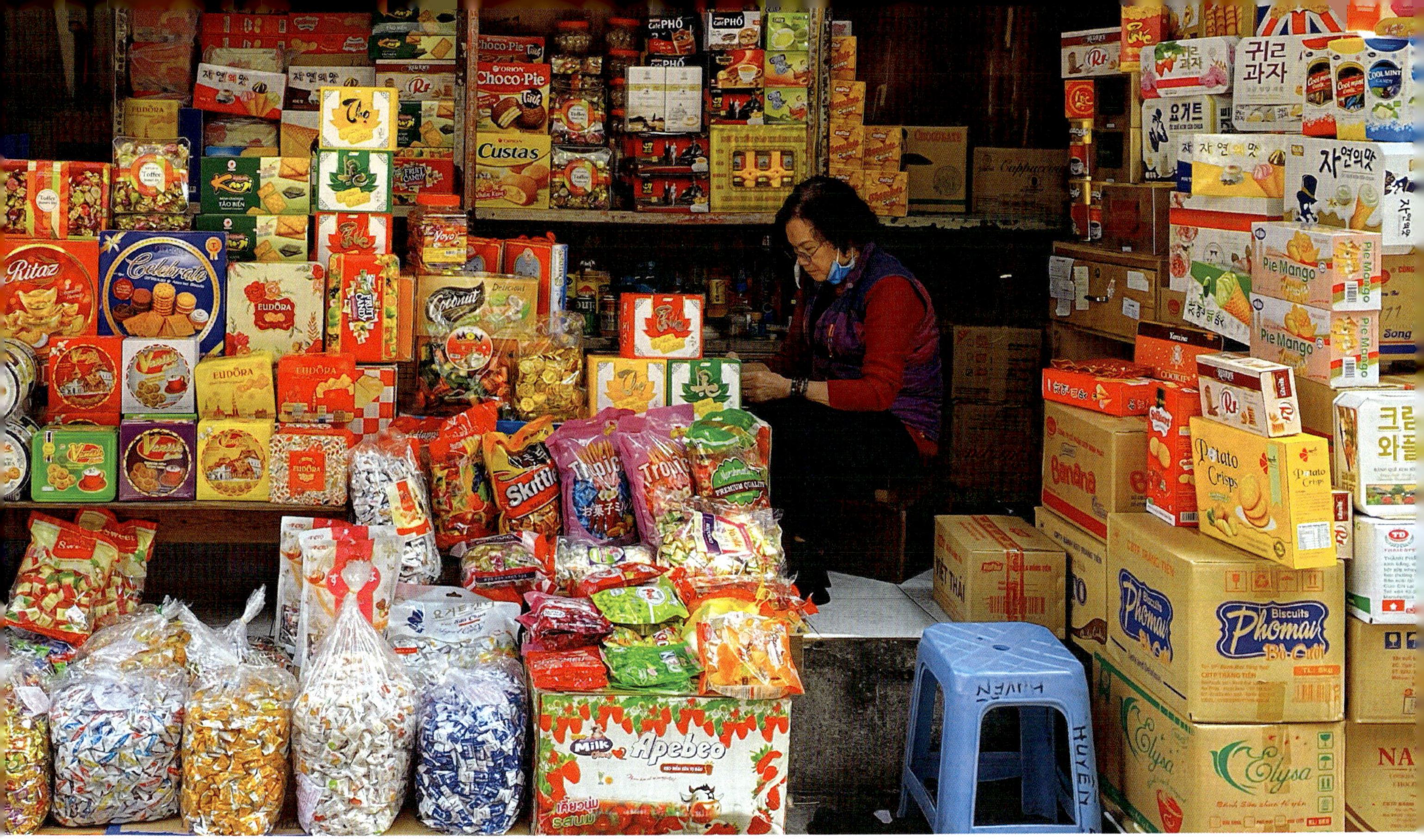

The food environment is the setting in which people choose what to eat, where they buy those foods, and where, when, and how they eat. It is more formally defined as the place where people interact with and access food within the wider food system.[1] Researchers have identified different types of food environments, which can be broadly grouped into either wild and cultivated food environments or built food environments (also referred to as market food environments).[2] This chapter focuses on the latter, using the term food environments. Key characteristics of food environments include types of foods available, their quality, safety, price, and convenience; the types of vendors; and promotional activities. How a consumer interacts with the food environment is determined by characteristics such as their access to foods, income, and preferences. Food environments are dynamic – they both shape and are shaped by consumers' food choices[3] – and consumers' interactions with the food environment are complex, with a range of factors influencing their decision-making when choosing foods. Policies and other interventions can be used to reshape food environments in order to promote healthier diets.

Food environments around the world are changing rapidly in response to the evolving needs and lifestyles of consumers, and as a result of transformations along agrifood value chains.[4] This chapter examines some of the key challenges and opportunities for food environments amid the rapid transitions occurring in low- and middle-income countries (LMICs). We present illustrative examples of evidence-based food environment policies and actions that are being implemented to promote diet quality in a diverse range of countries. Our conclusions reflect on potential policies for improving diets through changes in food environments, and discuss actions needed to move forward in strengthening the healthfulness of food environments in LMICs.

FOOD ENVIRONMENTS IN LOW- AND MIDDLE-INCOME COUNTRIES

Though many households in LMICs still produce much of their own food, they purchase most of the food they eat. Recent data from 11 African countries show that rural families purchase 56 percent of their food on average, challenging the notion that subsistence farming is the predominant source of food in rural areas.[5] This trend is well advanced among rural populations of other regions as well,[6] meaning that an increasing number of people rely on markets, and thus food environments, to access their food.

DEMAND FOR CONVENIENCE AND THE PENETRATION OF ULTRA-PROCESSED FOODS

Urbanization and rural transformation have led to profound changes in consumer preferences, with concomitant changes in food environments. Economic growth in urban areas has generated new income-earning opportunities for both men and women, which has increased demand for convenience foods, as consumers spend more time away from home and have less time for food preparation.[7] As rural economies transform, growth in nonfarm employment for rural men and women has led to a similar increase in demand for convenience.[8]

The food industry has responded by introducing new technologies that increase the shelf life of products and reduce preparation times[9] and increasing availability of ultra-processed foods (UPFs). These industrially formulated foods are energy-dense and contain added sugars, oils and fats, salt, and other additives (see Glossary).[10] Examples of UPFs include sugar-sweetened beverages, sweet and salty packaged snacks, ice cream, sausages, and instant noodles. While urban households consume more UPFs than rural households, consumption of these foods is now common even in remote rural areas (Box 1).[11] The penetration of these foods is commonly associated with the expansion of modern retail outlets such as supermarkets, but UPFs are also sold in small shops, kiosks, and by street vendors.[12] Their shelf-stable nature makes them suitable for the fragmented supply chains where these small and medium enterprises (SMEs) operate, as well as for long-distance transportation, often without temperature control.

AVAILABILITY OF FRESH FOODS IN INFORMAL RETAIL

Informal retail outlets, which include wet markets and many SMEs, have a larger market share than modern retail in many LMICs.[13] This is especially true for fresh foods, including fruits, vegetables, and animal-source foods.[14] In addition to offering these foods at lower prices, informal vendors offer several important advantages for consumers, including physical proximity (due to their density in poorer communities), the ability for customers to make purchases on credit, and the possibility of purchasing small quantities.[15] In contrast

BOX 1 ADOLESCENTS AND THE FOOD ENVIRONMENT

A study conducted in 2021 in 10 neighborhoods in Accra, Ghana, assessed how adolescents engage with their food environment. More than 60 percent of the total energy consumed by adolescents came from prepared and ready-to-eat foods obtained away from home, meaning directly from the food environment. Of these foods, two-thirds were consumed outside the home. Overall, foods consumed outside the home were much less micronutrient-dense than foods consumed at home. This pattern reflects the fact that the adolescents' food environment provided easier access to unhealthy options than to healthy ones. Nutrient-poor foods, ultra-processed foods, and sugar-sweetened beverages were consistently within closer proximity than healthy foods such as fruits.

In Viet Nam, a study conducted in an urban and peri-urban site and a rural town found similar results. Adolescents in all sites lived in a food environment that makes it challenging to avoid unhealthy options. In urban areas, for instance, most adolescents lived within 50 meters – or a 30-second walk – from the nearest vendor selling sugary drinks and ultra-processed foods. Across all sites, unhealthy foods were more accessible than healthy foods. Similar findings are also seen in recent research on adolescents and food environments in South Asia.

Source: Unpublished IFPRI research findings. For more on South Asia, see CGIAR, "Open-Access Agrifood Systems Data from 4,000 Households across Bangladesh, Inida, and Nepal," March 20, 2024. https://www.cgiar.org

to most UPFs, however, fresh foods are perishable. Supply chains are often long and fragmented, especially for informal retail, with poor temperature and storage conditions that result in losses in quantity and quality, which impact year-round availability.[16] Moreover, informal vendors may not adhere stringently to food safety standards. They typically operate without adequate access to electricity, water, or waste disposal, which leads to unhygienic food handling practices.[17] Though there are examples of positive engagement between governments and informal vendors on these problems, such as through training courses in hygienic practices, the relationship is often contentious. Informal vendors are subject to crackdowns, demolition of stalls, confiscation of goods, and financial penalties, which in turn affect food access for local consumers.[18]

ADVERTISING OF UNHEALTHY FOODS AND BEVERAGES

Food marketing around the globe – across all settings and forms of media – is largely geared toward promoting UPFs and sugary beverages.[19] Children and adolescents in particular are exposed to high volumes of such marketing.[20] An emerging body of evidence, mainly from high-income countries (HICs), suggests that this exposure, whether through traditional or digital media, influences children and adolescents' food preferences, choices, and diets.[21] There is some evidence that socioeconomically disadvantaged groups in HICs are disproportionately targeted with child- and adolescent-focused advertisements for unhealthy foods and beverages.[22] For LMICs, evidence on the effect of marketing of unhealthy foods and beverages on food choices and diets is still limited.

THE EXPANDING DIGITAL FOOD ENVIRONMENT

The internet has added a layer of complexity to food environments by opening new avenues for both the retail sale and marketing of food. Online grocery retail and mobile applications for food delivery are growing globally and accelerated especially during the COVID-19 pandemic.[23] These new digital access points for food increase convenience and reduce the time burden associated with food shopping. However, studies from HICs and Brazil suggest that most of the foods available through food delivery applications, which allow users to order from restaurants using their mobile phones, do not align with healthy eating recommendations.[24]

As with traditional media, social media platforms are increasingly used to advertise sugar-sweetened beverages, fast food, and other unhealthy foods, and they frequently target children and adolescents.[25] These platforms also provide food companies with new, sophisticated methods for gathering data on their target consumer groups and interacting with them at a low cost. A common strategy is the use of "influencers" who share positive reviews, photos, and other content, sometimes in return for payment from food and beverage companies.[26] Emerging evidence from several HICs suggests that adolescents exposed to food advertisements through social media are more likely to recall unhealthy food advertisements and those involving celebrities, and that this exposure influences their food choices.[27] The use of social media and other types of advertisement to create demand for healthy foods has been explored, but rigorous evidence on their effectiveness is missing.[28]

VULNERABILITY TO SHOCKS

Food environments, especially those that serve low-income consumers, are sensitive to shocks. The COVID-19 pandemic, for example, rapidly led to restrictions on the mobility of farmers, transporters, and other workers; closures of food processing facilities, which created stock shortages; reduced product offerings; and higher retail prices.[29] Some studies suggest that informal retail was disproportionally affected by the impacts of the pandemic. In a survey of informal milk vendors in Nairobi conducted four months after the pandemic's onset, for example, a third of respondents blamed difficulties in stocking milk on pandemic-related transportation issues and restrictions on business operations.[30] Higher prices resulting from these shocks have the most detrimental impact on poor households, who spend a large portion of their income on food and may lack sufficient coping mechanisms.[31]

MAKING FOOD ENVIRONMENTS MORE HEALTHFUL

Several policy options have been tested to make food environments more conducive to healthy eating.[32] These include providing information to consumers on the content of packaged foods, restricting advertising of unhealthy foods, and introducing fiscal measures to nudge consumers away from unhealthy foods and toward healthier options. Retail-level interventions to improve availability, access, safety, and promotion of healthy foods have also been tested. To enable dietary change, additional actions are needed that improve affordability of healthy options (see Chapter 4) and consumer knowledge about healthy eating (see Chapter 3).

FRONT-OF-PACKAGE LABELING

Clear and comprehensive labeling on food products can empower consumers to make informed choices. Strong evidence suggests that mandatory front-of-package labeling systems are most effective at guiding consumers toward healthier purchases, whereas voluntary labeling systems allow food companies to opt out of placing labels on products with poor nutrient profiles.[33]

The Americas have been at the forefront of mandatory front-of-package labeling policies. In Mexico and Chile, mandatory policies require that stop-sign-shaped warning labels be placed on products that exceed certain thresholds for energy, sugar, saturated fat, and salt content. These labeling requirements were implemented together with strong public awareness campaigns. Evaluations of the policies' impacts in both countries have shown positive results: households in Mexico and Chile are buying fewer unhealthy products,[34] and the food industry quickly responded by reformulating products to reduce energy, sugar, saturated fat, and salt content below the threshold requiring a label.[35] In addition, the cut-offs have helped guide government procurement policies at the institutional level (for example, in schools)[36] and informed decisions about which foods can be purchased or offered in food assistance programs.[37]

RESTRICTIONS ON MARKETING OF UNHEALTHY FOODS

In 2010 and 2023, the World Health Organization (WHO) approved recommendations to restrict the marketing of unhealthy foods and beverages to children,[38] but implementation of these recommendations at the country level has been slow. Evidence on the effectiveness of marketing restrictions is thus limited. As with food labeling, studies suggest that the best way to limit the marketing of unhealthy foods and beverages is through approaches that are mandatory, comprehensive (such as regulations on different media), and aligned with the WHO recommendations.[39]

Chile, Mexico, and Peru, among other countries, have used their front-of-package labeling guidance to mandate restrictions on child-directed food marketing. Products with warning labels cannot display cartoon characters, cannot be promoted or sold in schools, and cannot be marketed to children through traditional media such as TV and radio, in movie theaters, or online.[40]

With the global proliferation of digital services and their potential to reach wide audiences, especially through social media, regulation of digital marketing needs to be prioritized. However, the challenges in monitoring digital media are significant, especially considering the scope of digital marketing and the limited access to data for real-time monitoring.[41] Despite limiting advertisements of cigarettes and alcohol, social media platforms have yet to adopt restrictions on advertising unhealthy foods.[42]

FISCAL POLICIES

Fiscal policies seek to nudge consumers into healthier eating by increasing the price of unhealthy options and lowering the price of healthy foods. Taxes on unhealthy foods and beverages have been implemented in nearly 60 countries and smaller jurisdictions worldwide.[43] The vast majority of these have targeted sugar-sweetened beverages. Evidence suggests these policies reduce the purchase and consumption of unhealthy foods and beverages.[44] Two years after Mexico implemented its tax on sugar sweetened beverages in 2014, for example, purchases of taxed beverages decreased by 7.6 percent on average. The decline was even larger (11.6 percent) for low-income households.[45]

National policies designed to lower the price of healthy foods are rare. A meta-analysis of interventional and observational cohort studies, mainly from the United States, found that a 10 percent decrease in the price of fruits and vegetables (the most commonly targeted foods) increased purchases by 14 percent. Interestingly, this effect was larger than the effect of a 10 percent price increase on unhealthy foods, which decreased purchases by 6 percent.[46] It should also be noted that subsidies (which effectively reduce prices) in the reviewed studies were often combined with other interventions, such as changes in availability of healthy foods, labeling, or educational approaches, which may have contributed to their impacts.

The introduction of policies on front-of-package labeling, restricting marketing, and taxing unhealthy foods and beverages has been challenging. Concerned about reduced sales and rising costs related to reformulating foods, the food industry has used a diverse set of strategies to oppose these policies (Box 2) (see Chapter 8).[47] Coordinated, sustained efforts and expertise of stakeholders from civil society, international organizations, academia, and government agencies are needed to successfully implement, monitor, and evaluate policies.[48]

RETAIL-LEVEL INTERVENTIONS

Purchasing decisions in retail settings may be affected not only by price, but also by food availability, placement, and in-store promotions. Food manufacturers often seek placement of UPFs and snacks in prominent locations, for example, near store entrances or cash registers, at eye level on shelves, or in end-of-aisle displays, and may pay incentives to stores for this placement.[49]

A systematic review of studies from HICs examining the impact of interventions that include greater availability and more prominent placement of healthy foods, along with reduced availability and less prominent placement of unhealthy foods, could not draw firm conclusions due to methodological limitations

BOX 2 INDUSTRY TACTICS TO CHALLENGE FOOD ENVIRONMENT POLICIES

The food industry has adamantly opposed the development and implementation of food environment policies, including those related to front-of-package labeling, taxes on sugar-sweetened beverages, and marketing regulations. Key strategies used to challenge the introduction of these policies include the following:

Delay–Opponents push for longer consultation periods, demand more research and evidence, and argue that implementation is difficult.

Divide–Opponents develop and promote their own regulations (such as labeling, nutrient profiling, and marketing). These are usually less stringent than the ones proposed by governments and are voluntary as well as confusing or difficult to interpret. Opponents also privately lobby to stop regulation or make it less stringent.

Deflect–Opponents claim that the policy will have negative effects on trade and employment in manufacturing and agriculture. They argue that self-regulation is sufficient and that governments should not interfere with people's choices.

Deny–Opponents cast doubt on existing evidence or claim that the available evidence is inadequate, and they fund research that proposes less stringent alternatives.

Source: Based on World Cancer Research Fund International, *Building Momentum: Lessons on Implementing a Robust Front-of-Pack Food Label* (London: 2019).

of the included studies.[50] Adapation of such interventions to LMICs would need to consider the different types of vendors that consumers engage with, which are likely to be predominantly informal, and different store formats.

In Viet Nam and Nigeria, researchers have recently tested interventions that combine actions to improve the healthfulness of food environments with strategies to increase the affordability and accessibility of healthy foods.[51] The bundle of interventions included improvements in the display and marketing of fruits and vegetables; clean aprons for open-air fruit and vegetable vendors; delivery of nutritional information to consumers; distribution of coupons to purchase fruit; and campaigns to promote eating five servings of fruits and vegetables per day (400 grams). After the intervention, overall fruit and vegetable consumption did not significantly change in either country, but intake of specific fruits did increase.

IMPROVING THE AVAILABILITY OF NUTRITIOUS, SAFE FOOD

A few projects have sought to combine retail and demand-creation activities with supply chain reinforcement, especially related to improving food safety, a particularly relevant challenge in LMICs. Evidence on the effectiveness of these projects is forthcoming.

The Global Alliance for Improved Nutrition (GAIN)'s Vegetables for All project in Kenya connects last-mile vendors, known as *mama mboga*, in low-income urban and peri-urban areas to suppliers who are compliant with good agricultural practices. In combination with marketing (using the FitFoods brand developed by GAIN and its project partners) and training provided to vendors, the project aims to increase the desirability of vegetables among consumers, as well as their freshness and safety at point of sale.[52] Also in Kenya, the More Milk intervention, a project of the International Livestock Research Institute, provided in-person trainings on milk handling, hygiene, and business skills to informal dairy vendors. It also supported vendors with marketing materials to promote children's milk consumption. MoreMilk increased the uptake of good milk handling practices by vendors and increased milk intake in children.[53]

CONCLUSIONS

Food environments in both rural and urban settings in LMICs are undergoing a rapid transformation. Emerging evidence highlights the potential effectiveness of food environment interventions that influence people to limit their consumption of unhealthy foods and beverages. The rich experience of countries in the Americas in developing and implementing fiscal and mandatory front-of-package labeling policies should help countries in Africa and Asia to implement policies more efficiently, as consumption of unhealthy foods and beverages likewise presents an important challenge in these settings. However, important gaps remain in the evidence on effective strategies to promote fruits, vegetables, and other nutrient-dense foods as part of a sustainable healthy diet in LMICs. Other strategies, such as the prominent placement of healthy foods, have not been thoroughly studied in either HICs or LMICs.

The expansion of the digital food environment offers novel ways to acquire food but also presents new challenges, as it creates new threats to healthy eating and adds complexity to implementing and enforcing regulations. Valid metrics to monitor the digital food environment – such as assessing the nutritional content of foods promoted, the marketing techniques used, and exposure to marketing across different platforms – and research to assess its impact on dietary habits are urgently needed.

It is unlikely that interventions aimed only at increasing consumers' nutrition knowledge or at increasing the affordability of healthy foods will lead to a significant improvement in healthy diets. Tackling individual- and household-level barriers to healthy eating, in combination with mandatory policies and actions that improve the healthfulness of food environments and hold corporations accountable, will be essential.

"Food environments are dynamic – they both shape and are shaped by consumers' food choices."

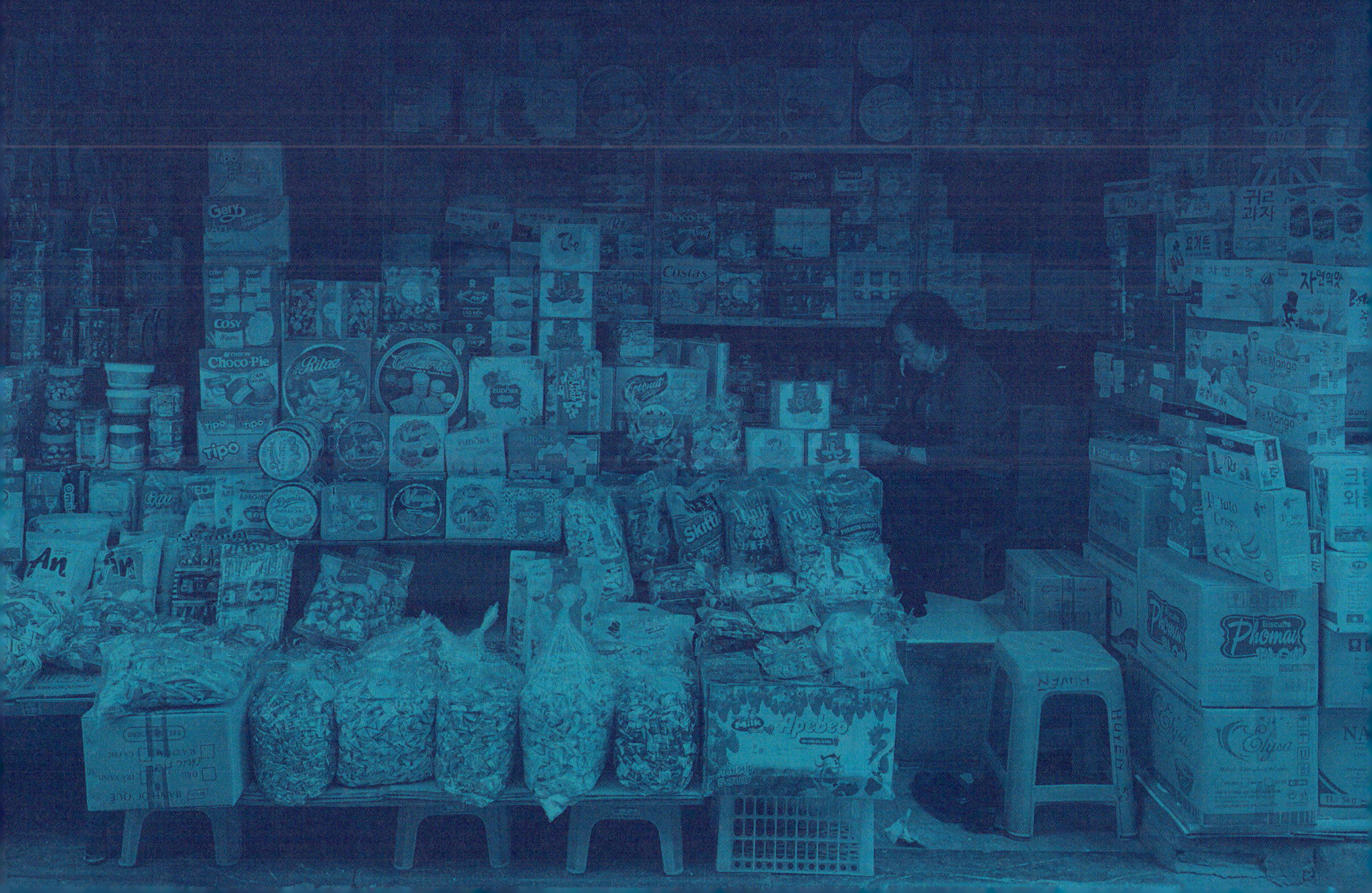

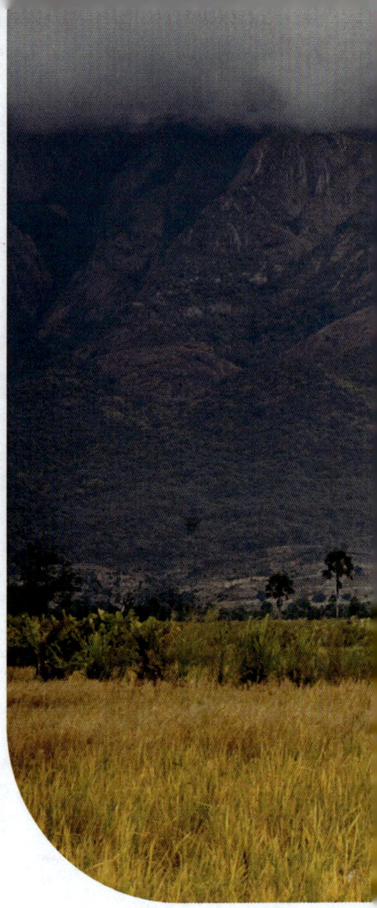

CHAPTER 6

Plant-Source Foods
Leveraging Crops for Nutrition and Healthy Diets

ERICK BOY, INGE D. BROUWER, JEN FOLEY, NATALIA PALACIOS, SAMUEL SCOTT, AND VICTOR TALEON

Erick Boy is chief nutritionist, HarvestPlus, Innovation and Policy Scaling Unit (IPS), International Food Policy Research Institute (IFPRI). **Inge Brouwer** is a senior research fellow, Nutrition, Diets, and Health Unit (NDH), IFPRI. **Jen Foley** is a senior program manager, HarvestPlus, IPS, IFPRI. **Natalia Palacios Rojas** is principal scientist and cereal nutritional quality lead, International Maize and Wheat Improvement Center (CIMMYT), Mexico. **Samuel Scott** is a research fellow, NDH, IFPRI. **Victor Taleon** is a research fellow, HarvestPlus, IPS, IFPRI.

KEY MESSAGES

- Food crops are key components of sustainable healthy diets. These crops, which include fruits, vegetables, and nutrient-enriched and whole grain staples, deliver energy and high concentrations of health-promoting vitamins, minerals, phytochemicals, and dietary fiber.
- Unhealthy diets are the leading behavioral risk factor for diet-related noncommunicable diseases (NCDs) and a major contributor to globally prevalent micronutrient deficiencies. Dietary improvements can meaningfully reduce NCD-related deaths and help address deficiencies in essential nutrients.
- Consumption of fruits and vegetables remains inadequate among many at-risk populations due to limited availability, affordability, and taste preferences, among other factors.
- Access to affordable and high-quality food crops for the poor in low- and middle-income countries is a global equity, health, and sustainability challenge. Seasonality, perishability, price instability, and household incomes, among other factors, shape the production of and access to non-staple food crops; consumption of staple crops remains relatively stable.
- Proven technologies, such as biofortification and some postharvest food processing techniques, can be scaled up to leverage crops for sustainable healthy diets.

To improve the contribution of plant-source foods to sustainable healthy diets, it is important to:

- Promote policies and accessible technologies that produce and supply more nutritious crops and foods, along with behavioral strategies that shift demand and consumer actions toward a sustainable healthy diet.
- Promote production and consumption of biofortified or fortified staple foods as complementary nutrition strategies where needed. These foods can be an equitable and affordable means of delivering nutrients to especially vulnerable populations, including women and children.
- Prioritize investments in crop diversity that can lead to increased accessibility, affordability, and appeal of safe and healthy diets when carried out alongside upgrades to market infrastructure and nutrition and hygiene education among farmers, value chain actors, and consumers.
- Create an enabling environment, supported by government and financial commitments, for scaling up crop-focused initiatives that can achieve nutrition and climate goals through holistic and context-specific multisectoral interventions that span agriculture, food, trade, and social protection.

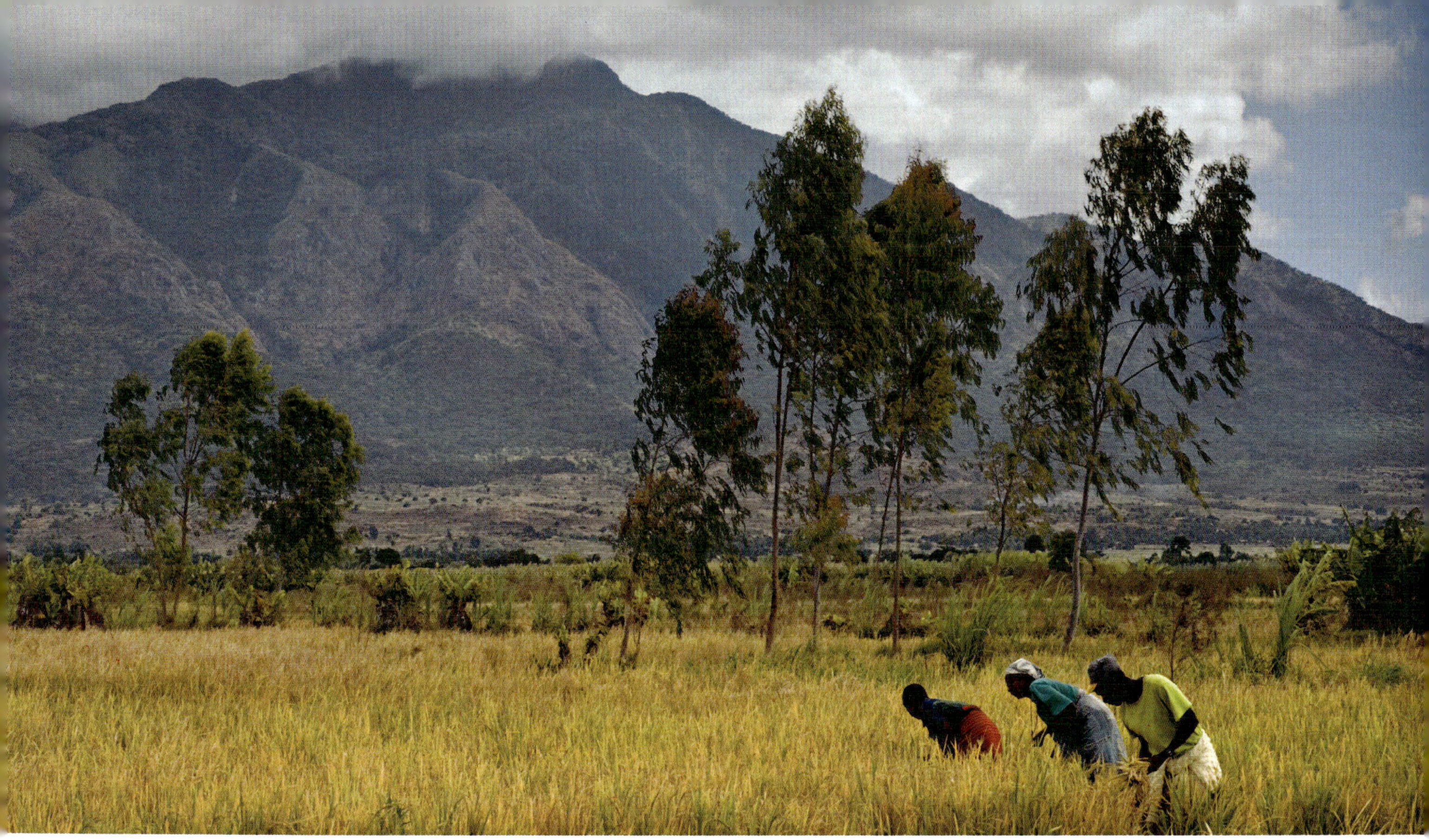

Addressing the urgent need for food systems to support sustainable healthy diets will require a major improvement in the availability of and access to affordable, nutritious foods in low- and middle-income countries (LMICs), along with increased consumer demand for healthy diets. Plant-source foods are key components of sustainable healthy diets. This chapter examines food crops that could be leveraged to improve health outcomes; describes production systems and their role in providing populations access to highly nutritious crops; and presents examples of evidence-based technologies that improve the nutritional content of crops, especially for vulnerable populations. Together, these approaches can be leveraged to help vulnerable populations attain healthy diets and support planetary sustainability.

Sustainable healthy diets are nutritionally adequate, meaning they are health-promoting and disease-preventing, protecting against all forms of malnutrition and noncommunicable diseases (NCDs), and they are environmentally sustainable, meaning they must be produced and consumed within the safe limits of our planet's boundaries. Sustainable healthy diets provide the energy and essential nutrients required for growth and development, and to promote well-being; are accessible, affordable, safe, equitable, and culturally acceptable; and preserve biodiversity and have low impact on the environment.[1]

Diets should provide affordable nutritional adequacy year-round.[2] Crops that deliver energy and high concentrations of vitamins, minerals, phytochemicals, and dietary fiber – such as fruits, vegetables, whole grains, legumes, and roots – are among the principal components of healthy diets essential for well-being[3] (for a discussion of the role that animal-source foods play in sustainable healthy diets, see Chapter 7). The individual foods that make up a healthy diet vary with local food availability, as well as cultural context, which influences acceptability; and with individual characteristics, including age and other factors that determine an individual's particular nutrient requirements (see Chapter 3). The health outcomes associated with diets relate to patterns of eating, rather than to specific foods.[4]

More than a third of the world's population cannot afford to buy a selection of foods that constitute a healthy diet (see Chapter 4).[5] Unhealthy diets underpin all forms of malnutrition and are the leading behavioral risk factor for diet-related NCDs; overall, NCDs are responsible for over 73 percent of deaths.[6] Insidious and largely preventable micronutrient deficiencies alone affect half of all children and two-thirds of women, limiting human potential, especially in LMICs.[7]

Dietary improvements such as increasing fruit and vegetable intake can reduce NCD-related deaths by 20 percent.[8] However, the nutritional content and availability of foods eaten in LMICs are projected to deteriorate because of the effects of climate change and unsustainable resource use, including increasing temperatures and CO_2 levels,[9] soil degradation, freshwater scarcity, and decreasing biodiversity, as well as food price volatility and limited access to high-quality seeds and fertilizers caused by civil and public health crises – thus compromising diet quality.[10]

To deliver sufficient calories to populations experiencing hunger and undernutrition, international and national agricultural research centers have historically focused their efforts on traditional staples, such as white maize, cassava, rice, and wheat. These crops are high in energy (calorie-dense) but lack the nutrient density needed for optimal health, particularly after milling. In many settings, this focus on caloric sufficiency has impeded a shift toward policies and food systems that can also deliver the nutrient-rich or nutrient-enriched food crops required to improve diets. Nevertheless, efforts to leverage crops for sustainable healthy diets are now underway in many LMICs. These include promoting the production (and consumption) of fruits, vegetables, and whole grains, as well as improving the nutrient contribution of plant-source foods through biofortification of staple crops and fortification in postharvest food processing.

CROPS THAT CONTRIBUTE TO SUSTAINABLE HEALTHY DIETS

Fruits, vegetables, and whole grains (as well as other crops not specifically addressed in this chapter) are essential for sustainable healthy diets, but consumption of fruits and vegetables remains low because of limited availability and affordability. Whole grain consumption is also limited due to taste preferences, among other impediments. Addressing these challenges requires expanding supply and increasing demand (see Chapter 3).

AVAILABILITY AND AFFORDABILITY OF FRUITS AND VEGETABLES

Fruits and vegetables are a rich source of vitamins, minerals, fiber, and antioxidants that protect against numerous diseases. They also contribute significantly to agrobiodiversity: 1,097 cultivated vegetable species have been identified worldwide, and 1,250 fruit species have been identified in Latin America alone.[11] Yet, the global availability of fruits and vegetables remains too low to support the level of consumption that populations need to be healthy.

Projections based on forecasted impacts of economic, demographic, and technological change show that no countries in sub-Saharan Africa and few countries in Asia and the Pacific will be able to supply the World Health Organization's minimum recommended daily per capita intake of 400 grams of fruits and vegetables in 2050.[12] Given that national data are sparse or absent in LMICs on common factors that influence food supply and utilization (such as food waste, meals consumed outside of the home, smallholder farmer production, and foods obtained from non-retail or informal markets), this availability gap could be even larger than projected.[13]

Affordability is another obstacle. Purchasing fruits and vegetables from markets is beyond the financial means of many, despite being a relatively cheap source of diverse micronutrients compared with, for example, animal-source foods (see Chapters 4 and 7). Many families' food choices, especially economically disadvantaged households, prioritize calories over nutrients.

Even when fruits and vegetables are available and affordable, many people do not consume an adequate quantity due to factors such as food safety, taste preferences, convenience, cultural appropriateness, or limited knowledge and awareness of the associated health benefits (see Chapters 3 and 5).[14] Moreover, foodborne diseases caused by biological contamination of food are also an important threat to public health, particularly in LMICs and settings where value chains are long. Fruits and vegetables, as well as livestock and fish products, are among the riskiest foods for biological hazards.[15]

The CGIAR Research Initiative on Fruit and Vegetables for Sustainable Healthy Diets (FRESH) is using end-to-end food systems approaches to address desirability, affordability, accessibility, and availability constraints to increasing fruit and vegetable intake.[16] For example, in northern Tanzania, FRESH partners are implementing an end-to-end approach that includes scaling up good agricultural practices via production hubs, with a focus on training farmers of staple crops to incorporate vegetables through intercropping and other mixed farming systems, and training commercial vegetable producers to improve their resource use efficiency. FRESH is also linking with midstream value chain actors (collectors, traders, wholesalers, and retailers) to reduce postharvest losses and improve food safety. In addition, FRESH researchers are designing and testing food environment and demand-side interventions to address accessibility, affordability, and desirability constraints.

WHOLE GRAIN STAPLES

Whole grains are a "complete package," meaning they provide carbohydrates, a small amount of healthy fat, protein, vitamins, minerals, and dietary fiber. Cereal grains like wheat, maize, and rice constitute more than half of the caloric intake of vulnerable populations globally, but they are frequently eaten in refined form to increase their palatability, functionality, and shelf stability. Compared to refined grains, whole grain cereals offer substantially higher levels of nutrients. Essential nutrients such as zinc and iron can be lost from staple crops during processing. For example, milling can unintentionally strip off the outer parts of the grain that contain essential amino acids, fatty acids, iron, zinc, B vitamins, tocopherols, dietary fiber, and health-promoting phytochemicals.[17]

Investing in more nutritious staple foods, as part of a strategy to improve diets and health, is an equitable way to deliver essential nutrients sustainably. Staple foods are consumed as an everyday source of food by all members of households, including young children, adolescent girls, and women; they can offer a gender-equitable vehicle for enriching diets when these foods are naturally high in nutrients, biofortified, or industrially fortified. In many contexts, social norms dictate unequal food distribution among household members of especially nutrient-dense foods such as animal-source foods.[18] As a result, women and young children, who often eat least and last, suffer the greatest burden of malnutrition. For young children, who have high requirements for nutrients but small stomach capacity for foods, staples can only deliver adequate and safe nutrition when appropriately combined with other nutrient-dense foods and/or foods fortified with multiple micronutrients.[19] Supporting the development and promotion of more productive, resilient, and nutritious varieties of staple crops preferred by smallholder farmers and consumers across LMICs will be a key component of sustainable healthy diets and greater nutrition security.

Plant breeding efforts carried out by CGIAR focus on more than 20 high-priority staple crops – including cereals, legumes, and root and tuber crops – to jointly address the impacts of climate change, environmental degradation, and other challenges to agricultural productivity and nutrition, such as pests and plant diseases, while meeting the varietal preferences of producers and other value chain actors. Food crop technologies developed through CGIAR in collaboration with national agricultural research systems had been adopted on nearly 221 million hectares of land across LMICs as of 2020.[20]

CROP PRODUCTION FOR SUSTAINABLE HEALTHY DIETS

Multiple factors shape the production and utilization of plant-source foods, including seasonality, perishability, price instability, household incomes, and combinations of these factors. Making use of local production and traded food products, increasing production of lesser-known nutritious crops, and increasing the nutrient content of staple crops will all be important for a shift toward sustainable healthy diets.

GLOBAL OR LOCAL FOOD PRODUCTION

Local food production is increasingly viewed more favorably than national or global food production that requires long-distance trade.[21] This shift has been driven by the COVID-19 pandemic, other global crises, and the unsustainable nature of existing food systems. However, the local versus global debate is misleading. Although it is often assumed that local food systems produce higher-quality, fresher, and more sustainable foods, and that they reduce vulnerability to shocks that disrupt international markets, being (un)sustainable or (un)healthy is not unique to either local or global food systems, and resilience to shocks is not directly related to where food comes from. In each geographical context, efforts should be made to secure access to healthy foods through direct links with local producers where possible and useful, while giving consideration to the efficiency (productivity, price, seasonality, safety, and sustainability) of the whole system. Where efficiency is low, the price of food increases to the detriment of low-income populations. Trade through regional or global markets, therefore, can play a key role in bringing healthy, affordable foods to markets and populations in need.[22] However, globally, there is also an economic incentive to trade commodities that are ultra-processed and/or have a longer shelf life and stability over long distances – qualities lacking in fruits and vegetables.[23]

In some contexts, "orphan crops" – locally produced crops that have been neglected or underused by communities as well as plant breeders and policymakers – and wild edible species can be promoted to help fill nutritional gaps. Within this highly variable pool of plant products are fruits (for example, papaya, pumpkin, and mulberry) and vegetables (kale, okra, and sweet potatoes, among others) with exceptionally high nutritional value.[24] These crops are typically not traded internationally but are important for local and regional food security (including mitigation of shocks), locally available, often produced or harvested by farm households exclusively for home consumption or informal trade, and contribute to year-round healthy diets and agrobiodiversity.[25]

In any context, several challenges and trade-offs exist related to the choice of which crops to produce. First, it is vital to identify and address the challenges and hazards for local farmers, consumers, and the environment[26] entailed by increasing crop production. These challenges can include high water, chemical, and labor requirements, which could be addressed by introducing labor-saving techniques and increasing access to irrigation; and losses of fruits and vegetables due to perishability, which could be addressed with cold-chain technology.[27] Second, especially for underutilized crops, cultivars with enhanced pest and disease resistance must be developed, and postharvest technologies must be improved, for example to lengthen shelf life and increase protein digestibility. Third, promoting orphan crops (for example, through breeding, marketing, subsidies, conditional cash transfers and vouchers, and other strategies) may lead to a rapid expansion of external markets and development of large-scale and intensive production, which increases local incomes. As seen in the case of teff in Ethiopia, however, the growth of external markets can limit availability of these crops for local consumption, if appropriate political and economic protections are not put in place.[28]

CROP DIVERSIFICATION

Crop diversification – the practice of growing more than one crop in an area – can be accomplished by adding a new crop species or a new variety to a farm either spatially (for example, through a shift from monocropping to intercropping) or temporally (for example, by adding more varieties or crops to an existing rotation system).[29]

Crop diversification can improve human nutrition and sustainability through multiple, interlinked pathways.[30] Diverse crop systems such as intercropping and other regenerative agriculture intensification practices improve soil quality,[31] which promotes mineral uptake, crop yields, and better plant and planetary health. Growing a greater array of crop species on-farm through spatial crop diversification can improve dietary diversity and ecosystem resilience. Intercropping (growing more than one crop simultaneously on the same plot) not only enhances resource-use efficiency but also promotes agrobiodiversity. For example, in Guatemala, intercropping combinations, like maize-bean-potato, demonstrated the highest potential for nutrient adequacy per area unit of cultivated land and promoted soil health and cross pollination.[32]

For smallholder farmers, diversification has been linked with dietary diversity, although other factors, notably good market access and increasing availability of diverse foods at markets, are more strongly associated with improvements in nutrition status.[33] However, the benefits of crop diversification extend beyond diets. Increasing the variety of crops grown can help reduce smallholder vulnerability to production losses and improve household food security, particularly as climate change, and associated extreme heat, floods, and droughts, put unpredictable stress on agriculture. And when crop diversification is linked to markets, it can create income-generating opportunities that improve farmer livelihoods.[34]

The nutritional contributions of diverse agricultural systems could be enhanced further with a combination of modern technologies, scientific progress, and traditional knowledge. For example, fusing available technologies like nutrient-enriched crops (biofortified crops with nutritional qualities that have been enhanced during plant growth)[35] with traditional crop diversification farming systems could address dietary and food security challenges, especially for smallholder farmers.[36] Breeding for improved nutrition also introduces otherwise untapped genetic variation for additional and non-negotiable farmer-preferred traits into new crop varieties, contributing to agricultural diversity.[37] Further research is needed to examine how integrating these diverse knowledge and technology systems along with nutrition education programs can impact diets in target populations (see Chapters 3 and 5).

Challenges to improving diet quality through crop diversification include farmers' reluctance to embrace the complexity of growing additional crops, limited market demand for new crops due to the absence of supportive government policies, and insufficient access to inputs, suitable equipment, technical expertise, and storage and transportation infrastructure.[38]

TECHNOLOGIES TO IMPROVE SUSTAINABLE HEALTHY DIETS

Food fortification and biofortification are well-established, proven strategies to address micronutrient deficiencies in vulnerable populations. These technologies can be further scaled up to improve access to critical nutrients.

BIOFORTIFICATION

Biofortification improves diet quality by enhancing the micronutrient density of widely consumed staple food crops through plant breeding, modern biotechnology, or agronomic practices such as fertilizers or foliar sprays.[39] Plant scientists screen for genetic variation in global plant gene banks to develop nutrient-dense cultivars and, through breeding, develop nutrient-dense cultivars of a particular food crop. Biofortified seeds are bred to also be high-yielding and with farmer-preferred traits that help offset climate-induced declines in agricultural productivity and nutrition. Once added nutrients are incorporated into a variety, they remain year-on-year as seeds are replanted. Hybrid seeds of any crop, biofortified or not, are not as productive if replanted from a previous harvest, so common practice is to purchase new hybrid seed every year.

Biofortified crops can be sustainably and readily integrated into existing cropping systems and programs that support healthy food systems. Therefore, plant breeding is a continuous forward-looking process that requires alignment of nutritional, climate-resilient, and pest-resistant traits with sufficient investment to maintain a healthy food supply.

More than 450 varieties of 13 nutrient-enriched biofortified crops have been released as public goods in more than 40 countries, where they are being eaten by more than 100 million people in LMIC farming households and millions more who purchase them through markets. These efforts have been led by HarvestPlus (IFPRI) and other CGIAR Centers in collaboration with national agricultural research systems and public and private sector partners in host countries, with strong evidence of positive impacts on nutrition (Box 1).

Increasing consumption of biofortified crops and foods is a highly cost-effective public health intervention, and among the highest value-for-money investments for economic development,[40] based on the World Bank criteria of cost per disability-adjusted life years (DALYs) saved.[41] Socioeconomic and sensory

BOX 1 PROVEN BENEFITS OF BIOFORTIFICATION

Randomized controlled studies consistently show positive effects of eating biofortified crops on nutrition and health across age groups and diverse geographies.

- Children in India who ate zinc-enriched wheat daily experienced a significant reduction in the number of days they spent with common infections.[a]
- Women in Rwanda and schoolchildren in India experienced improvements in iron status, cognition, and physical activity after regularly eating beans and pearl millet enriched with iron.[b]
- Children under five years of age in Kenya, Mozambique, Uganda, and Zambia had improved vitamin A status after eating vitamin A-enriched cassava, orange-fleshed sweet potato, or vitamin A-enriched maize, respectively, as main components of their diets.[c]
- Menus incorporating nutrient-rich biofortified foods were highly acceptable among Indian children attending childcare centers and schools and provided a significant portion of their daily nutrient requirements.[d]
- Consumers are highly accepting of biofortified varieties.[e]

Source: HarvestPlus, https://www.harvestplus.org/wp-content/uploads/2021/12/Biofortification_The-Evidence.pdf

evaluation studies examining farmers' and consumers' acceptance of biofortified crops show that farmers like their various agronomic and consumption attributes, are willing to buy them, and sustain adoption of nutrient-enriched varieties.[42]

CGIAR has committed to mainstreaming biofortification to scale up its impact and integrate breeding for improved micronutrient density across all its programs. Doing so takes investment and time (it takes 6 to 10 years to breed, test, and release a new biofortified variety of a crop), and scaling requires more than safeguarding seed supply and building consumer demand. Key market constraints need to be addressed with relevant stakeholders to enhance the competitiveness of biofortified value chains; businesses require support with tools for commercialization; and an enabling environment needs to be established through policies, standards, and regulations to increase consumer access. Adoption of seed standards is essential for identifying and aggregating biofortified seed along the supply chain, and certification provides official assurance of the genetic purity and quality of nutrient-enriched seeds produced.[43]

Successfully leveraging biofortified crops for sustainable healthy diets comes with challenges. National financial and political commitments are required to ensure the prioritization of nutrition traits within agricultural systems and a continual pipeline of nutrient-enriched seeds. Smallholder farmers need ready access to affordable high-quality biofortified crops, as well as training on how to grow and process biofortified crops after harvest. Additional evaluations of biofortification's impact, investment in biofortification businesses by the private sector, and timely implementation of policy frameworks and regulatory guidance are needed to enable this technology to deliver on its full potential to improve the quality of diets.

POSTHARVEST FOOD PROCESSING

Most foods are processed after harvest to reduce losses caused by pests (such as drying cereals, parboiling rice), remove toxic compounds to make foods edible (grating and heat treatment of cassava), preserve or enhance the flavor or texture of foods (refining cereals into flour or fermenting milk), remove pathogens (pasteurizing milk and fruit juices), and increase shelf life (decorticating and degerming cereals). Processing can improve the nutrition contribution of crops to healthy diets, but it can also do the opposite. Most notably, industrialized milling has led to the widespread removal of the most nutritious parts of grains, largely to prolong shelf life and improve palatability.

Large-scale food fortification (LSFF) is a proven and cost-effective nutrition strategy that adds vitamins and minerals during processing at industrial facilities to commonly consumed foods and suitable condiments. LSFF provides nutrient-dense, sustainable options to increase the diet quality of staple crops, particularly for populations that may not be able to access or afford a diverse diet, or where nutrients need to be restored due to processing losses. Because fortification can provide key minerals, such as iron and zinc, that have lower bioavailability in plant-based diets than in animal-based diets,[44] LSFF will remain an important technology even if global consumption of plant-based food increases.

When mandated by law and when coverage is high, LSFF has proven effective in significantly reducing the prevalence of micronutrient deficiencies, with greater impact among adults than in younger children, likely due to the larger amounts of the fortified food consumed.[45] Many countries have adopted mandatory fortification strategies, especially for maize, wheat, rice, oil, and salt, yet compliance varies. In LMICs, processing is mostly handled by small and medium enterprises.[46] Thus, developing enabling environments to increase the involvement of these enterprises in food fortification could enhance competition and increase the number, quality, and affordability of healthy diet components accessible to marginalized populations, including smallholder farmers.[47]

In addition, prioritizing the use of less-refined flours for cereal flour fortification could better leverage LSFF to enrich the quality of diets and protect against obesity and diet-related NCDs.[48] Shifting a significant portion of global grain consumption toward whole grains using both supply- and demand-side approaches would be a pivotal and achievable enhancement for diets and global food systems.

RECOMMENDATIONS

Diet quality is deteriorating and projected to worsen, with widespread implications for human and planetary health. Sustainable healthy diets should remain the global aspiration of food systems transformation, and nutritious crops are the fundamental currency of food systems that deliver sustainable healthy diets. Access to affordable and high-quality crops such as fruits, vegetables, and nutrient-enriched staples and other whole grains for the poor in LMICs is a global equity, health, and sustainability challenge.

To leverage crops for sustainable healthy diets, policymakers should:

- Combine policies and accessible technologies – intercropping, biofortification, and postharvest processing techniques such as LSFF – to produce and supply more nutritious crops and foods along with behavioral strategies to shift demand and behaviors toward sustainable healthy diets (see Chapters 3 and 5).
- Promote production and consumption of biofortified or fortified staple foods where needed. These foods are a major component of diets of all household members, including women and children, and thus can be an equitable and affordable means of delivering nutrients.
- Prioritize investments in crop diversity, including nutrient-rich crops such as fruits and vegetables, that in combination with upgrades to urban market infrastructure and nutrition and hygiene education among farmers, value chain actors, and consumers could lead to increased accessibility, affordability, and appeal of safe and healthy diets.
- Create an enabling environment, supported by government and financial commitments, for scaling up crop-focused initiatives that can achieve nutrition and climate goals through holistic and context-specific multisectoral interventions that span agriculture, food, trade, and social protection (see Chapter 8).

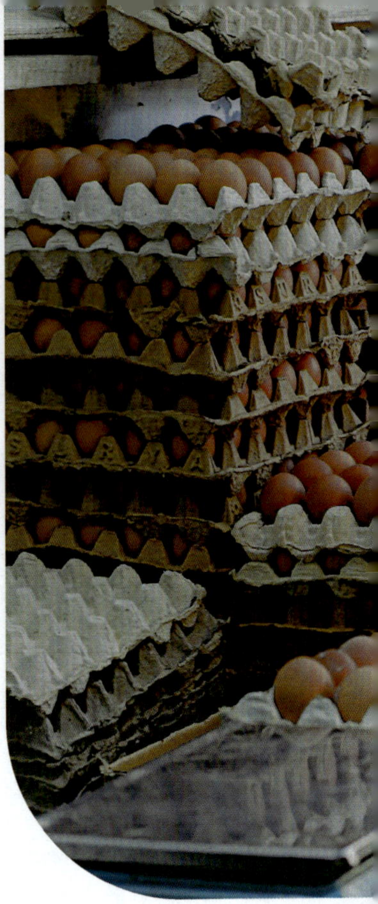

CHAPTER 7

Animal-Source Foods
Their Role in Sustainable Healthy Diets

JEF L. LEROY AND SILVIA ALONSO

Jef L. Leroy is a senior research fellow, Nutrition, Diets, and Health Unit, International Food Policy Research Institute (IFPRI). **Silvia Alonso** is a principal scientist epidemiologist, International Livestock Research Institute (ILRI).

The authors thank Iain Wright, deputy director general for research and development–Integrated Sciences, International Livestock Research Institute (ILRI), and Siboniso Moyo, deputy director general for research and development–Biosciences, ILRI, for their input to this chapter.

KEY MESSAGES

- Animal-source foods (ASFs) are an excellent source of high-quality proteins and bioavailable micronutrients that can be difficult or impossible to obtain from plant-source foods. ASFs are particularly important for individuals with high nutrient requirements, such as young children.
- ASF consumption can contribute to negative health outcomes. Processed meat is known to be carcinogenic; however, the association between noncommunicable diseases and consumption of unprocessed red meat and saturated fatty acids continues to be debated. Unsafe animal products are an important contributor to foodborne disease worldwide.
- Global livestock production has substantial negative effects on the environment, but the impact varies widely by type of ASF, production system, and region. The largest impacts are seen with ruminant production.
- Demand for ASFs is growing and expected to grow further, particularly in low- and middle-income countries (LMICs), due to urbanization, changes in dietary preferences, and population growth.

More sustainable and healthy consumption of ASFs can be encouraged in various ways:

- Promote a shift toward more plant-based diets in high-income countries and other populations with excess intake of ASFs through, for example, public awareness campaigns and adjusting prices to include environmental costs.
- Support increased ASF consumption among populations with deficient diets in LMICs, for instance by making ASFs more affordable through increased farm productivity, improved market efficiency, and by raising household income, for example, using social safety nets.
- Address foodborne disease with better monitoring and food safety systems, especially in informal markets.
- Invest in sustainable ASF production systems to benefit human health and keep global livestock production within planetary boundaries.
- Develop and test food system and food environment innovations that promote moderate ASF consumption in countries at all income levels.

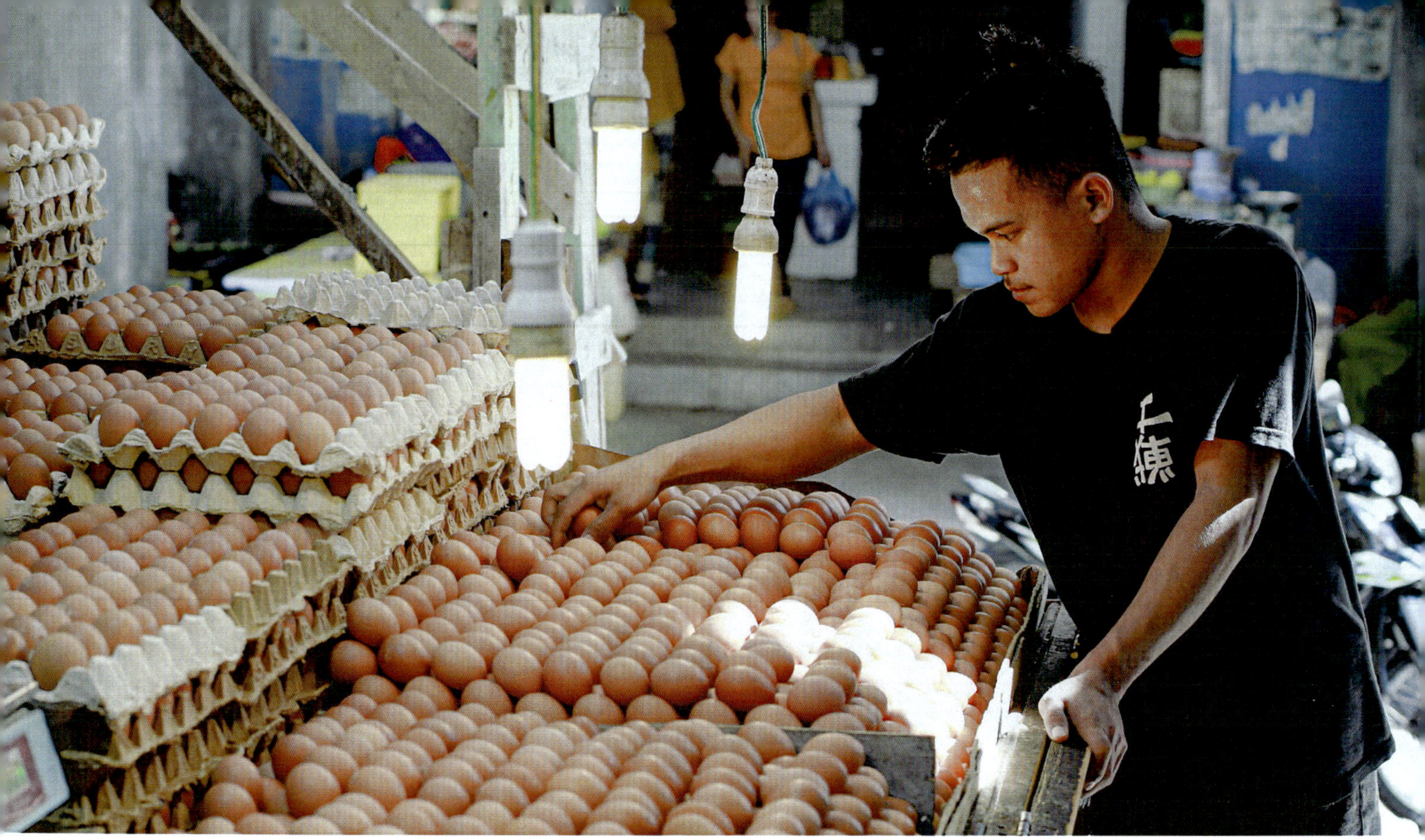

Diets are rapidly evolving in low- and middle-income countries (LMICs) due to changes in income, women's employment, and urbanization, as well as developments in technology, food marketing, and public policy.[1] As part of this change, consumption of animal-source foods (ASFs) (Box 1) has increased sharply in recent decades. Between 1990 and 2015, global annual per capita demand for ASFs increased by more than 40 kilograms (kg). Global estimates, however, obscure differences in consumption levels between and within regions. Per capita intake of red meat in 2018, for instance, varied from 7 grams (g) per day in South Asia to 87 g per day in Southeast and East Asia, and and 114 g per day in Central and Eastern Europe and Central Asia (Figure 1). ASF intake is higher among people in urban areas and those with higher levels of education and lower among rural residents and those with lower levels of education.[2]

Global demand for ASFs is expected to continue growing due to changes in dietary preferences and population growth in LMICs, though only minimal changes are expected in high-income countries (HICs). By 2050, global demand for meat and dairy is expected to be 57 and 48 percent higher, respectively, than in 2005.[3]

ASFs are an excellent source of high-quality proteins and bioavailable micronutrients that can be difficult or impossible to obtain from plant-source foods (PSFs), especially for individuals with high nutrient requirements, such as young children.[4] Excessive consumption of certain types of ASFs, however, increases the risk of cancer and is associated with cardiovascular and other noncommunicable diseases (NCDs).[5] Globally, livestock production is detrimental to the environment, but impacts vary across types of ASFs, production systems, and regions.

This chapter examines ASFs as part of a sustainable healthy diet.[6] We examine the beneficial role of ASFs in providing essential micronutrients in some age cohorts and populations in LMICs; the potential negative health impacts, including the risk of diet-related NCDs and foodborne disease; and the environmental impacts associated with livestock production. We conclude with some recommendations for ASF consumption, including policies and interventions for reducing excess consumption and promoting consumption where ASFs could play a larger role in sustainable healthy diets.

FIGURE 1 Regional ASF intake (grams/day) in 185 countries, 2018

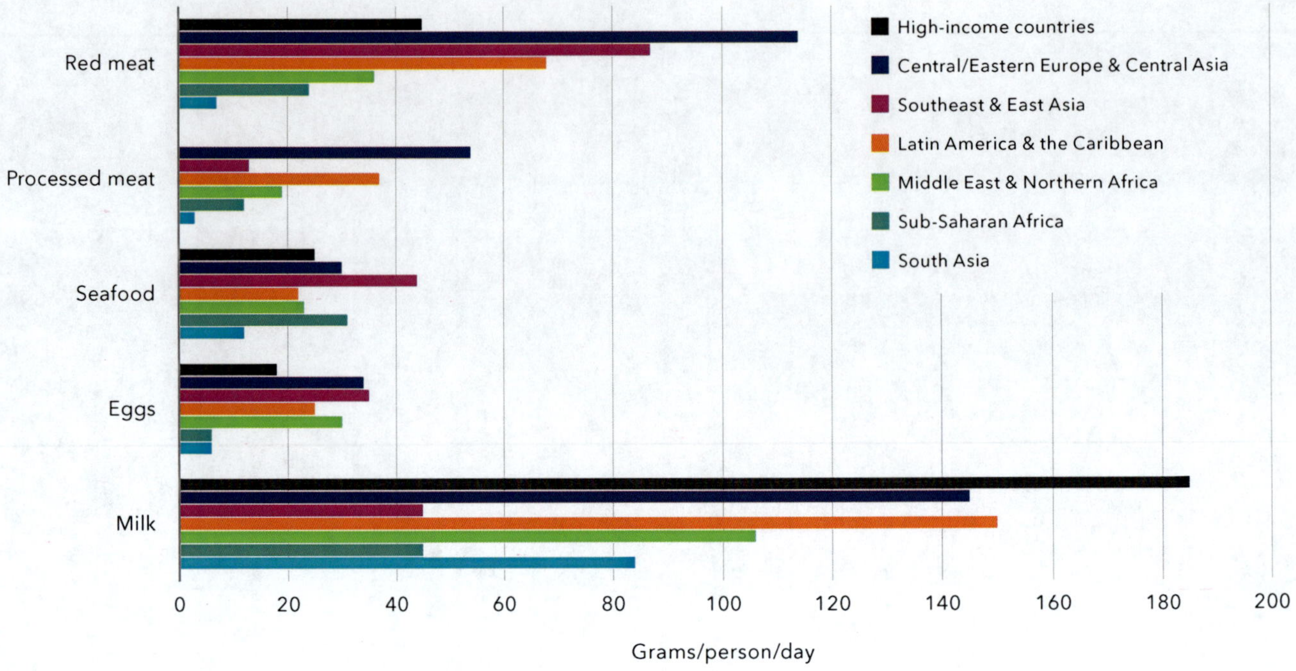

Source: Based on V. Miller, J. Reedy, F. Cudhea, et al., "Global, Regional, and National Consumption of Animal-Source Foods Between 1990 and 2018: Findings from the Global Dietary Database," *Lancet Planetary Health* 6, 3 (2022): e243-256.

BOX 1 DEFINITIONS

ANIMAL-SOURCE FOODS: Animal-source foods (ASFs) are categorized into meat (such as flesh foods and organs), fish (aquatic ASFs, including fish, crustaceans, and bivalves), dairy products (milk and foods derived from milk such as butter, yogurt, and cheese), and eggs.[a]

ALTERNATIVE PROTEINS: Alternative proteins include food products made from plants, microorganisms, insects, and cultivated proteins. Although insects are consumed in many parts of the world, they are typically considered an alternative protein.[b]

PROCESSED MEATS: Processed meats broadly include any type of meat that has been salted, cured, fermented, or smoked, or that has undergone other processes to enhance flavor or improve preservation.[c]

RED MEAT: Red meat refers to mammalian muscle meat, such as beef, pork, mutton, and goatmeat.

NUTRITIONAL ATTRIBUTES OF ASFs

ASFs are both energy and nutrient dense, meaning that they provide significant amounts of calories and nutrients even if only small quantities are consumed. Some nutrients, such as vitamin B12, are unique to ASFs and cannot be obtained from PSFs.[7] Other vitamins and minerals are available in fruits, grains, tubers, seeds and nuts, and legumes, but are less concentrated and bioavailable (meaning that less of the nutrient is absorbed). As a result, larger quantities of PSFs must be consumed to meet nutrient requirements.[8]

ASFs are also an excellent source of high-quality proteins that provide all essential amino acids, the "building blocks" that the human body needs to synthesize proteins.[9] These amino acids can be obtained from PSFs as well, but doing so requires combining foods from different food groups. Aquatic ASFs (as well as aquatic PSFs) are the only sources of long-chain n-3 fatty acids, which are essential to human health. These fatty acids can be synthesized by the body from fatty acids in terrestrial PSFs, but the conversion is inefficient and may not be sufficient to meet nutrient requirements.[10] Several bioactive compounds such as creatine, taurine, and anserine are also unique to ASFs and appear to play key roles in human health and cognition.[11] Small quantities of meat or fish not only provide considerable amounts of high-quality proteins and bioavailable micronutrients, but also increase the absorption of iron from PSFs.[12]

BENEFICIAL EFFECTS OF ASFs THROUGHOUT THE LIFE COURSE

Nutritional needs change throughout the life course. During pregnancy and lactation, additional nutrients are needed for fetal growth and milk production. Infants and young children are known to have particularly high nutrient requirements due to rapid growth and development (see Box 2, for previous misconceptions about the role of protein in children's growth). Around the age of six months, a child's energy and nutrient needs start to exceed what is provided by breast milk, and complementary (solid) foods need to be introduced into the child's diet to meet those needs. This complementary feeding period is a particularly vulnerable time for nutrient deficiencies. Recurring infections, common in children living in unsanitary conditions, further increase nutrient needs. Another important challenge in infancy and young childhood is limited gastric capacity, meaning that children's small meals need to be nutrient dense.

Adolescence marks a second period of rapid growth and development that requires higher nutrient intake. Adolescent girls and women of reproductive age need higher levels of dietary iron to compensate for menstrual iron loss. Dietary needs change again in old age, a time that is often characterized by loss of muscle mass and frailty.[13]

ASFs can play an important role in meeting the increased nutrient needs in these critical periods. Plant-based complementary foods by themselves, for instance, are insufficient to meet requirements

BOX 2 PROTEINS AND CHILD UNDERNUTRITION

In the 1950s, the development community widely believed that inadequate intake of dietary protein was the primary cause of child malnutrition in low- and middle-income countries (LMICs).[a] This was largely based on the false premise that kwashiorkor (a form of malnutrition characterized by edema), which responded to milk supplementation, was the predominant form of child undernutrition.[b] In 1968, the UN agencies declared a "protein crisis." Only a few years later, several researchers established the need to consider the combination of protein and energy in preventing malnutrition, rather than protein alone. An influential paper titled "The Great Protein Fiasco" subsequently buried the global focus on protein in the fight against child undernutrition,[c] and nutrition research shifted to the importance of micronutrients.

The role of protein has gained renewed attention with the recent finding that serum amino acid levels are significantly lower in stunted children than non-stunted children.[d] This finding does not imply, however, that higher protein intake would lead to improved linear growth. Among infants and young children in LMICs, protein intake generally exceeds required levels when diets are adequate in energy.[e] Protein supplementation trials have not shown impacts on linear growth.[f] The hypothesis that protein requirements in children are higher than previously estimated, due to frequent infections and related malabsorption and systemic inflammation,[g] has not been confirmed.

Based on current knowledge, low intakes of micronutrients and essential fatty acids, not protein, are the key dietary factors limiting child growth and development.[h]

for iron, zinc, and calcium in the complementary feeding period during infancy.[14] In the absence of micronutrient-fortified products, ASFs thus need to be included among complementary foods.[15]

Evidence on the beneficial effects of ASFs is limited to specific foods and a relatively small number of nutrition and health outcomes. Milk intake during pregnancy, for instance, is positively associated with birth weight and length, but the evidence is mostly from observational studies.[16] Adding ASFs to the diets of children ages 6 to 24 months in LMICs improves linear growth.[17] The consumption of milk and dairy in older children and adolescents leads to increased height (particularly in children with short stature, according to evidence from LMICs and HICs), increased bone mineral content and density (evidence primarily from HICs), and lower risks of overweight and obesity (evidence from HICs and China).[18] Evidence from HICs demonstrates that lean red meat consumption in older adults has positive effects on muscle health.[19] It is likely that other outcomes would benefit from increased ASF intake, especially when diets are deficient, but experimental evidence is largely absent, especially in LMICs. Few studies, for instance, have assessed the effect of ASF intake on cognition.[20]

HEALTH RISKS OF CONSUMING ASFs

Much of the debate about the negative health effects of eating ASFs relates to the association between NCDs and consumption of processed meat, unprocessed red meat, and saturated fatty acids. Foodborne disease is another health risk associated with ASF intake.

NONCOMMUNICABLE DISEASES. Each year, NCDs kill 41 million people, equivalent to 73 percent of all deaths globally, and this burden is increasing .[21] In 2018, the International Agency for Research on Cancer (IARC) categorized processed meat (Box 1) as "carcinogenic" to humans.[22] Processed meats are typically high in sodium, which has been associated with increased risk of hypertension, stroke, cardiovascular disease, and higher mortality.[23] High sodium intakes are particularly harmful to health in conjunction with low potassium intake.[24]

The IARC has classified red meat as "probably carcinogenic" to humans.[25] High intakes have been found to be associated with cardiovascular disease and type 2 diabetes.[26] Evidence suggests that cooking methods such as grilling, deep frying, and barbecuing might increase NCD risk, and that consuming a balanced diet (that is, a diet rich in minimally processed PSFs) may moderate the risk associated with red meat intake.[27] Importantly, the causal connection between red meat consumption and negative health outcomes continues to be heavily debated among health experts.[28]

The health impact of saturated fatty acids, primarily found in ASFs such as high-fat dairy and red meat, are clearer. Reducing consumption of these fatty acids has been shown to lower serum low-density lipoprotein cholesterol and the risk of cardiovascular disease, but the evidence on preventing coronary heart disease or reducing mortality is much weaker.[29]

FOODBORNE DISEASE. Unsafe foods are responsible for an estimated 600 million foodborne illnesses and nearly 500,000 deaths in the world annually.[30] This corresponds to an annual total of 33 million disability-adjusted life years (DALYs, which is the sum of years of life lost and years lived with disability), with children under five years old bearing 40 percent of this burden. The burden in Africa (over 1,200 DALYs per 100,000 people) and Southeast Asia (around 700 DALYs per 100,000 people) is considerably higher than that in HICs (35 to 50 DALYs per 100,000 people).[31] Foodborne diseases commonly manifest as enteric infections and diarrhea and contribute to undernutrition through lowered appetite, reduced nutrient absorption, and inflammation.[32]

Not all food products are equally important as sources of foodborne disease. Studies on food source attribution that estimate the relative importance of different foods as causes of foodborne illnesses are very limited due to the complex methodology and lack of surveillance data worldwide, and particularly in LMICs. The few available studies often rank ASFs among the top 10 foods implicated in foodborne disease outbreaks.[33] A recent study offers the first globally comparable estimates on regional differences in food sources for 11 common foodborne pathogens based on expert consensus.[34] Vegetables were deemed the main vehicle of foodborne *parasites*, responsible for 60–80 percent of parasitic foodborne infections, while ASFs appeared to be the most common source of foodborne *bacteria*.

It is unsurprising that ASFs would be an important source of foodborne illness, given that these foods are perishable in nature and offer a rich environment for microorganisms. Many foodborne pathogens are carried by livestock. Studies conducted largely in the global North show that most foodborne disease outbreaks are caused by zoonotic pathogens (organisms transmitted between animals and humans). For example, *Salmonella enteritidis* can subclinically colonize hens and be ingested by humans through eggs or poultry meat. Cattle are a reservoir for the life-threatening Shiga toxin-producing *Escherichia coli*, which has led to several deadly outbreaks in the United States and elsewhere. Even though vegetables are also an important source of foodborne illness, often when consumed raw and unwashed, the pathogens transmitted via vegetables mostly originate in livestock.[35] Despite limited robust data on source attribution, the consumption of unsafe food is an undeniable cause of illness in humans, and the consumption of unsafe animal products is certainly an important contributor to foodborne disease worldwide.

ENVIRONMENTAL EFFECTS OF ASFs

Global livestock production negatively affects the environment. The main impacts include greenhouse gas emissions (Figure 2), increased land and water use, and biodiversity loss. Globally, livestock production causes 14.5 percent of total human-induced greenhouse gas emissions, with beef and dairy cattle accounting for two-thirds of those emissions.[36] Emissions vary substantially between products, with ruminants having the largest impact, and within product groups depending on the production method.[37] Currently, about half of all global agricultural land, or 2.5 billion ha, is used for livestock and livestock feed production. Of this land, four-fifths is grassland, much of which (1.3 billion ha) is marginal or nonarable land; grazing is the only way to use these lands for food production. The remaining one-fifth of land devoted to livestock production is used to grow feed crops.[38]

Livestock production has a large water footprint, accounting for 41 percent of all water used in agriculture.[39] Most water used for livestock production (96 percent) is water from rainfall, which is also referred to as "green water" (as opposed to "blue water," which is surface and ground water).[40] In addition to the direct use of water, other aspects of livestock production, including animal manure, inputs for producing animal feed, and antibiotics and other veterinary medicines, can pose threats to water quality, such as eutrophication caused by nutrient leaching and runoff.[41]

Livestock production has also contributed to biodiversity loss as livestock and feed production have expanded into previously intact ecosystems and contributed to climate change through greenhouse gas emissions, deforestation, eutrophication of water, and overfishing.[42] However, well-managed livestock grazing can have positive impacts in some specific habitats, such as grassland habitats in Europe and (sub) tropical grasslands.[43]

Livestock production is thus a major cause of global environmental degradation, and these negative impacts are expected to increase with growing ASF demand. However, large differences exist across ASF types and production systems. For example, water use varies widely: layer hens require an estimated 38 liters (L) of water (3.8 L of which is blue water) per g of protein, while bovines require 200 L (8 L of blue water and 34 L of green water falling on nonarable land) per g of protein. Importantly, green and blue water use varies widely depending on the production type, even for the same type of ASF.[44] Greenhouse gas emissions also differ substantially. Emissions from beef production vary from less than 15 kg CO_2-equivalent per kg of carcass weight in northern Europe to more than 75 kg in South Asia, with a global average of 46.2 kg. A key factor explaining these differences is the digestibility of feed, with more fibrous rations leading to higher methane emissions from enteric fermentation. Emissions from production of pork and chicken

FIGURE 2 Greenhouse gas emissions of selected foods

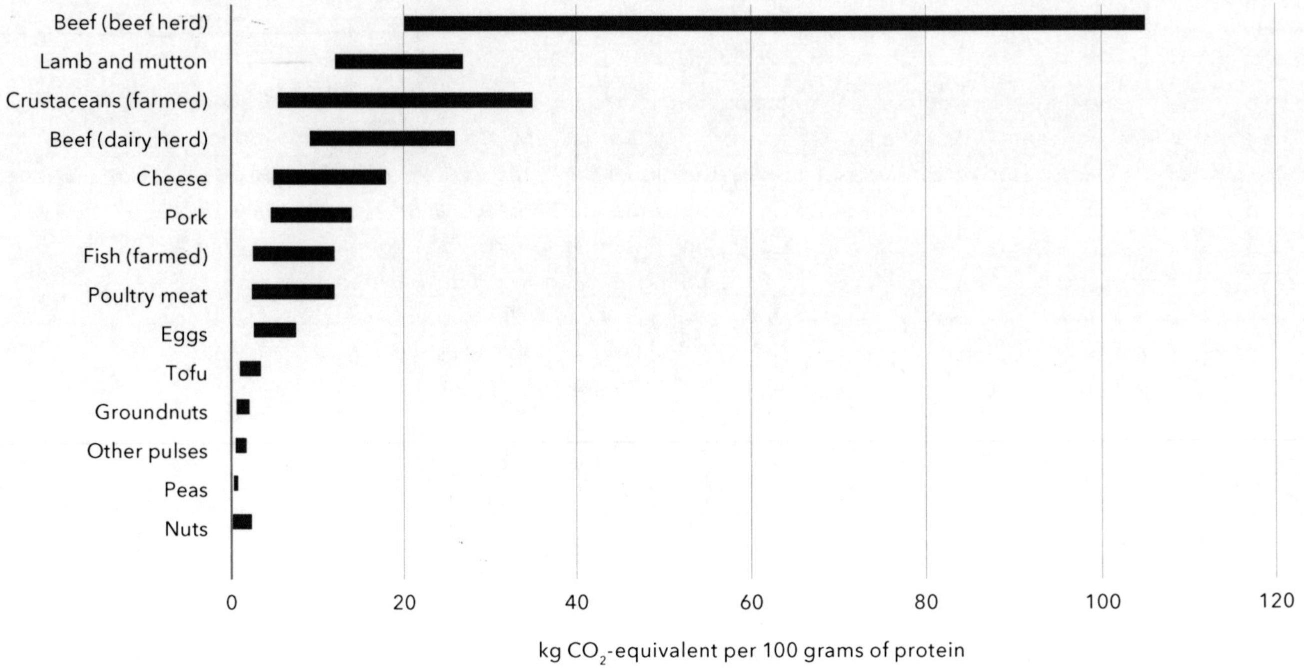

Source: Based on J. Poore and T. Nemecek, "Reducing Food's Environmental Impacts through Producers and Consumers," *Science* 360, 6392 (2018): 987-992. Reprinted with permission from AAAS.

Note: Greenhouse gas emissions include a range from low-impact producers (10th percentile) to high-impact producers (90th percentile).

(6.1 and 5.4 kg CO_2-equivalent per kg of carcass weight, respectively) are substantially lower and vary less across regions.[45]

In mixed crop-livestock systems, which remain common around the world, especially among smallholders, animals deliver nutrient-rich manure that improves soil fertility and increases soil organic matter. In turn, crops and their residues can be used to feed animals. The separation of cropping and livestock increases the need to use chemical fertilizers and import feed. It also leads to problems with management and excessive application of manure, which subsequently degrades soils and leads to emissions, leaching, and runoff.[46]

SHIFTING TO SUSTAINABLE HEALTHY DIETS: MODERATE ASF CONSUMPTION

ASFs are rich in bioavailable nutrients and can contribute to healthy diets. Global production of animal products, however, has important negative effects on the environment. It is impossible to determine an overall average amount of ASFs for all of the world's consumers that is both beneficial to human health and environmentally sustainable, given the wide-ranging differences in nutritional needs and production methods.[47]

In general, ASFs should be consumed in moderate amounts that correspond with nutritional requirements. Consumption will need to increase in groups with high nutrient needs, such as infants and young children, who currently do not have sufficient access to ASFs and consume nutrient-deficient diets, a situation still common in many LMICs. In Africa south of the Sahara and southern Asia, healthy diets are too expensive for 85 percent and 70 percent, respectively, of the population (see Chapter 4).[48] ASFs are considerably more expensive (relative to starchy staples) in lower-income countries than in HICs, making them much less affordable for those who would benefit most from consuming them.[49] Making ASFs affordable in

BOX 3 IMPROVING MILK QUALITY IN AN URBAN SETTING IN KENYA: THE MOREMILK PROJECT

The informal sector is the primary source of food for billions of people in LMICs. The MoreMilk intervention, implemented from February to September 2022, targeted informal dairy vendors in Eldoret, a secondary city in Kenya, with in-person trainings on milk handling, hygiene, and business skills. It included presentations and discussions of laboratory results on milk safety, and a carefully designed marketing campaign to promote children's milk consumption. The intervention increased the uptake of good milk handling practices by vendors and increased milk intake in children. MoreMilk vendors and their customers reported improvements in nutrition and milk hygiene knowledge and practices. These improvements in hygiene and cleanliness, as well as nutrition messages provided by vendors, led to increases in both customer trust and purchases of milk.

Source: Unpublished findings from an evaluation of the MoreMilk project. See also: www.ilri.org/research/projects/moremilk-making-most-milk

low-income settings will require a combination of increasing livestock productivity, improving market efficiency to reduce prices, and increasing household income through, for instance, social safety nets.[50] Cash transfers to poor households in Mexico, for example, increased household consumption of fruits and vegetables and ASFs, and improved the overall nutrient density of the household diet. The transfers, however, also increased energy consumption (even though diets were not energy deficient) and led to excessive weight gain.[51] Inclusion of education focused on healthy diets in safety net programs is thus needed to limit potential negative effects on the diet.[52]

In populations with excess ASF intake and a high risk of diet-related NCDs, consumption will need to be drastically reduced.[53] In addition, shifting to ASFs with a smaller negative impact on the environment would be beneficial. Options to explore for accomplishing this objective include public awareness campaigns, front-of-package labeling to highlight health risks (see Chapter 5), inclusion of meat-free days in institutional catering, and price corrections to include the full environmental costs, including all externalities. Rigorous evidence on the effectiveness of interventions aimed at moderating ASF intake is currently missing.

For ASFs to benefit human health and nutrition, the foodborne disease risks associated with their intake must be addressed. Country or regional risk assessments need to be conducted to identify the most important food safety hazards and the high-risk foods in order to inform and prioritize food safety efforts.[54] Countries must continue to upgrade their food safety systems and promote best practices in food storage, preparation, and consumption. To do this, greater attention is required in the global South to improve food safety in informal and often unregulated markets, where most people buy from food vendors.[55] These markets can be leveraged to be both a source of safe food and a way to promote nutrition awareness and information among low-income households (Box 3).

Reducing global ASF consumption, while ensuring adequate consumption among communities with nutritionally deficient diets, and investing in sustainable livestock production systems will result in large reductions in the environmental footprint of food production. In a hypothetical scenario where global consumption of animal products is halved by replacing livestock production that generates above-median greenhouse gas emissions with vegetable equivalents, food-related greenhouse gas emissions and land use would decline by 36 percent and 51 percent, respectively.[56]

While the environmental footprint of producing alternative proteins is considerably lower than that of ASFs,[57] most of the market growth to date has been in HICs. High production costs and limited consumer acceptance are important barriers that need to be overcome to expand the role of these proteins.[58]

Moreover, little evidence exists on the nutritional effects of adding alternative proteins to diets in LMICs. Given the high prevalence of micronutrient deficiencies in these regions, the primary concern with these products is whether they provide the same amounts of bioavailable micronutrients as do ASFs.

In sum, shifting toward more plant-based diets in HICs and increasing ASF consumption among populations with deficient diets in LMICs would benefit human health and result in a more equitable distribution of ASFs produced within planetary boundaries.[59] Accomplishing this goal will require developing and testing innovations for food systems and food environments that promote moderate ASF consumption in countries at all income levels.

“Animal-source foods can play an important role in meeting increased nutrient needs during critical periods of the life course.”

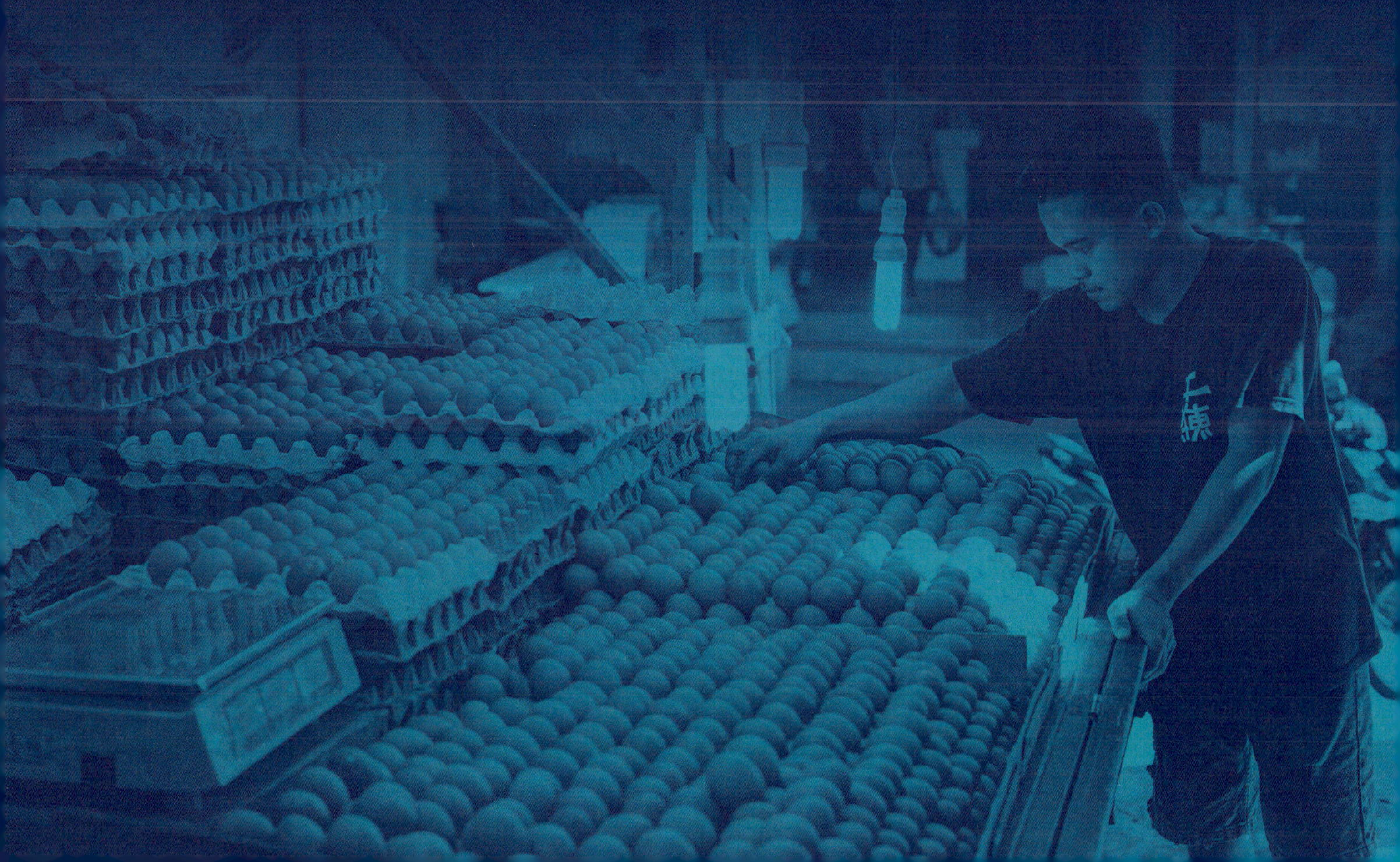

CHAPTER 8

Improved Governance
Creating Supportive Environments for Diet and Nutrition Policies

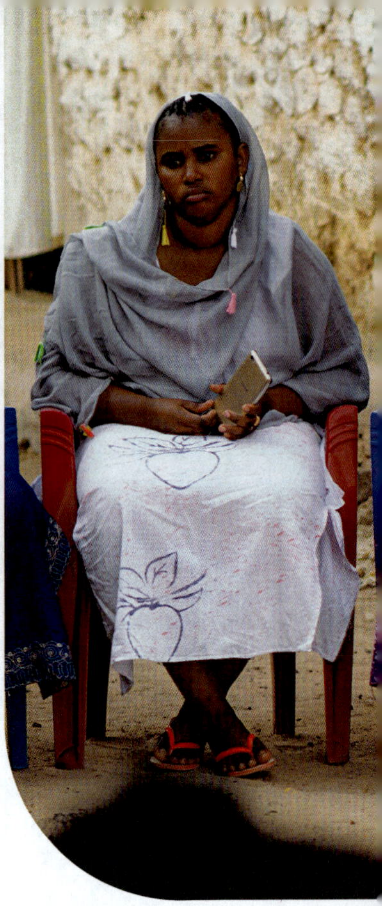

DANIELLE RESNICK AND MARIA-TERESA NOGALES

Danielle Resnick is a senior research fellow, Development Strategies and Governance Unit, International Food Policy Research Institute, Washington, DC. **Maria-Teresa Nogales** is the founder and director, Fundación Alternativas, La Paz, Bolivia.

KEY MESSAGES

- Sound governance is essential for successful policy interventions that contribute to improved diet quality and nutrition – these include fiscal and transfer policies, subsidies, regulations, and investments in technology and research.
- Improving diets and nutrition depends on a state's administrative capacity to develop policy, regulate commercial activities, and deliver public services; and on its ability to raise taxes and mobilize funds for food system investments. Low state capacity limits policy choices.
- Bundling different policies together is often recommended but may not be feasible given different government incentives. Addressing diverse administrative needs for different policies and managing trade-offs across nutrition goals and other objectives require substantial state capacity.
- State capacity and political incentives also shape government engagement with food companies and other interest groups, which may either oppose or support government goals. Policies are more likely to be contested when powerful actors lack incentives to implement them.
- Citizen engagement and grassroots movements can play a transformative role in reshaping food systems. These are most likely to flourish when there is sufficient civic space and committed political leadership.

Good governance can be fostered by activities to:

- Complement economic analyses of policies for diets and nutrition with governance assessments to ensure policies are sustainable and scalable from both capacity and political economy perspectives.
- Identify and address government constraints, such as insufficient financing, poor data, and corruption or demoralization in bureaucracy that limit capacity and influence.
- Build government accountability to citizens – for example, through online transparency tools.
- Provide an enabling governance environment that fosters the growth of successful grassroots movements that can support better diets and nutrition.

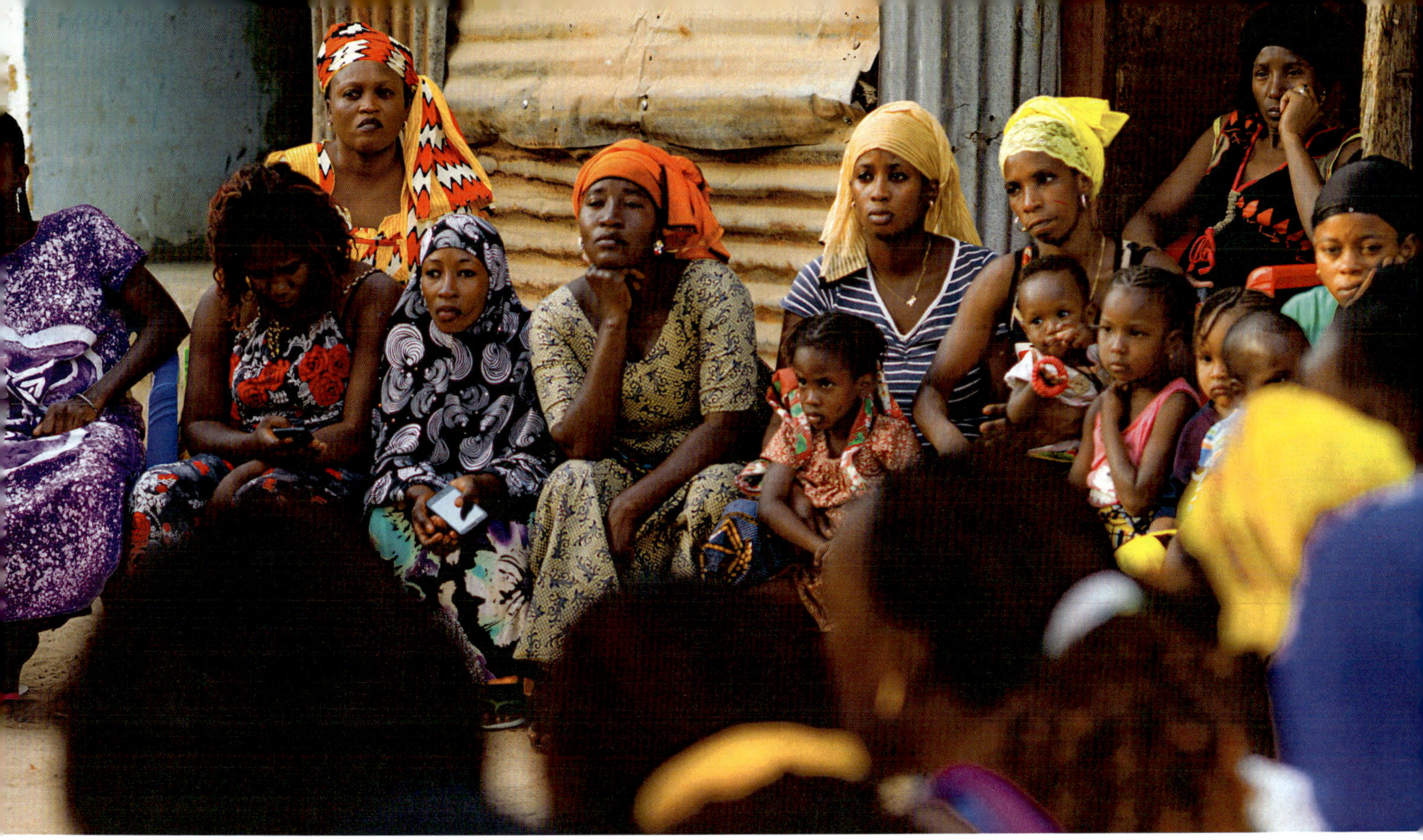

Most policy interventions to improve diet quality and nutrition require sound governance to be successful. In fact, the role of governance increasingly has been acknowledged as fundamental to achieving healthy food systems.[1] Governance encompasses the interrelationships between formal institutions and informal modes of power, across different geographic scales, and among state and non-state actors. This chapter examines how multilevel and multistakeholder governance can be strengthened to improve diets, with a focus on enhancing state capacities, navigating corporate influence, and fostering citizen agency. Throughout, the chapter highlights existing challenges in each of these areas while also discussing approaches that have potential to improve the governance environment at national and local scales.

STATE CAPACITIES AND POLITICAL INCENTIVES FOR BETTER NUTRITION POLICIES

Several policy approaches, including fiscal and transfer policies, regulations, and targeted investments, are frequently advocated to address different sets of diet and nutrition challenges. Fiscal policies are a common tool for addressing noncommunicable diseases (NCDs). For instance, taxes on sugar-sweetened beverages (SSBs) have been adopted in more than 40 countries as well as several regions and US states (see Chapter 5).[2] Transfer policies, such as consumer subsidies and cash transfers, have been used to help poorer households improve their food security or diversify their diets. Historically, governments have allocated subsidies to cereal-based products, such as bread, rice, and maize meal (see Chapter 6). More recently, national and local governments, especially in high-income countries, have begun adopting subsidies on nutritious foods to increase dietary diversity, and existing review studies suggest they can improve healthy eating choices.[3] Almost 25 US states participate in the Double Up Food Bucks program, which doubles the value of benefits for recipients of food stamps under the Supplemental Nutrition Assistance Program (SNAP) every time recipients spend on fresh fruits and vegetables.[4] Cash transfers, vouchers, and in-kind transfers likewise have demonstrated positive impacts on dietary diversity and nutrition outcomes in many low- and middle-income countries (LMICs).[5] Regulations are an important tool for establishing healthy food environments. For instance, regulations on the food industry's marketing and labeling of unhealthy foods have long been deemed necessary to change consumption behaviors (see Chapter 5).[6] Investments in technology and research are another key policy instrument, increasing the affordability of healthy foods. For example, investments in both biofortification and large-scale food fortification are frequently cited as among the most cost-effective means of addressing micronutrient deficiencies (see Chapter 6).[7]

Bundling these different policy options together is often most effective for addressing nutrition problems but may not be feasible given existing state capacities or political incentives. There are multiple facets to state capacity, but two are central to nutrition. The first is *administrative capacity*, which refers to a state's ability to develop policy, regulate commercial activities, and deliver public services. Achieving these goals depends on having sufficient technical staff, transparent and updated data and recordkeeping, coordination mechanisms, and reach across geographic territory and different social constituencies.[8] The ability to provide these functions impartially and autonomously from political interference is the hallmark of a meritocratic civil service.[9] The second key dimension of state capacity is *extractive power* – that is, the ability to raise tax revenue. Extractive power is important not only because it reflects whether states can reach the totality of their populations and exert compliance and oversight, but also because tax payments often serve as a mechanism by which citizens can demand accountability for service provision.[10] Moreover, revenue mobilization is critical to provide funds for sustainable investments in the food system, which is pivotal given that debt accumulation in LMICs has outstripped economic growth over the past decade.[11]

State capacity defined in these terms is essential for improving diets and nutrition for several reasons. First, many scholars advocate combining policy interventions to create the largest impact on nutrition outcomes, such as allocating cash transfers along with nutritional supplements[12] or with behavior change communication programs to change eating habits.[13] Similarly, subsidies for healthy foods are considered most powerful when tied to taxes or regulatory restrictions on unhealthy foods.[14] Yet, these policies have different administrative requirements and political constituencies that can thwart implementation. SSB taxes, for instance, are often implemented through value-added, excise, or import taxes, which can be levied uniformly on specific unhealthy foods or beverages and generate revenue for indebted governments. In contrast, in the constrained resource environments facing many LMICs, subsidies for healthy foods need to be targeted to the poorest to ensure they have the greatest impact on the diets of this population; this targeting requires a higher level of technical competence and recordkeeping. Relatedly, the design of market regulations for the food industry is more complex for the public to understand, and enforcement involves an outlay of state resources for oversight and compliance officers. For both these reasons, regulations are often less galvanizing for the public and less desirable in the view of governments. These intricacies are highlighted in a study that explains why India, Mexico, and South Africa adopted SSB taxes in the mid-2010s but failed to adopt marketing and labeling regulations on ultra-processed foods.[15]

Second, trade-offs across nutrition goals and other economic development objectives can stress state capacity for coordination. For instance, some countries have levied import bans and tariffs on fruits and vegetables to both decrease the size of their import bill and build up their own horticulture producers, but these policies also increase the cost of such healthy foods for domestic consumers. Botswana, for instance, traditionally depends on South Africa for about 80 percent of its fresh produce but implemented a ban in 2022 on 16 such products to protect domestic producers along with an Impact Accelerator Subsidy to support horticultural farmers.[16] The ban has since been extended until 2025 and the number of products doubled, even though it has led to retail shortages in Botswana, as well as price increases for horticulture products and spoilage of domestically cultivated fresh fruits and vegetables, due to a lack of complementary investments in refrigerated storage facilities.[17] Industrial policy and employment goals have likewise been used as a justification to protect sectors producing unhealthy foods – such as sugar, which is protected through sugar master plans in places like Nigeria and South Africa, even while those governments simultaneously implement SSB taxes to reduce sugar consumption.[18] Ultra-processed food industries have major impacts on the food environment (see Chapter 5) but also generate large numbers of manufacturing and distribution jobs in LMICs,[19] which provide citizens with incomes that help them afford more diverse diets. Trade-offs also exist among nutrition goals, such as when food fortification advocates choose products like sugar or bouillon – a seasoning high in sodium content – as vehicles for industrial fortification, based on consumer behaviors and economic organization. In several cases, this has required ministries of health to have sufficient capacity to convey a complex message to their publics that stresses the value of micronutrient-enriched products while simultaneously discouraging overconsumption of such products.

Third, states need capacity to manage the movement from "easy" to "hard" stages of policy reforms.[20] Easy stages occur when policies have just been put in place, sometimes through "stroke of the pen" decisions and with donor support, and interest groups have yet to identify how their costs and benefits will be affected or threatened. Hard stages emerge over time when impacts are assessed, amendments are needed, donor program support may dwindle, and divisions among interest groups may emerge. The efficacy of SSB taxes, for instance, declines over time if they are not constantly adjusted for inflation to avoid eroding their real value.[21] Regulations and standards must shift as new data emerge about their efficacy and in alignment with changes in regional or global economic bodies and standards. For instance, Chile's adoption of a comprehensive law in 2016 to mandate restrictions on marketing of ultra-processed foods to children and requiring front-of-package labeling for foods high in sugar, salt, and transfats reflected recognition that SSB taxes alone were insufficient to tackle obesity[22]; many Latin American countries have now followed suit (see Latin America section). Similarly, a review of almost two decades of large-scale food fortification policies in LMICs reveals that while such programs may initially take off with donor subsidies for vitamin premixes, they are hampered by a lack of sustainability planning, including ensuring continuous quality assurance and control, monitoring, and corrective measures as consumption patterns change over time.[23]

As an example of how state capacity matters, one cross-country analysis of 194 World Health Organization (WHO) member states between 2014 and 2021 uncovered highly variable implementation of the 19 WHO-recommended policies for combatting diet-related NCDs.[24] Policies with the lowest implementation rates were related to unhealthy food, as well as alcohol and tobacco. Figure 1 maps NCD policy implementation vis-à-vis state capacity as measured by the World Bank's government effectiveness index, highlighting that policy implementation is higher where state capacity is also higher. At the same time, Figure 1 suggests that implementation is not entirely driven by capacity; indeed, a recent study finds that ideological resistance in some high-income countries, as well as powerful corporate financial interests in others, also explains differential levels of implementation.[25]

These issues are equally relevant at the subnational level, especially with respect to cities. Rapid urbanization is often identified as one of the drivers of increasing NCDs in LMICs, as people eat away from home more and prefer ready-to-eat, prepackaged foods or prepared meals that may include excessive oil and sodium.[26] Poorer urban settings in LMICs often experience food safety challenges affecting fresh fruits and vegetables as well as animal-source proteins (see Chapter 7).[27] Ultra-processed foods have filled the demand niche for more convenient, safer foods, but with negative effects on morbidity and mortality. City government responses to address these challenges and promote a shift toward healthier consumption patterns vary considerably across the global South and, like national responses, are contingent on subnational capacity constraints, including policy autonomy in the health and agriculture domains and revenue-raising powers. Integrating the voices of city leaders into national nutrition and health policy discussions is critical to ensure that appropriately targeted interventions are identified across diverse urban locales. One approach for doing so is the Partnership for Healthy Cities, through which mayors from 73 cities across the globe have committed to supporting at least 1 of 14 possible policy options to prevent NCDs and enhance safety.[28] If cities are poised to be important partners in tackling the unique nutrition issues caused by urbanization, it will be important to identify subnational sources of financing, including municipal investment funds and municipal bonds.

FIGURE 1 Average implementation of 19 WHO-recommended NCD policies by level of state capacity, 2020

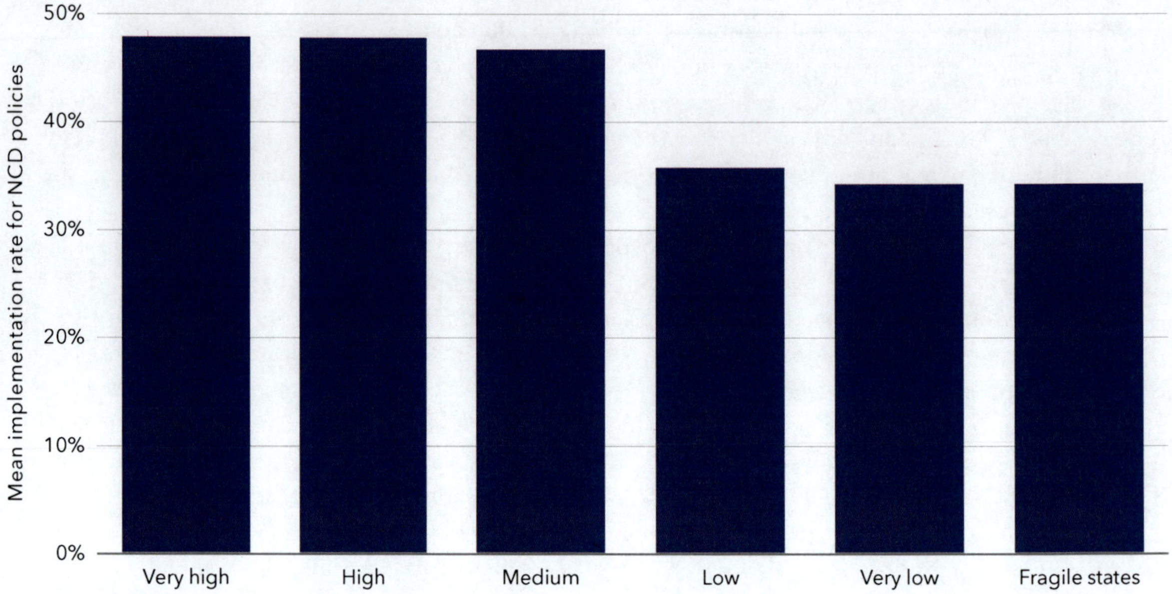

Source: Data on noncommunicable disease (NCD) policy implementation is from L.N. Allen, S. Wigley, and H. Holmer, "Assessing the Association between Corporate Financial Influence and Implementation of Policies to Tackle Commercial Determinants of Non-Communicable Diseases: A Cross-Sectional Analysis of 172 Countries," *Social Science & Medicine* 297 (2022): 114825. Fragile states classification is from The Fund for Peace's Fragile States Index (https://fragilestatesindex.org), and capacity is measured from the World Bank's Data Bank (https://databank.worldbank.org/).

Note: The NCD policy implementation measure captures 19 policies. Capacity is measured using the World Bank's government effectiveness index, which refers to "perceptions of the quality of public services, the quality of the civil service and the degree of its independence from political pressures, the quality of policy formulation and implementation, and the credibility of the government's commitment to such policies." Capacity-level classifications are based on five equal cut-offs along the metric's range of values, which span −2.5 to 2.5. "Most fragile states" are those ranked 90 to 100 on the Fragile States Index.

NAVIGATING CORPORATE INFLUENCE IN THE FOOD SYSTEM

State capacity and political incentives not only affect the degree of successful policy implementation but also shape the nature of engagement between food companies and governments. In settings of weak capacity, as well as those where political elites have close ties to the business community, "Big Food" – the term given to multinational companies producing ultra-processed foods and beverages – is likely to have more leverage. Indeed, corporate influence throughout the food system and particularly in the ultra-processed food sector is well documented.[29] One study identified six strategies used by the food industry to promote its influence, including shaping the narrative, providing financial incentives to politicians, building constituencies with credible professionals and community leaders, threatening legal actions, engaging in policy substitution (that is, proposing self-regulation or voluntary initiatives), and fragmenting or destabilizing industry opponents.[30] Other studies have developed frameworks related to how food industry actors shape preferences and alter the political, knowledge, legal, and extralegal environments to their benefit.[31] In some cases, the influence of business has undermined the policy interventions discussed earlier, such as, for instance, the reduction of taxes on SSBs in Ecuador in 2023, which were originally implemented only in 2016.[32]

At the same time, not all corporate actors are behemoth ultra-processed food industries. Many possess multiple motivations beyond profit, and some have led the way in reducing malnutrition where weak state capacity to act is otherwise a major hindrance (see Box 1 on Madagascar). Moreover, improving diets and nutrition through the food system inevitably requires partnerships among governments, researchers, and corporate actors to stimulate innovations in producing, processing, and distributing healthy foods.

BOX 1 PRIVATE SECTOR PUSH FOR VOLUNTARY FORTIFICATION STANDARDS IN MADAGASCAR

Madagascar has among the highest malnutrition rates in the world, with child stunting prevalence averaging 39.8 percent nationally and more than 45 percent in almost half of the country's 22 regions. A drought in 2021 in the southern part of the country caused almost 2 million people to be declared vulnerable to famine conditions. At the same time, the government is plagued by frequent political volatility, including a crisis from 2009 to 2014 precipitated by a military coup, and weak state capacity. In fact, based on 2022 data from the World Bank's government effectiveness index, the country's percentile rank is 14.6 percent out of a possible 100.

Within this context, private sector and civil society actors have filled an important void. A large-scale food manufacturer, TAF foods, partnered with a civil society association, known as GRET, and the University of Antananarivo to produce a fortified infant flour for children from 6 to 24 months of age. Called Koba Aina ("flour of life"), it is distributed through Nutri'zaza, a social enterprise. The flour is sold at an affordable price of about 400 Malagasy ariary per bag (US$0.09) and targeted at low-income urban neighborhoods through Nutri'zaza's system of Hotelin-jazely ("restaurants for babies"). Nutri'zaza's sales agents are exclusively women who share best practices with customers about infant and child feeding and monitor babies' growth at no charge to families. In 2019, Nutri'zaza, GRET, and TAF pushed for Madagascar's first voluntary standard for infant flour, leading to the development of Madagascar's own fortified foods logo. One indirect benefit of this initiative is that it strengthened capacity within the Madagascar Standards Agency, which previously lacked any experience with creating a voluntary fortification standard.

Source: Scaling Up Nutrition (SUN), "The Case of Madagascar: Scaling Up Nutrition Movement In-Depth Country Studies" (Geneva: 2019); Institut National de la Statistique and DHS Program, ICF, "Enquête Démographique et de Santé à Madagascar" (Antananarivo and Rockville, Maryland: 2022); World Bank, "The Urgency of Reforms: Structural Transformation and Better Governance at the Heart of the Strategy to Reduce Poverty," Systematic Country Diagnostic Update for Madagascar (Washington, DC: 2022).

Indeed, investments in R&D and risk-taking by private sector actors have been critical to, for instance, discovering plant- and insect-based alternative proteins that may address nutritional, animal welfare, and environmental concerns simultaneously.[33] Similarly, private sector investments in e-commerce and logistics – catapulted by the COVID-19 pandemic – have increased access to fresh foods for a broader range of consumers in many LMICs who previously were limited by options in their immediate physical neighborhoods.[34] E-commerce in food retail, for instance, grew by more than 100 percent in Brazil, Indonesia, and South Africa in 2020 (see Chapter 5).[35]

The fact remains, though, that the food industry holds tremendous power over consumer food choices, with limited public awareness of its intentions and modalities of influence. Several tools to promote transparency and accountability are emerging. From industry itself, there are initiatives like the Zero Hunger Pledge, whereby 43 companies have publicly declared their financial pledges and progress toward meeting Sustainable Development Goal 2 on eradicating hunger and promoting nutrition.[36] In large-scale food fortification, there have been tools such as the micronutrition fortification index in Nigeria, whereby companies annually publicize their efforts toward meeting national fortification mandates based on a standardized template and receive recognition through a prize ceremony intended to create positive peer pressure.[37] At the global level, the nongovernmental organization Feed the Truth developed the Food and Agriculture Corporate Transparency (FACT) index, which tracks how major multinational food companies engage in four activities: corporate spending to affect electoral outcomes; lobbying to influence decisions of officials, legislators, or regulatory agencies; spending to influence scientific studies and institutions; and donating to charitable organizations to gain favor from potential critics. Companies that are engaging in these activities and publicly disclosing them receive better scores on the index because they are at least demonstrating a commitment to transparency.[38]

One finding from the FACT is that the same company may have differing levels of accountability in different countries. As such, there is also potential to use alternative tools, such as the Corporate Financial Influence Index (CFII),[39] to examine the degree to which corporations can use their financial leverage to influence policymaking given a country's legal and institutional setting. Importantly, the CFII tends to be worse in countries with more autocratic systems, suggesting that political regime type may have important associations with transparency over business practices.[40]

FOSTERING CITIZEN AGENCY IN DECISIONS ABOUT HEALTHY FOODS

While the private and government sectors are key for shaping diets and nutrition policies, citizens play a critical role as well. In recent years, citizen agency has been recognized as a pivotal dimension of food security, along with access, availability, utilization, stability, and sustainability.[41] *Agency* refers to the ability of different groups and individuals to exert some autonomy over food policy decisions, such as by having equal opportunity to exercise their voice in decision-making structures.

The concept of agency underpins several transnational movements that have emerged in recent years that aim to make food systems more equitable. For instance, the *food sovereignty* movement, which gained ground in the 1990s and then reemerged during the 2007–2009 food price and land grab crises, promotes local control over markets, food cultures, resources, and modalities of production.[42] Reforms to the FAO's Committee on World Food Security in 2009 were partially driven by the importance of incorporating the views of food sovereignty activists into its dialogues and as a means of accountability to civil society through the creation of the Civil Society and Indigenous Peoples' Mechanism, which facilitates direct engagement of these groups with UN agencies and governments. The People's Summit, held in parallel to the UN Food Systems Summit in 2021, was largely driven by those supporting food sovereignty principles.[43]

The *right to food* is often subsumed within the food sovereignty movement but is conceptually distinct. While food sovereignty relies on listening to and respecting "voices from below," the right to food requires action from above, namely the state. Moreover, the right to food draws on a human right recognized in the International Covenant on Economic, Social and Cultural Rights (ICESCR). Within the ICESCR, the right to adequate food is achieved "when every man, woman and child, alone or in community with others, has physical and economic access at all times to adequate food or means of procurement."[44] Upholding the right relies on states fulfilling their obligations, including adopting legislative and financial measures to ensure people are protected from hunger and avoiding discrimination in food allocation, including food aid from international actors. Rights approaches signify an important departure in state-citizen relations because they empower citizens to demand social welfare and service provision by mobilizing universal rights recognitions rather than through the programmatic appeals of political parties or via employers.[45] Twenty-nine countries, including LMICs, have explicit constitutional provisions, while another 16 have implicit provisions for the right to food.[46]

Because of their expansive goals, neither movement necessarily prioritizes diets or nutrition; rather, they emphasize adequate food intake and food that respects and reflects local customs, which can sometimes be mobilized to assert individual rights to consume even unhealthy foods.[47] Moreover, obligating a state to uphold the right to food again requires a capable state, citizen awareness of this right (where it exists), and public knowledge about how to access the legal system to compel the state to act – all of which are likely to be most lacking in lower-income countries.

Notwithstanding these challenges, the principles of these movements – people-centered development, rights, and sovereignty – are often embedded to different degrees within hybrid forms of citizen-led or citizen-supported governance structures. Some of these initiatives to support diets and nutrition emerge organically from homegrown enterprises. For instance, in Peru, Lima's food policy roundtables emerged from community soup kitchens that expanded to help the poor during the COVID-19 pandemic.[48] Others include multistakeholder food platforms that typically bring together civil society with the private sector and local and national governments to develop a vision for the food system, draft and monitor policies, and help oversee intersectoral cooperation.[49] In contexts of weak state capacity, such platforms can enhance the agency of those directly involved in the food system.[50] Still another approach is to embed such platforms within transnational city networks that revolve around high-level initiatives, such as the Milan Urban Food Policy Pact, the C40 Cities initiative, and the CityFood Initiative.[51] Box 2 discusses citizen-led efforts that span these different structures across several Bolivian cities, where they were intended to enhance access to healthy diets in ways that help strengthen local communities.

Although there are some important instances of civil society participation on food safety in more authoritarian settings,[52] the potential for citizen-led engagement in food systems to succeed typically depends on the existence of freedom of expression and association. These have become more constrained globally over the last decade of democratic backsliding, which has coincided with growing restrictions on civil

BOX 2 BOLIVIA'S CITIZEN-LED FOOD SYSTEMS TRANSFORMATION

Bolivia, like many other countries, is currently experiencing a rapid urbanization process that has significant impacts on food systems, diets, food security, and the environment. Despite these challenges, the government has often upheld conventional business practices and investments; in many cases, it does so at the expense of reaching sustainability objectives.

Consequently, citizens and local stakeholders have taken the lead in orchestrating local initiatives to drive strengthened food systems governance, while also promoting the adoption of healthy and sustainable diets. These initiatives encompass a wide spectrum of activities ranging from policy advocacy and food systems research to the expansion of urban agriculture initiatives, the promotion of local food supply chains, the development of agrotourism, and the establishment of the country's first food banks, among others. While these endeavors differ in scale, the sum of these efforts is fueling a thriving food movement committed to ensuring the country's constitutional right to food.

The La Paz Food Security Committee (CMSA-LPZ), established in 2013, has gained national and international recognition for its citizen-led food systems advocacy work. This committee has been instrumental in drafting and instigating the adoption of municipal food security legislation; promoting the integration of food systems approaches into metropolitan development and planning documents; and ensuring the inclusion of food security and food systems in Bolivia's newly developed Urban Agenda. With more than 40 active member organizations, CMSA-LPZ is a diverse and multidisciplinary platform, spearheaded and facilitated by the local organization Fundación Alternativas and supported by various international agencies. Its members include representatives from market vendor associations, food entrepreneurs, municipal and departmental authorities, NGOs, academia, local universities, the private sector, and environmental and food activists, among others.

In addition to the policy and advocacy efforts of CMSA-LPZ, other local initiatives are contributing significantly to the creation of local supply chains, the reduction of food waste, the revalorization of local culinary heritage, and awareness building around healthier dietary practices. Notably, in La Paz, EcoTambo has emerged as a community-supported organic farmers market, offering both in-person and online purchasing options. This initiative not only stimulates citizen engagement in supporting local agroecological family farmers, but also introduced a traceability system that enables consumers to learn about the origins of their food and the individuals behind its production. Initially launched by the local nonprofit organization Semilla EcoSocial, EcoTambo has evolved into a self-governing entity led by its female farmer members.

Similarly, in 2017, a group of university students pioneered the country's first food bank, Banco de Alimentos de Bolivia, in Cochabamba, one of the country's three major metropolitan areas. This initiative follows global best practices by rescuing surplus food from various sources, including farming associations and supermarkets, which would otherwise go to waste. The rescued food benefits more than 15,000 people. Meanwhile, in Sucre, Bolivia's capital, Manq'a is a culinary school and restaurant that embraces a farm-to-table approach in collaboration with local farmers. The core interest of this initiative lies in preserving the nation's culinary heritage and fostering a new generation of food entrepreneurs. Their work has already inspired replicas in other countries in Central and South America. Initially supported by ICCO Cooperation, Manq'a has since become an independent local organization.

These collective efforts, from small-scale grassroots projects to metropolitan-area-wide initiatives, underscore the power of community-driven change and the capacity of individuals to influence policy, challenge conventional practices, and reinvigorate culinary heritages.

society groups that disproportionately advocate for rights, including rights to food.[53] Moreover, multistakeholder efforts can be vulnerable to shifts in government administrations with different partisan ideologies. Indeed, in several cases, multistakeholder food system strategies and food policy councils in urban locales have seen their momentum curtailed as a result of political turnover in leadership.[54] More generally, multistakeholder platforms have sometimes been accused of power asymmetries in composition or interest articulation, potentially translating into inequalities within the food system,[55] which suggests the need for built-in and frequent mechanisms of self-reflection among members.

RECOMMENDATIONS

Numerous policy levers exist to enhance access to affordable, healthy, and diverse diets, but the enabling governance conditions for adopting and implementing these – across public, private, and civil society stakeholders as well as between national and subnational scales – vary significantly. Indeed, policy choices are much more limited in contexts of constrained state capacity and much more contested where powerful actors lack material or ideological incentives to implement them. Consequently, there are several recommendations for providing a more holistic approach to diet and nutrition interventions.

First, economic analyses of the impacts of fiscal, transfer, regulatory, or investment policies on diet outcomes should be complemented by governance assessments to ensure such interventions are sustainable and scalable from a capacity and political economy perspective. Simple options that result in second-best outcomes for nutrition might be first-best from the viewpoint of feasible implementation. Second, to expand the set of first-best feasible policy options, binding governance constraints need to be identified and tackled. For instance, by uncovering whether insufficient financing, opaque data, corruption among frontline service providers, or demoralization in the bureaucracy are the main hindrance to policy uptake, necessary governance reforms and financial resource mobilization strategies can be identified to build a comprehensive action agenda for diets and nutrition. Third, improved and equitable access to information is a fundamental enabler for improved food systems governance overall.[56] To build accountability to citizens over time, there are opportunities for developing online transparency tools, such as keeping scorecards of the corporate food industry's political influence; monitoring government commitments to nutrition goals; and tracking budgets of nutrition-policy investments.[57] Fourth, grassroots movements are playing a key role in reshaping food landscapes from below and demonstrating the transformative potential of an engaged citizenry. These movements are most likely to flourish when sufficient civic space and committed political leadership also exist. Their growth and embodiment in multistakeholder platforms and food policy councils provide a unique natural experiment to identify when, why, and how they lead to improved nutrition policy decisions, thereby providing the basis for more cumulative learning about these increasingly popular modalities.

These and other potential interventions could ensure that diet and nutrition policies are not only properly targeted to the specific needs of different population groups but also appropriately calibrated to the underlying governance environment.

"State capacity and political incentives not only affect the degree of successful policy implementation but also the nature of engagement between food companies and governments."

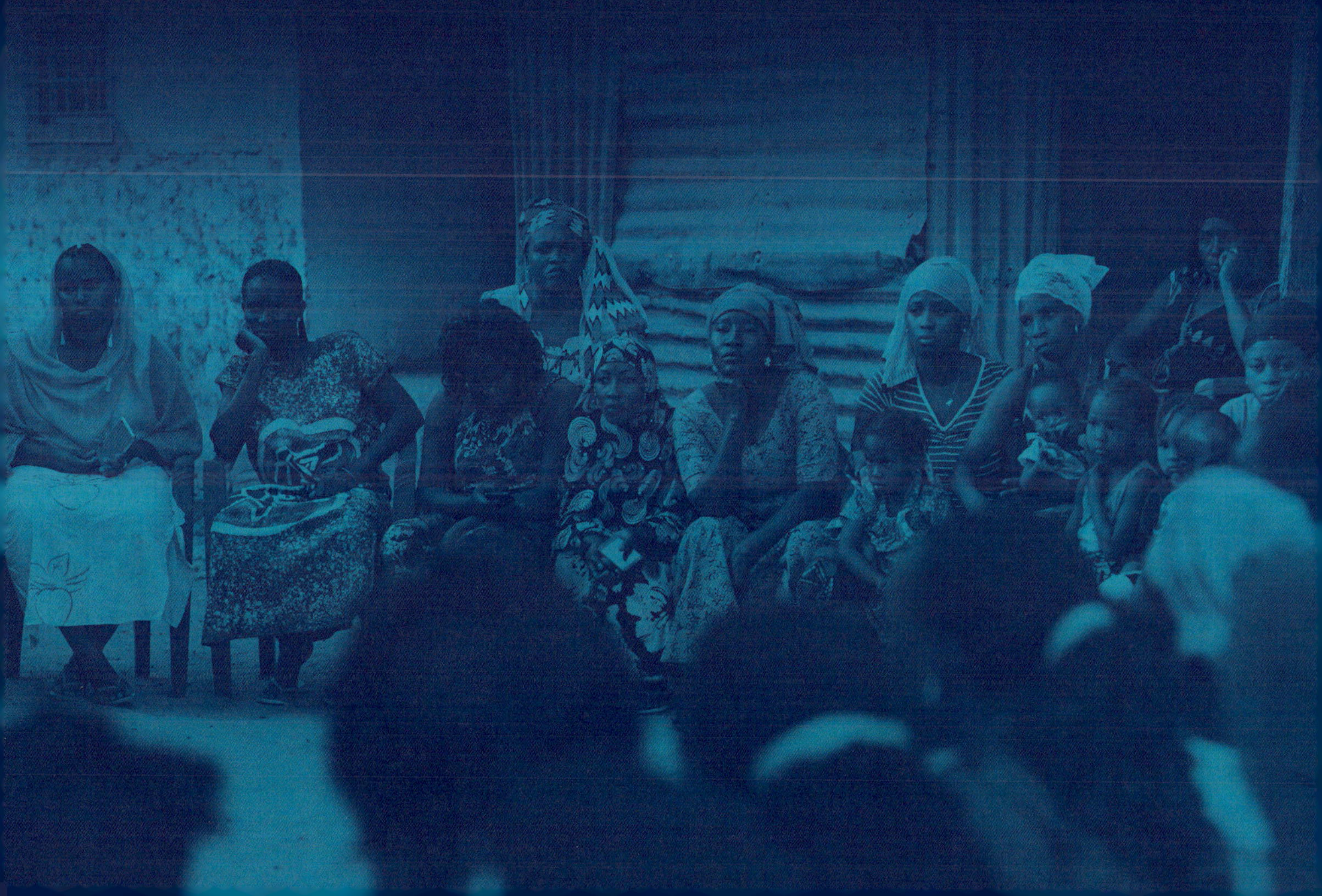

REGIONAL DEVELOPMENTS

MALNUTRITION AND UNHEALTHY DIETS ARE A GLOBAL PROBLEM, BUT THE challenges, responses, and potential solutions vary across low- and middle-income regions. Recent shocks have compounded long-term problems of undernutrition, and demographic, socioeconomic, and marketing trends are making obesity increasingly common. This section examines the evolving problem of malnutrition as well as policy interventions designed to make healthier, more diverse diets more affordable, accessible, and desirable, including these topics:

- Increasing production of fruits, vegetables, and animal-source foods in Africa to address micronutrient deficiencies.
- Boosting resilience of food systems to frequent shocks in the Middle East and North Africa.
- Increasing nutrition knowledge in Central Asia to address the double burden of malnutrition.
- Making healthy foods more affordable through fiscal reforms in South Asia.
- Managing the nutrition transition in the rapidly urbanizing context of East and South East Asia.
- Promoting intraregional trade in Latin America and the Caribbean to increase availability of diverse healthy foods.

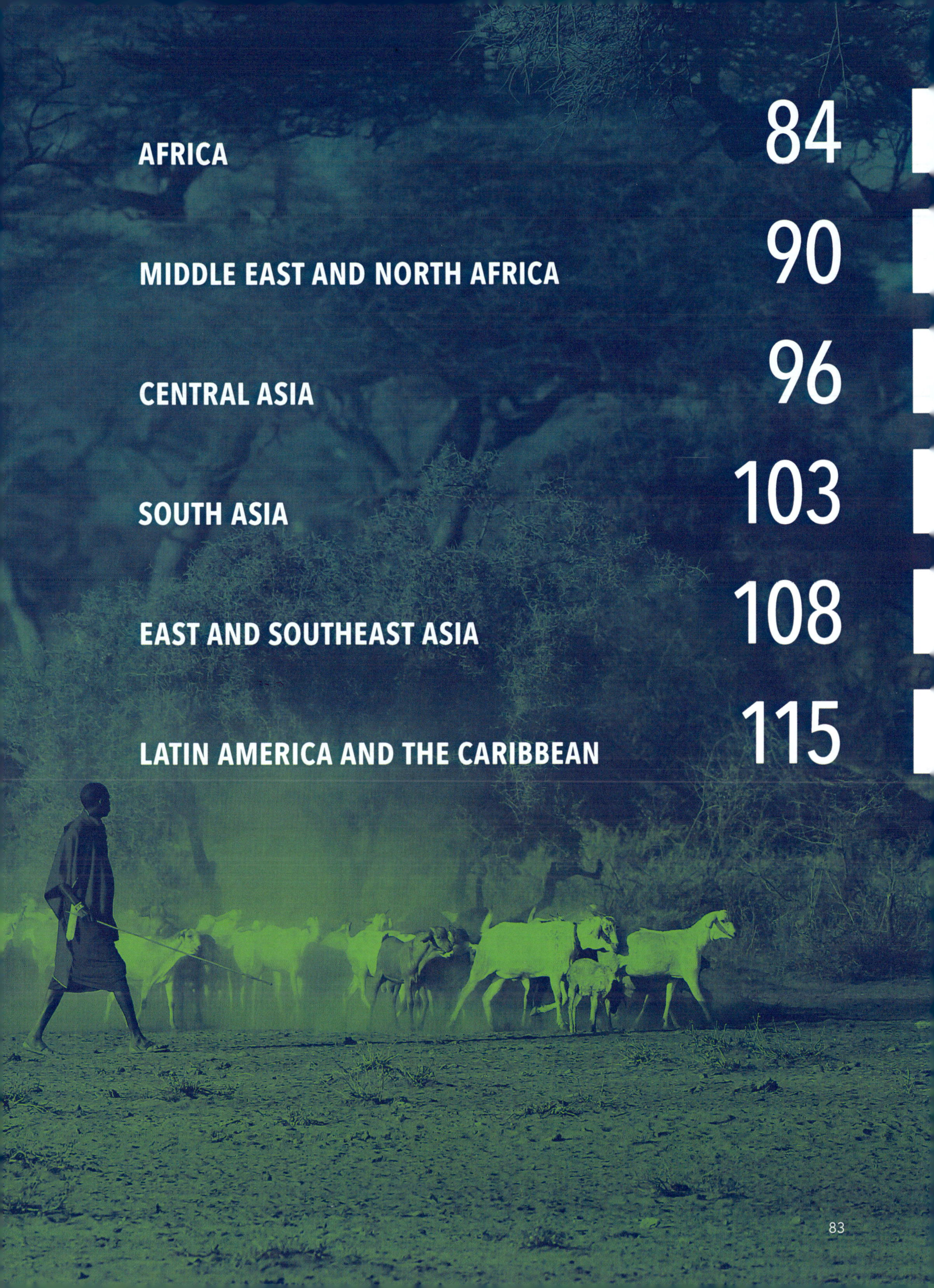

AFRICA

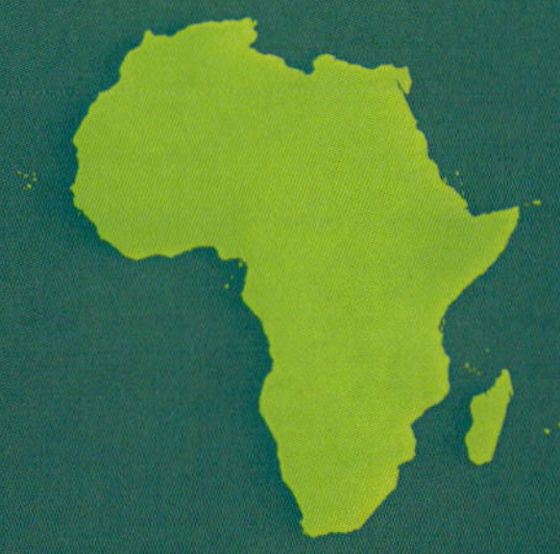

ELODIE BECQUEY, SAMUEL BENIN, WIM MARIVOET, AND AULO GELLI

Elodie Becquey is a senior research fellow, Nutrition, Diets, and Health Unit, International Food Policy Research Institute (IFPRI). **Samuel Benin** is the acting director for Africa, Development Strategies and Governance Unit, IFPRI. **Wim Marivoet** is a research fellow, Development Strategies and Governance Unit, IFPRI. **Aulo Gelli** is a senior research fellow, Poverty, Gender, and Inclusion Unit, IFPRI.

African food systems are dominated by cereals production, leaving them unable to supply sufficient nutrient-dense foods, such as animal-source foods, pulses, nuts and seeds, vegetables, fruits, and fats and oils.[1] The resulting high cost of nutrient-dense foods puts healthy diets out of reach for most Africans (Figure 1, panel A). A fifth of the region's population is undernourished,[2] and for many more, dietary diversity is inadequate (Figure 1, panels B and C), particularly in western and central Africa, where dietary diversity in young children is the lowest in the world.[3] Poorly diversified diets, together with poor health and sanitation conditions, increase the risk of maternal and child undernutrition and of various micronutrient deficiencies across population groups, which in turn heighten the risk of illness, disability, and death.[4] Poor nutrition has not only a high human cost but also a high economic cost. A study in 21 African countries estimates that about US$30.4 billion is lost in one year due to lower labor productivity and higher healthcare and education costs attributable to child wasting and stunting.[5] Overall, Africa faces a high burden of undernutrition, with prevalence of vitamin A and iodine deficiencies and of inadequacy of iron intakes among the highest in the world,[6] and with maternal anemia (39 percent) and child stunting (30 percent) well above global averages (30 and 22 percent, respectively).[7] Though child wasting (5.8 percent) gradually decreased in recent decades, child overweight (4.9 percent) and adult obesity (13 percent) gradually increased, reaching average levels on par with those observed globally. However, these averages hide important cross-regional and urban/rural disparities, with northern and southern Africa generally performing better in terms of undernutrition and worse on child overweight or adult obesity, compared with poorer regions in Africa.

The changing and diverse diet and nutrition conditions in Africa call for context-specific and evidence-based strategies to increase the supply, affordability, and consumption of healthy foods overall, and of nutrient-dense foods for the most vulnerable, while curbing the rising consumption of unhealthy foods. Integration of effective strategies into policy is key to their sustainable implementation at scale.

SUBNATIONAL GAPS IN NUTRITIOUS FOODS

Intake of adequate nutrients to meet recommended levels varies regionally within countries, depending on total food production, marketing, and consumption. Spatial nutrient adequacy profiles were derived for Burkina Faso, Ghana, Kenya, Rwanda, and Uganda, looking at six globally scarce micronutrients (calcium, folate, iron, vitamin A, vitamin B12, and zinc). The profiles show that both the nature and underlying causes of micronutrient gaps in household consumption vary widely between and within these countries.[8] In general, intake gaps for calcium, iron, vitamin B12, and zinc are greater than those for folate and vitamin

FIGURE 1 Affordability and diversity of women and young children's diets, by country and region

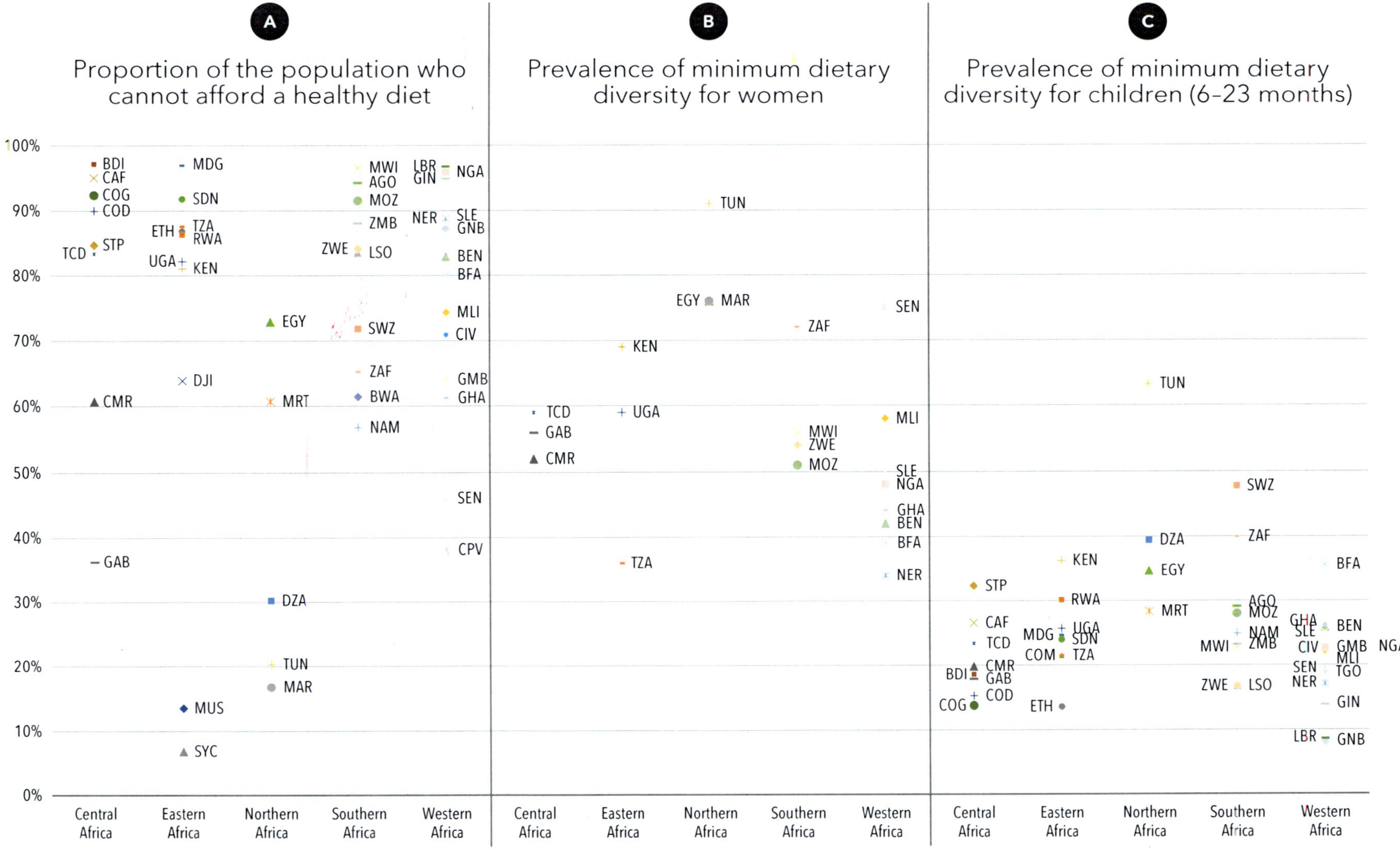

Source: Based on data from the *Food Systems Dashboard*, accessed December 2023. www.foodsystemsdashboard.org

Note: Central Africa: BDI = Burundi, CMR = Cameroon, CAF = Central African Republic, TCD = Chad, COG = Congo, COD = Democratic Republic of the Congo, GNQ = Equatorial Guinea, GAB = Gabon, STP = Sao Tome and Principe; Eastern Africa: COM = Comoros, DJI = Djibouti, ERI = Eritrea, ETH = Ethiopia, KEN = Kenya, MDG = Madagascar, MUS = Mauritius, RWA = Rwanda, SYC = Seychelles, SOM = Somalia, SSD = South Sudan, SDN = Sudan, UGA = Uganda, TZA = United Republic of Tanzania; Northern Africa: DZA = Algeria, EGY = Egypt, LBY = Libya, MRT = Mauritania, MAR = Morocco, TUN = Tunisia; Southern Africa: AGO = Angola, BWA = Botswana, SWZ = Eswatini, LSO = Lesotho, MWI = Malawi, MOZ = Mozambique, NAM = Namibia, ZAF = South Africa, ZMB = Zambia, ZWE = Zimbabwe; Western Africa: BEN = Benin, BFA = Burkina Faso, CPV = Cabo Verde, CIV = Côte d'Ivoire, GMB = Gambia, GHA = Ghana, GIN = Guinea, GNB = Guinea-Bissau, LBR = Liberia, MLI = Mali, NER = Niger, NGA = Nigeria, SEN = Senegal, SLE = Sierra Leone, TGO = Togo.

A, with the more serious gaps in calcium, iron, vitamin B12, and zinc often due to low domestic production of foods rich in those micronutrients. Nutrient losses observed between domestic production and markets, which may relate to postharvest losses or food trade, appear most critical in Burkina Faso and Ghana, and mainly affect foods rich in calcium, iron, and zinc. Limited demand is another cause of micronutrient inadequacy, particularly the limited consumption of foods rich in folate (in Burkina Faso, Kenya, and Uganda), vitamin A (in Ghana, Kenya, and Rwanda), and vitamin B12 (in Ghana, Kenya, and Uganda). The limited demand for folate-rich and vitamin A-rich foods is likely rooted in a lack of nutrition knowledge, while low demand for foods rich in vitamin B12 likely reflects the fact that animal-source foods are unaffordable for many households.

Despite these general observations, and given the diverse pattern of nutrient inadequacies within countries, food and nutrition security policies should devote more attention to addressing the context-specific drivers of poor diets through interventions that increase production, facilitate trade, and increase affordability and awareness of nutritious foods.[9]

LESSONS FROM SUCCESSFUL PROGRAMS

Strategies and programs that address gaps in the production, marketing, and consumption of diversified healthy foods have potential to improve nutrition outcomes.

NUTRITION-SENSITIVE AGRICULTURE PROGRAMS. Generally, nutrition-sensitive agriculture programs (see Chapters 2 and 3) can improve maternal and child diet adequacy, health, and care practices in rural areas by increasing micronutrient-dense food production for consumption, agricultural income to support household expenditures on health and food, nutrition-related knowledge, and/or women's empowerment, as well as by strengthening local institutions.[10] Enhanced homestead food production (EHFP), implemented by Helen Keller International, is one example of a nutrition-sensitive agricultural model that has proved effective in Africa. Targeted to women, EHFP integrates inputs and training to help farmers produce a variety of local micronutrient-dense crops and raise small animals, while also providing counseling on child nutrition, health, and hygiene. Rigorous impact evaluations of EHFP in Burkina Faso show positive impacts on child dietary diversity, nutrition, and health, and on maternal nutrition and empowerment.[11] Implementation of EHFP across four African countries showed that such complex programs require careful design, flexible and sequenced implementation, and cross-sectoral integration and coordination (see Chapter 2).[12]

Programs that provide livestock as a productive asset in low- and middle-income countries are generally associated with higher consumption of animal-source foods and higher overall dietary diversity, with mixed effects on child growth.[13] Examples of such livestock transfer programs in Africa that improved dietary outcomes include Heifer International's Passing on the Gift program in Rwanda and Zambia,[14] through which beneficiaries receive either a dairy cow, two draft cattle, or eight goats, with the requirement that they "pass on" the same number of female offspring to new beneficiaries. In Ethiopia, successful livestock transfer programs include a transfer of two egg-laying chickens (recognized through a public ceremony as child owned)[15]; a poultry production package with inputs and 16 vaccinated, improved-breed chickens in lieu of the same value in cash to beneficiaries of Ethiopia's Productive Safety Net Programme[16]; or 25 improved-breed chicks, with or without accompanying nutrition counseling.[17]

NUTRITION-SENSITIVE SOCIAL PROTECTION PROGRAMS. Nutrition-sensitive social protection programs (SPPs) involve transfers of cash, food, or vouchers; can be conditional or unconditional; and are generally designed to support access to food for the most vulnerable.[18] These programs can potentially reduce malnutrition directly, for example by improving diet quality, or indirectly, by increasing household food security,[19] although their impacts on nutrition outcomes for women and children in low- and middle-income countries have been mixed.[20] For example, systematic reviews on the effects of cash transfers on maternal and child nutrition outcomes find consistent positive effects on dietary outcomes and less consistent evidence on micronutrient status and anthropometric outcomes that suggests effects are small or non-existent.[21] Globally and in Africa, expenditures on SPPs have grown rapidly. Countries in sub-Saharan Africa spend on average 1.5 percent of gross domestic product (GDP) on SPPs, close to the global average, though the African programs are largely donor funded.[22] Also, the level of spending on SPPs varies across the continent. African countries include some of the world's top spenders, notably Lesotho (7 percent of GDP) and South Sudan (10 percent), as well as many countries that spend very little.

School feeding programs are one common type of SPP (see Chapter 3). Considered the world's most extensive safety net in terms of the number of countries implementing them,[23] school feeding programs can improve nutrition outcomes for school children and their younger siblings, and they are particularly effective for the most vulnerable children.[24] These programs have the additional benefit of improving school enrollment, attendance, and learning.[25] For example, the Ghana School Feeding Program (GSFP), Ghana's largest assistance program, operates in 11,000 schools and serves 3.6 million children. A rigorous impact evaluation found that the GSFP improves children's nutrition status, as well as cognition and learning, with larger effects accruing in girls and in children from poorer households.[26] When foods are grown locally, school feeding programs have the potential to also improve food security of smallholder farmers, though the evidence on these benefits is limited.[27] However, these programs face challenges in supplying a sufficient amount of quality food in a timely way, as well as in accessing the infrastructure needed to prepare food hygienically.[28]

FOOD FORTIFICATION. Fortifying food with key micronutrients is another cost-efficient food-based strategy to improve diets and nutrition (see Chapter 6). In Africa, food fortification mainly relies on the release of biofortified crops and on the fortification of industrially processed foods. Microbial-based biofortification is an emerging strategy in the region; it relies on the production of micronutrients by microorganisms through traditional or optimized fermentation of local foods.[29]

Crops biofortified with vitamin A, including maize, cassava, and sweet potato, have been shown to improve vitamin A status among children and women in several African countries[30] in a highly cost-effective way (see Chapter 6).[31] To date, 284 biofortified crop varieties have been released in 20 African countries, mostly in eastern and southern Africa.[32] Testing is ongoing in 16 other African countries and includes new crops and nutrients such as Irish potato, lentil, rice, sorghum, and wheat, fortified with zinc and combined iron and zinc.[33] Challenges to scaling up biofortification in Africa include supply interruptions, lack of evidence on efficacy, and the unwillingness of farmers and consumers to grow and eat biofortified foods, in addition to difficulties coordinating among other key actors.[34] Because of Africa's great diversity of staple crops, compared with those of Asia or Latin America and the Caribbean, more biofortified crops and varieties within crops are needed to reach a wide population, thus increasing the relative cost and decreasing economies of scale for biofortification.

Industrial food fortification is also an effective strategy for tackling poor micronutrient status (see Chapter 6).[35] For example, a study conducted in urban Cameroon found that mandatory wheat flour fortification led to an improvement in iron, zinc, folate, and vitamin B12 levels among women and children.[36] A study in Abidjan, Côte d'Ivoire, found that fortified oil provided 37 percent of recommended vitamin A intake for women and 27 percent for children under age two.[37] In Africa, food fortification is expanding and is now mandatory in many cases: salt fortification is mandatory in 45 countries,[38] most often with iodine; wheat flour in 30 countries[39] and maize flour in 12 countries,[40] most often with iron and folate; and oil in 25 countries,[41] most often with vitamin A.[42] Successful scale-up of fortification generally relies on strong multisectoral action involving the food industry, research institutes, and the government for coordination, regulation, enforcement, and monitoring (see Chapter 8). In addition, regional authorities such as the Economic Community of West African States (ECOWAS) typically play a key role in ensuring program impact and scale-up through the establishment of fortification standards and regulation.[43]

FIGURE 2 Overview of key African Union milestones to improve food security and nutrition

1987

Establishment of the African Task Force on Food and Nutrition Development
Guides and supports the development of food, nutrition, and nutrition-sensitive policies and programs

2003

Maputo Declaration on Agriculture and Food Security in Africa and establishment of the Comprehensive Africa Agriculture Development Program (CAADP)

2005

African Regional Nutrition Strategy

2014

Malabo Declaration on Accelerated Agricultural Growth and Transformation for Shared Prosperity and Improved Livelihoods
Major focus on ending hunger in Africa by 2025

Mainstreaming of nutrition in the National Agriculture Investment Plans begins as part of CAADP and the Malabo Declaration

Proclamation of October 30th of each year as Africa's Day for Food and Nutrition Security
Takes stock, celebrates achievements, and charts the way forward

2015

Renewal of African Regional Nutrition Strategy

2018

Establishment of the African Leaders for Nutrition initiative
Catalyzes high-level political engagement to advance nutrition in Africa

2021

Africa Common Position Paper on Food Systems
Identifies 12 game-changing solutions critical for ensuring access to safe and nutritious food for all

2022

Declaration of 2022 as the Year of Nutrition for Africa

Declaration on scaling up food fortification and biofortification

Source: Based on African Union documents.

REGULATION AND TAXES. ECOWAS and partners have also led efforts to regulate complementary foods for infants and young children, including providing support to member countries to adapt and adopt international regulations and guidelines.[44] More broadly, regulations are used both to improve the availability and affordability of nutrient-dense foods in the food environment, and also increasingly to protect consumers from poor dietary habits that lead to obesity and related noncommunicable diseases, like hypertension and diabetes (see Chapter 5). For example, African national policies occasionally include bans on the sale of sugar-sweetened beverages, products high in saturated fats, and ultra-processed foods in the vicinity of schools, and likewise, mandatory or voluntary regulations on food labeling and marketing.[45] In South Africa, the Health Promotion Levy – a tax on sugar-sweetened beverages – has increased prices for carbonated drinks and corresponded to reductions of added-sugar intakes, especially among the largest consumers of these beverages.[46] This positive impact is consistent with global evidence that taxes and subsidies are generally effective at changing consumption of targeted items (see Chapter 5), although evidence of ultimate impact on health is lacking.[47]

FOSTERING A CONDUCIVE ENVIRONMENT

Incorporating successful programs into policy is key to their scale-up and sustainability. In recent decades, political commitment to food security and nutrition has grown at all levels across the continent, along with the coherence of multisectoral nutrition action.[48] For example, 42 of the 66 countries participating in the global Scaling Up Nutrition (SUN) movement are African countries.[49] The African Union has adopted numerous declarations, strategies, and programs to improve food security and nutrition (Figure 2).

Associated with these developments are the Continental Nutrition Accountability Scorecard (CNAS) and the Africa Agriculture Transformation Scorecard (AATS) led by the African Union, which aim to provide actionable information to African governments and stakeholders on country-level

BOX 1 NATIONAL NUTRITION POLICY ENVIRONMENTS: THE WEST AFRICAN CASE

A review of nutrition-relevant policies in West Africa found that, as of September 2020, all countries in the region had adopted a comprehensive or specific nutrition policy, strategy, or action plan. Most policies reported on mechanisms to coordinate nutrition across multiple sectors and bodies that support nutrition governance, and they are often placed in high-level and influential offices, such as the office of the president or the prime minister.

In the agriculture, economic, and social sectors, about half of the sectoral policy documents were oriented toward nutrition, meaning that they met the basic criteria of having a nutrition objective, indicator, or a budget for nutrition.

The situational analyses conducted for the policies generally described World Health Assembly nutrition targets, with under-five stunting and wasting most often covered. Macronutrient and energy deficiencies were rarely described as an issue, while micronutrient deficiencies were frequently cited (by order of importance: vitamin A, iodine, iron, zinc, folate, other B vitamins) and clearly linked to health consequences. Overweight and obesity was also described as a growing issue, although it was less well addressed with related activities and indicators than undernutrition.

Overall, the report points to several policies among those reviewed where more internal coherence is recommended to better align policy objectives, activities, and indicators with nutrition-relevant situational analyses. It also highlights the untapped potential of leveraging sectors that have known potential to contribute to better nutrition. For example, in the environment sector, only 5 of 45 documents were nutrition oriented.

Source: L. Casu, A.D. Diatta, I. Uzhova, M. Dramé, J. Kaboré, F. Touré, E. Becquey, and R. Verstraeten, *Nutrition-Relevant Policy in West Africa: A Comprehensive Review* (Dakar: TNWA; Washington, DC: IFPRI, 2022); L. Casu, I. Uzhova, A.D. Diatta, M. Dramé, and R. Verstraeten, *Guidance for Improving Nutrition-Relevant Policy in West Africa*, TNWA Evidence Note No. 25 (Dakar: IFPRI, 2021).

progress in achieving nutrition targets.[50] The CNAS shows that most countries have made progress in passing legislation on food fortification and breastfeeding and in developing multisectoral action plans on nutrition,[51] although gaps remain in mainstreaming nutrition into national policies (Box 1). However, most countries are not on track to achieve other CNAS or AATS targets, such as those focused on stunting and anemia or on access to key services such as water, sanitation, and agricultural extension.[52]

CONCLUSION

Addressing the high burden of micronutrient deficiencies and undernutrition in Africa will require leveraging local, national, regional, and continental food systems to increase the supply and reduce the cost of nutritious foods. In addition, this will require appropriately contextualizing evidence-based multisectoral policy and program approaches, including agriculture, health, nutrition, and social protection. The sustainability of these efforts also requires a focus on the food environments of growing urban areas and related dietary transitions, as well as on strengthening people's resilience and capacity to cope with global threats posed by climate change, conflicts, and other shocks that reduce access to and availability of the foods needed for a healthy diet.

MIDDLE EAST AND NORTH AFRICA

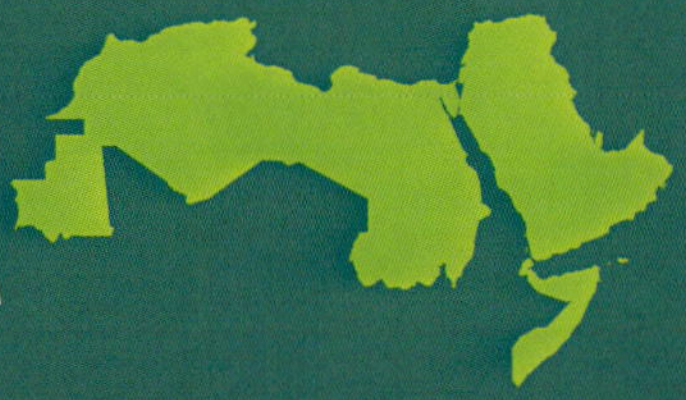

KIBROM A. ABAY, LINA ABDELFATTAH, SIKANDRA KURDI, AND MOHSEN SARHAN

Kibrom Abay is a senior research fellow and **Lina Abdelfattah** is a senior research associate, Development Strategies and Governance Unit, International Food Policy Research Institute (IFPRI). **Sikandra Kurdi** is a country program leader for Egypt and a research fellow, Development Strategies and Governance Unit, IFPRI. **Mohsen Sarhan** is the chief executive officer, Egyptian Food Bank.

Over the past several years, global and regional trade shocks have triggered rampant inflation and spikes in food and fuel prices in the Middle East and North Africa (MENA). These shocks have disrupted domestic food systems, affecting the accessibility and affordability of nutritious diets. The MENA region is always vulnerable to such shocks, but the trade shocks triggered by the Russia-Ukraine war came at a crucial juncture, as the region is experiencing a rise in the double burden of malnutrition, characterized by the concurrence of micronutrient deficiencies and undernutrition with overweight and obesity. Even before the Russia-Ukraine war, the cost of a healthy diet was increasing in the region. In 2020, more than half the population – about 162.7 million people – could not afford a healthy diet,[1] with a slightly higher share in low-income countries and those affected by conflict and political instability, and the number of people suffering undernutrition reached 59.8 million.[2] At the same time, the overweight/obesity rates in the Arab countries are among the highest in the world.

FIGURE 1 Food import dependency in the MENA region, kilocalories, 2017–2019 average

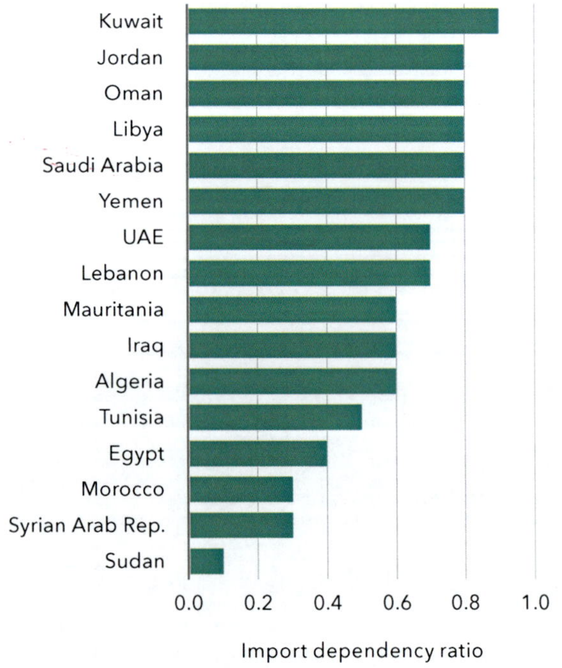

Source: Data from FAOSTAT, https://www.fao.org/faostat/

The MENA region's heavy dependence on food imports leaves it particularly vulnerable to world food prices and trade shocks.[3] Most of the region's countries are sizable net importers of food (Figure 1). This is especially true for Gulf Cooperation Council countries, including Oman, Qatar, Saudi Arabia, and Yemen, where more than 80 percent of domestically available calories are provided through imports. In addition, MENA countries rely heavily on food imports to supply essential nutrients. In countries such as Egypt, Jordan, Libya, and Yemen, the average domestic food supply does not meet the recommended daily intake for some nutrient categories. Because of these dependencies, the recent global trade shocks have created strong inflationary pressures across the region. For example, food inflation in Egypt tripled over this period, rising from about 20 percent immediately before the Russia-Ukraine war to 63 percent in March 2023.[4]

The MENA region is also marked by political instability, fragility, and persistent conflicts that contribute to large refugee populations, many hosted by countries within the region, and to food insecurity more broadly. The region's protracted humanitarian crises triggered by natural disasters (for example, the 2023 earthquake in Morocco) and political instability in neighboring countries (the ongoing civil war in Sudan) are forcing major population displacements. In 2022, more than two-thirds of the region's undernourished people were from conflict-affected countries.[5] Projections show that by 2024 the region will host 15.8 million forcibly displaced and stateless people.[6] The recent Israel-Gaza conflict, which started in October 2023, is adding further pressure to an already fragile situation. The conflict has created a major humanitarian crisis and increased the influx of refugees to neighboring countries. MENA is also among the world's regions most vulnerable to climate change and water scarcity.[7] The compound crises arising from conflict, climate change, and trade shocks pose a long-term threat to national food security in many MENA countries.

AFFORDABILITY OF NUTRITIOUS DIETS

Rising food prices threaten the affordability of nutritious diets, especially for poor households, throughout the MENA region. Recent estimates find that the number of poor in MENA has increased by more than 20 million since the outbreak of the Russia-Ukraine war and the associated surge in food prices.[8] The World Bank estimates that a 1 percent increase in the price of food items in the region is likely to push about half a million more people into poverty.[9]

The impact of food inflation varies across countries and households, depending on their exposure to food prices and trade shocks. Poor and net-consumer households are the most vulnerable to inflation, mainly because they allocate a larger share of their income to food purchases. In response, these households are likely to increase their already heavy reliance on cereals and cheaper energy-dense foods because the cost per calorie is lower.[10]

Immediately following the outbreak of the Russia-Ukraine war, IFPRI launched a phone survey of about 6,000 households in Egypt to assess how poor and near-poor households were responding to the economic stresses.[11] Households were asked about how their consumption habits had changed since the start of the war and the perceived drivers of these changes. A large share of households reported (1) a decrease in consumption of unsubsidized foods such as meat, chicken, and eggs, which are key protein sources, and (2) either a slight increase or no change in the consumption of subsidized foods, which are often calorie-dense staples. Some households reported increasing their consumption of less nutritious food groups to reduce food spending. For instance, households increased their consumption of starchy foods such as potatoes and pasta that, while filling, tend to have fewer nutrients. In response to questions about why they reduced their consumption of certain foods, more than two-thirds of households cited price increases as the main cause. Overall, these patterns suggest a shift from unsubsidized to subsidized products, highlighting the importance of Egypt's national food subsidy program (Figure 2).

The MENA region is very diverse, and although some oil-exporting countries (including Bahrain, Kuwait, Oman, Qatar, Saudi Arabia, and the United Arab Emirates) continue to benefit from the surge in oil prices, other countries are facing multiple shocks. Fragile and conflict-affected countries, such as Iraq and Yemen, witnessed deterioration in food security over the last couple of years (Figure 3). These countries continue to grapple with compounding effects of conflict and high food and fuel prices that ultimately increase food insecurity. For example, the share of households experiencing moderate or severe food insecurity in Yemen increased from about 53 percent in 2022 to 70 percent in 2023.

FISCAL POLICY RESPONSES TO SHOCKS

The recent inflationary and supply shocks have triggered important public policy responses in the MENA region. However, most of these responses add to existing fiscal pressures and have not been nutrition-sensitive, as they generally aim to ensure a minimum adequate level of calorie intake rather than diet quality. Most countries adopted and expanded conventional subsidies and price controls on calorie-dense staple foods rather than putting greater focus on supporting more diverse diets that would meet nutritional needs.

FIGURE 2 Consumption of subsidized and unsubsidized foods in Egypt, March–November 2022

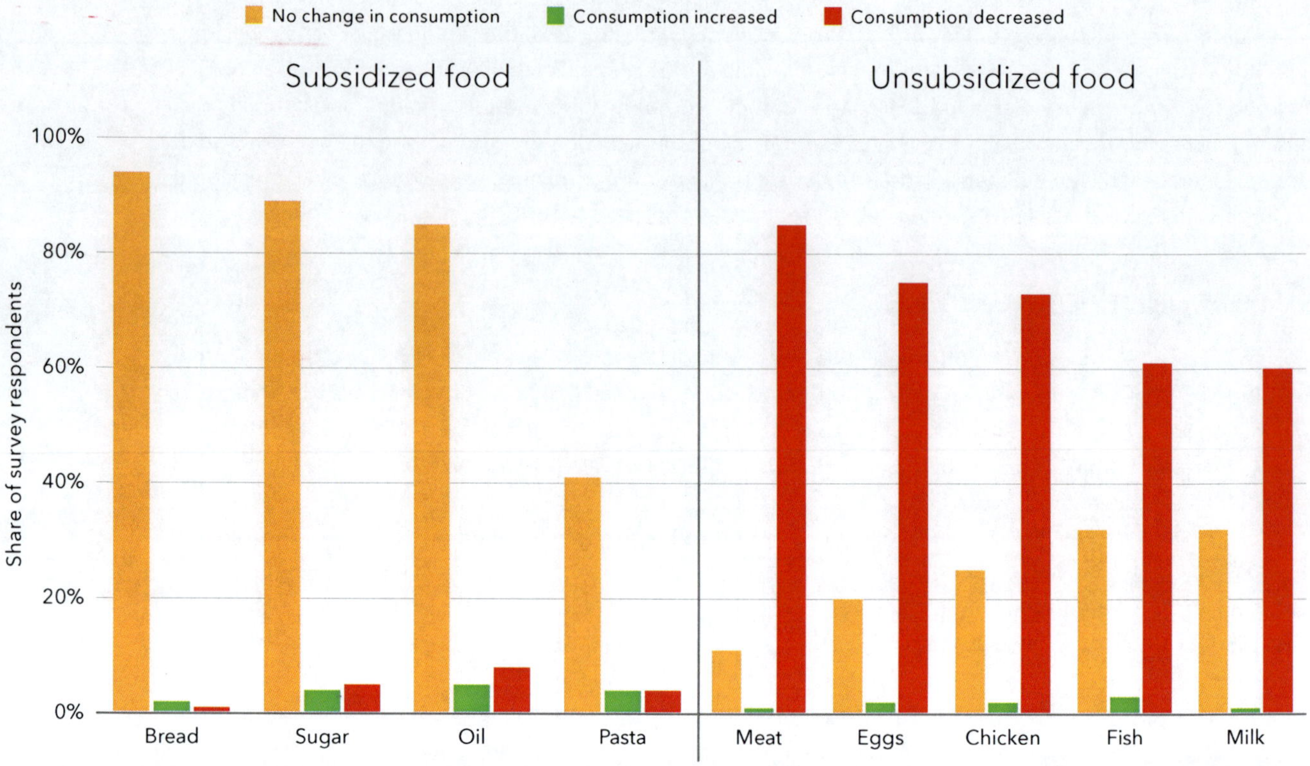

Source: Based on phone survey data reported in K.A. Abay, N. Karachiwalla, S. Kurdi, and Y. Salama, "Food Price Shocks and Diets among Poor Households in Egypt," *IFPRI Blog*, Dec. 29, 2022.

FIGURE 3 Share of households experiencing moderate or severe food insecurity

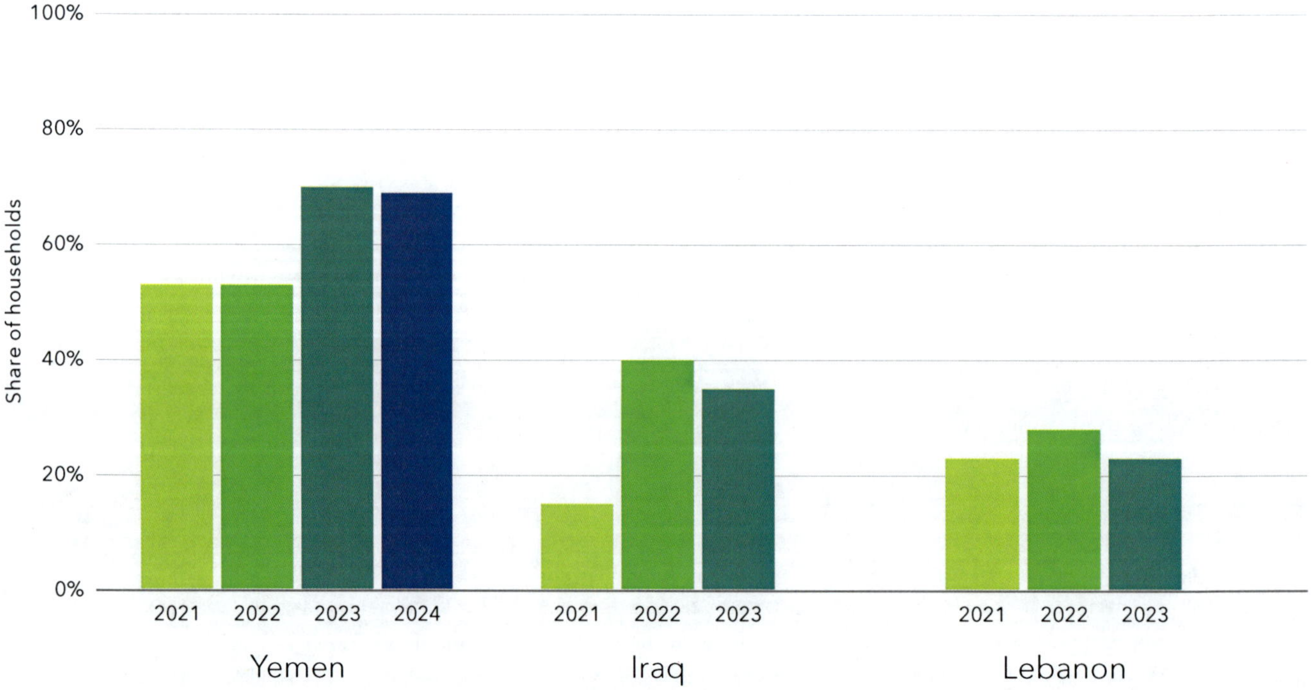

Source: Data from Data in Emergencies Hub (DIEM), FAO, accessed March 2024, https://data-in-emergencies.fao.org

Most MENA countries introduced a variety of fiscal policies to cushion the adverse impacts of these inflationary pressures.[12] These included increases in food and fuel subsidies, new price controls, incentives to boost domestic agricultural production, trade regulations, indirect tax exemptions, product-specific exchange rates, and the introduction or expansion of cash transfers and financial support for vulnerable households, including utility coverage. Some policies were introduced immediately after the outbreak of the Russia-Ukraine war, while others have been introduced more recently. While some fiscal measures have helped to contain inflation, the medium-term impact on households and diets remains to be evaluated.

INTERVENTIONS TO IMPROVE DIETS AND NUTRITION

Existing social protection programs and related public policy responses can play an important role in limiting the impacts of rising food prices on diet quality and nutrition in the MENA region.

FOOD SUBSIDY PROGRAMS – THE CASE OF EGYPT

TARGETING FOOD SUBSIDY PROGRAMS TO THOSE MOST IN NEED. Egypt's long-standing bread subsidy program, the Tamween ration card system, reaches about 70 percent of the country's households. Recent assessments find that the coverage of this subsidy program is not sufficiently progressive; only a third of its total costs in 2015 were directed to households in the lowest two quintiles. Modeling work shows that replacing this staple-heavy food subsidy with targeted cash transfers of roughly equivalent fiscal cost could improve the welfare of the poorest households.[13] Consistent with this, another recent impact evaluation shows the importance of targeting food subsidy programs to the most vulnerable, as those households not covered by Tamween reported disproportionally greater deterioration in diet diversity after the recent inflationary shock (Figure 4).[14] Among these nonbeneficiaries, ultra-poor households reported a reduction in dietary diversity of about one food group, compared with a 0.56 reduction reported by program beneficiaries.[15]

FIGURE 4 Impact of subsidies on dietary diversity in Egypt, 2022–2023

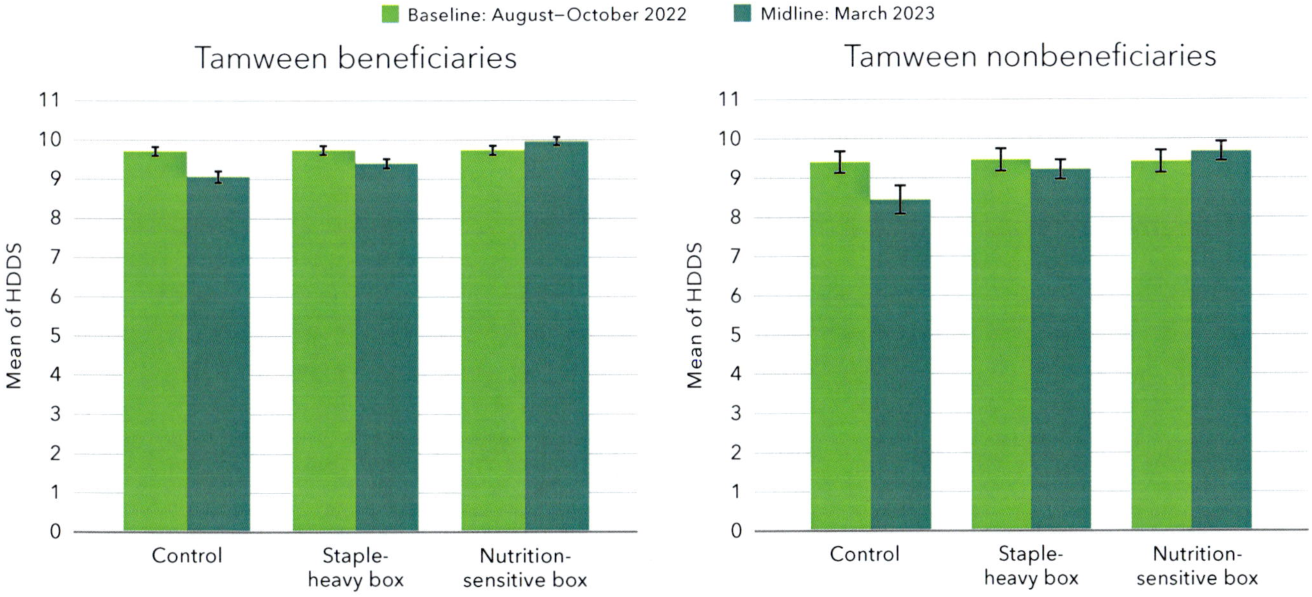

Source: K.A. Abay, L. Abdelfattah, M. Elkaramany, D. Elsabbagh, and S. Kurdi, "Nutrition-Sensitive Food Distribution amidst Inflationary Shock: Evidence from a Randomized Intervention in Egypt," IFPRI Discussion Paper 2218, IFPRI, Washington, DC, 2023.

Note: HDDS = household dietary diversity score (range of 0-12; higher score is more diversity). For a description of this scale, see www.fao.org/nutrition/assessment/tools/household-dietary-diversity/

In addition, Egypt's food subsidy programs in the last decade have not been sufficiently nutrition-sensitive and have tended to encourage overconsumption of calorie-dense staples. Studies show that households participating in Tamween, and hence consuming energy-dense subsidized food items, exhibit higher rates of obesity.[16]

NUTRITION-SENSITIVE FOOD DISTRIBUTION. In early 2023, amid a period of inflationary shocks in Egypt, IFPRI conducted an impact evaluation of a direct food distribution program introduced by the Egyptian Food Bank.[17] The program offered two modalities: a standard "staple-heavy" food box and a "nutrition-sensitive" food box. The nutrition-sensitive food box represents an attempt to address micronutrient deficiencies and poor diet quality[18] by including more diverse and nutrient-dense food items.

The nutrition-sensitive food box improved dietary diversity and food security[19] among ultra-poor households (Figure 5), and led to better outcomes in diet quality. Household dietary diversity increased by about 9 percent, and iron, protein, and energy intake increased by 19, 13, and 12 percent, respectively. In contrast, the staple-heavy food box did not significantly increase macro- or micronutrient intake. This evidence suggests that well-designed and nutrition-sensitive food transfers can effectively offset the adverse impacts of inflationary pressures on diet quality and food security.

SCHOOL FEEDING PROGRAMS

School feeding programs are gaining popularity in the MENA region (see Chapter 3). These programs not only deliver direct benefits for nutrition but also have potential to improve school participation; strengthen general diet quality by changing habits and improving food environments; promote gender equity; and improve learning and health outcomes.

School feeding programs generally take two forms in the region: humanitarian-type interventions, which rely on packaged, shelf-stable snacks, and more varied, complete programs, which offer sandwiches, fruits,

FIGURE 5 Impact of nutrition-sensitive food distribution on dietary diversity and food insecurity in Egypt

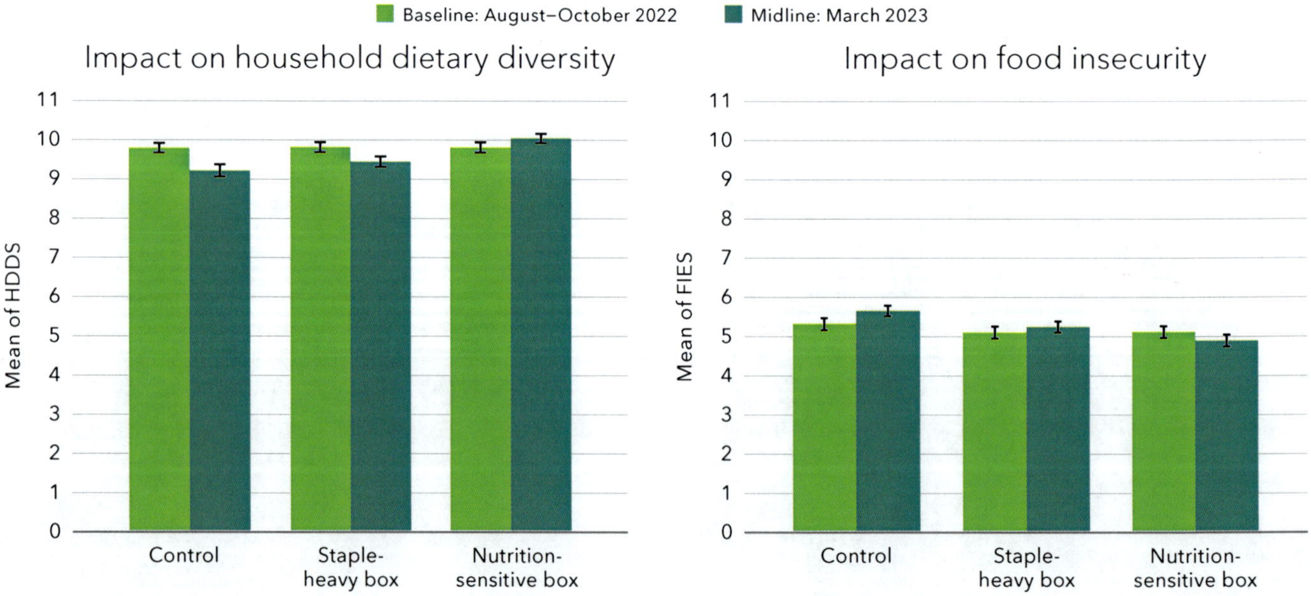

Source: K.A. Abay, L. Abdelfattah, M. Elkaramany, D. Elsabbagh, and S. Kurdi, "Nutrition-Sensitive Food Distribution amidst Inflationary Shock: Evidence from a Randomized Intervention in Egypt," IFPRI Discussion Paper 2218, IFPRI, Washington, DC, 2023.

Note: HDDS = household dietary diversity score (range of 0-12, higher score is more diversity); FIES = food insecurity experience (range of 0-8, higher score is more insecurity). For description of these scales, see www.fao.org/nutrition/assessment/tools/household-dietary-diversity/; and FAO, *FIES Basics: The Food Insecurity Experience Scale: Measuring Food Insecurity through People's Experiences* (Rome: 2014).

vegetables, and/or milk. Humanitarian school feeding has become increasingly common, especially in conflict-affected countries including Iraq, Syria, and Yemen. These programs are primarily implemented by governments in partnership with the World Food Programme and distribute high-energy biscuits or date bars, which are a cost-effective means of delivering nutritional benefits. In recent years, complete school feeding programs have been initiated in other countries, such as Jordan. These programs generally cost three to four times more per child per day than humanitarian interventions and have much higher operational costs. While relatively expensive, these programs offer more varied food options and are more likely to be preferred by students. They also generate greater benefits for the local economy, as food items are usually sourced locally and local women are employed in preparing and packaging the meals.

CONCLUSION

National policy responses to global food crises need to consider the region's double burden of malnutrition along with other vulnerabilities, including climate change, water scarcity, conflict, and rising public debt resulting from government spending. Countries in the MENA region need to reinforce their investments and efforts to increase the resilience of their food systems. To this end, countries should consider diversifying their food imports and exports while continuing to invest in social protection programs that protect poor and vulnerable households from food price hikes. Social protection needs to effectively target the most vulnerable groups, including women, who account for a large share of the poor. In addition, countries should consider reforming their food subsidies both to improve diets and reduce vulnerability to shocks. Investments in these subsidies, which have historically prioritized consumers over producers, need to be better integrated into national food systems. Rethinking consumer policies and encouraging the production of healthier and more sustainable diets are equally important.

Longer-term policies in the region should include strategies to mitigate vulnerability to trade shocks, climate change, and water scarcity. While some countries have the potential to increase domestic production, compounding crises arising from climate change and water scarcity could limit these ambitions. For example, in some countries, such as Egypt, adapting farming systems to become more resilient to water shortages and climate change should be the priority, rather than expanding production. The region's strong potential to develop wind and solar energy could facilitate a transition toward a greener future. Renewable energy expansion could reduce vulnerability to oil price shocks and climate change, while also generating additional revenues by diversifying exports. Most importantly, countries affected by prolonged conflict should focus on restoring livelihoods while also laying the groundwork for longer-term investment to support diversification and resilience to shocks.

Overall, the MENA region's food security challenges require a multifaceted policy approach that addresses immediate vulnerabilities to trade shocks and price fluctuations while also tackling long-term issues of climate change, water scarcity, and malnutrition. Strengthening social protection, diversifying food production and trade, and enhancing resource management and climate adaptation strategies are critical for building resilience against future crises.

CENTRAL ASIA

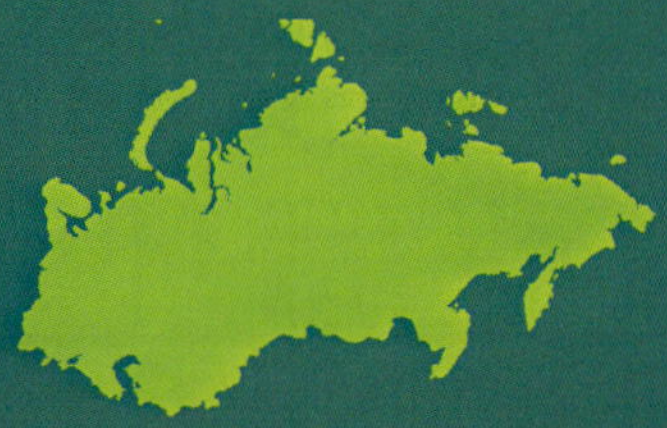

KAMILJON AKRAMOV, ISABEL LAMBRECHT, AND SARAH PECHTL

Kamiljon Akramov is a senior research fellow, **Isabel Lambrecht** is a research fellow, and **Sarah Pechtl** is a visiting fellow, Development Strategies and Governance Unit, International Food Policy Research Institute.

Food systems in Central Asian countries face serious challenges related to diet quality and nutrition, which are compounded by the growing effects of climate change, unstable commodity markets, and a heavy reliance on remittances and undiversified trade flows. In the 1990s, these countries experienced a significant drop in gross domestic product, as well as high levels of inflation, poverty, and food insecurity. Over the past two and a half decades, however, economic growth in the region has rebounded due to the transition from centrally planned to more market-oriented economies. Central Asia includes five countries in economic transition: Kazakhstan and Turkmenistan are now classified as upper-middle-income economies; and the Kyrgyz Republic, Tajikistan (recently a low-income country), and Uzbekistan are now lower-middle-income economies. Economic growth has been accompanied by substantial increases in incomes, leading to noticeable progress in reducing poverty, food insecurity, and undernutrition among all population groups, including low-income people, youth, and women. Yet, micronutrient deficiencies are increasingly common, and the prevalence of overweight and obesity is rapidly rising in the region.

NUTRITION AND DIET QUALITY IN CENTRAL ASIA

FOOD SECURITY AND DIET QUALITY

The prevalence of undernourishment among the total population declined significantly from 2004/2006, when it was highest or close to highest, to 2020/2022 in almost all of the region's countries. While the most significant reductions were achieved in Tajikistan (from 37.6 percent to 9.3 percent), the country still reports the highest prevalence of undernourishment, just above the world average of 9.2 percent. Substantial reductions were also seen in Uzbekistan (from 14.8 percent to less than 2.5 percent), Kazakhstan (from 7.2 percent to less than 2.5 percent), and the Kyrgyz Republic (from 8.0 percent to 4.8 percent).[1] Only Turkmenistan saw a slight increase in undernourishment, from 4.2 percent to 5.7 percent, as the country faced a food crisis due to declining income from hydrocarbons, poor harvests caused in part by climate change, and government inaction in response to the economic impact of the COVID-19 pandemic.[2]

Beginning in 2020, the economic fallout of the COVID-19 pandemic increased food insecurity in Central Asia. The latest estimates suggest that 2.4 percent of the population in Kazakhstan and 6.9 percent in the Kyrgyz Republic were moderately or severely food insecure in 2020/2022, up from 2.1 percent and 6.3 percent, respectively, since 2016/2018. In Uzbekistan, however, the increase was much larger – the share of the population experiencing moderate or severe food insecurity rose from 14.9 percent before the pandemic to 26.1 percent in 2020/2022.[3] Comparable country-level data on food insecurity are not available for Tajikistan and Turkmenistan, both of which have a high prevalence of undernourishment. Moreover, patterns of food insecurity are highly context specific and can differ widely within countries, by subpopulation, and by time of year. An example from recent survey findings during winter, the lean season between harvests, in the Khatlon Region of Tajikistan is described in Box 1.

BOX 1 FOOD SECURITY AND DIETARY DIVERSITY IN KHATLON REGION, TAJIKISTAN

In 2015 and 2023, IFPRI surveyed 2,000 households in Khatlon, a region of Tajikistan that is predominately rural and historically the country's poorest. Data were collected during the winter in both years, the season when food insecurity is typically most prevalent in Tajikistan. The survey showed that food security improved substantially over this eight-year period: in 2023, 27.0 percent of households reported that they did not have food in their home at least once in the past month, as compared to 40.2 percent in 2015.

Hunger levels also improved, with the share of households reporting moderate to severe hunger falling by 1.7 percentage points to reach 12.1 percent in 2023. However, while 11.6 percent of households experienced improvements in their hunger status from 2015 to 2023, 9.7 percent reported a worsened hunger status, underscoring the tenuous food security situation for many families in Khatlon.

The findings on dietary diversity were also mixed. In both 2015 and 2023, only 31 percent of adult women achieved minimum dietary diversity. Women had less diverse diets than men, and lower consumption of meat, chicken, and fish (43 versus 53 percent) and dairy (45 versus 50 percent). Over the same period, diets shifted from less expensive protein sources (such as pulses) toward more expensive options (such as meat, chicken, and fish). Additionally, household consumption of vitamin-A-rich fruits and vegetables declined, and food consumed away from home increased more than threefold. Food expenditures increased from 2015 to 2023 but were directed toward purchasing more expensive food items that did not necessarily improve dietary diversity.

FIGURE B1 Minimum dietary diversity for women (24-hour recall), Khatlon Region, Tajikistan

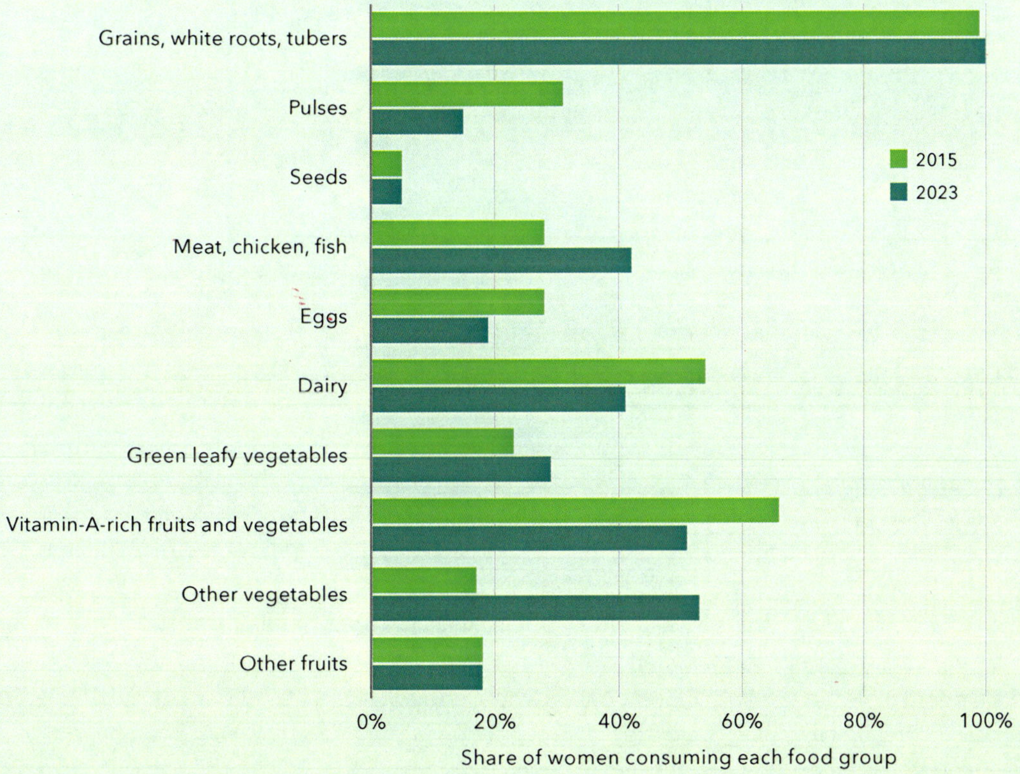

Source: I. Lambrecht, M. Mardonova, and K.T. Akramov, "Welfare and Vulnerability in Tajikistan: Evidence from Twelve Districts in Khatlon Province, 2015-2023," Central Asia Working Paper 2, IFPRI, Washington, DC, 2023.

FIGURE 1 Prevalence of stunting among children under 5 years of age (2000–2022)

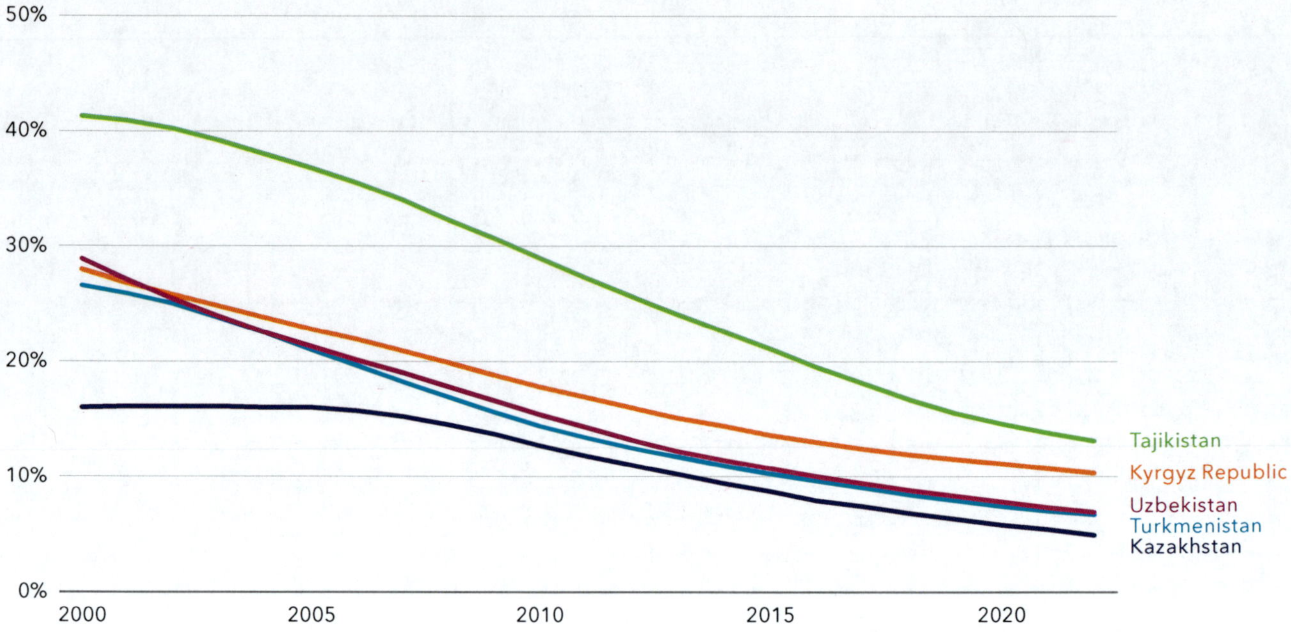

Source: Data from FAOSTAT, accessed March 18, 2023. https://www.fao.org/faostat

In the past decade, the prevalence of stunting in children under five years of age in Central Asia has fallen by about half (Figure 1), with the highest rates in 2022 found in Tajikistan (13.1 percent) and the Kyrgyz Republic (10.3 percent), and the lowest in Kazakhstan (4.9 percent).[4] The prevalence of wasting in the region has fallen below the world average of 6.8 percent, with the highest rates reported in Tajikistan (5.6 percent) and Turkmenistan (4.1 percent).[5] Based on these estimates, Tajikistan is considered a "medium" prevalence country for both stunting and wasting, the Kyrgyz Republic a "medium" prevalence country for stunting, and Turkmenistan a "low" prevalence country for wasting.[6]

OVERWEIGHT AND OBESITY

The prevalence of overweight and obesity has increased rapidly in Central Asia (Figure 2). Based on data from 2022 for the region as a whole, more than half of the adult population is estimated to be overweight or obese. Rates vary by country, however, with 62.7 percent overweight or obese (BMI ≥ 25) in Uzbekistan (30.0 percent obese), 58.8 percent in Tajikistan (23.8 percent obese), 58.1 in the Kyrgyz Republic (26.6 percent obese), 53.1 percent in Kazakhstan (18.4 percent obese), and 27.0 percent in Turkmenistan (21.4 percent obese).[7]

A major driver of the increasing prevalence of overweight and obesity among adults is the shift in dietary patterns toward higher intakes of meat, fat, sugar, and processed foods.[8] Across the region, obesity disproportionately affects women,[9] which may be explained in part by women's lower levels of physical activity in Central Asia.[10] These differences are particularly notable in Tajikistan (27.5 percent of women and 19.8 percent of men are obese), Turkmenistan (23.5 percent and 18.8 percent), and Uzbekistan (32.7 percent and 26.8 percent), with a smaller difference seen in the Kyrgyz Republic (28.3 percent and 24.0 percent). Both men and women appear to be more active in Kazakhstan compared to the rest of the region, where obesity affects 18.0 percent of women and 18.3 percent of men.[11]

The prevalence of overweight (including obesity) is significantly lower among children under five years of age, but is high enough that some countries are categorized as "moderate" prevalence countries (5-10 percent).[12] Among children, 7.7 percent were estimated to be overweight in Kazakhstan, 6.4 percent in

FIGURE 2 Prevalence of overweight and obesity among adults (2000–2022)

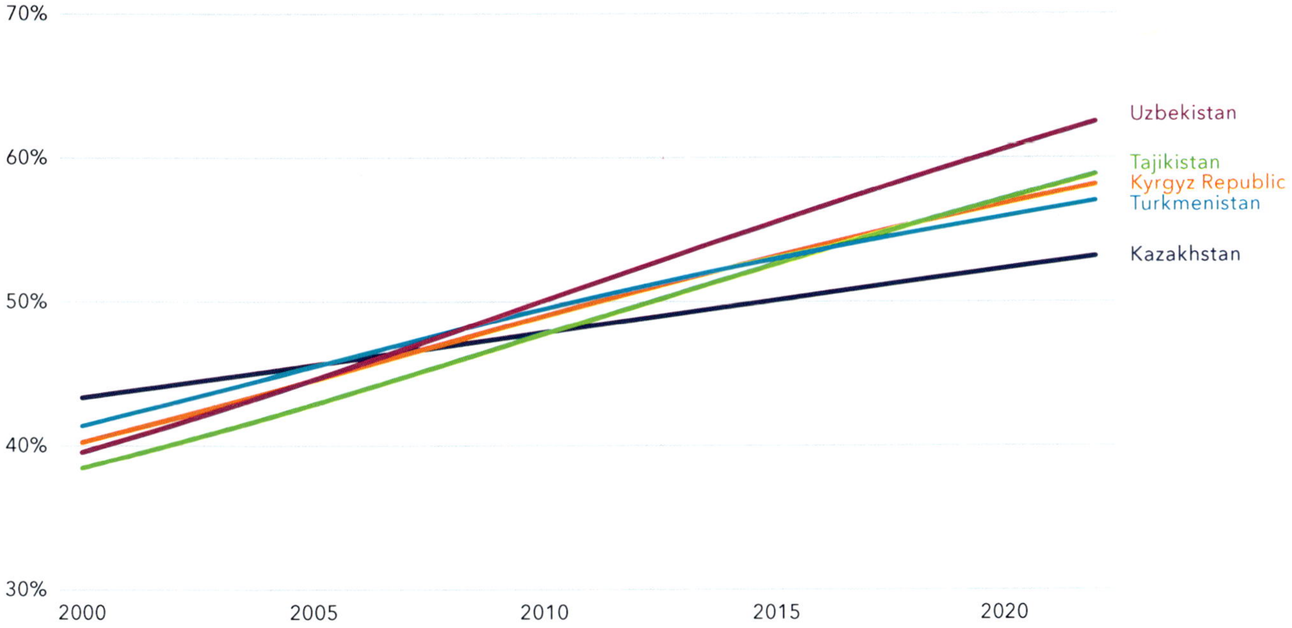

Source: Data from FAOSTAT, accessed March 18, 2023. https://www.fao.org/faostat

the Kyrgyz Republic, 4.2 percent in Uzbekistan, 3.6 percent in Turkmenistan, and 3.0 percent in Tajikistan in 2022. Moreover, overweight among children (measured based on the child's weight for height) has declined in all Central Asian countries since 2012.[13] This decline in overweight may be explained in part by reductions in stunting over the period, which occurred from an early age (under six months) and perhaps began in utero, resulting in taller children. Other factors, such as improvements in infant and young child feeding (IYCF) practices, may also have contributed to this decline. The Kyrgyz Republic witnessed significant improvement in applying adequate IYCF practices between 2012 and 2018.[14] In contrast, a worsening trend in IYCF practices was observed in both Tajikistan (between 2012 and 2017) and Turkmenistan (between 2015 and 2019). Recent longitudinal data are unavailable for Kazakhstan and Uzbekistan.

Traditional cuisine and recently introduced foods are contributing to overweight and obesity. Traditional food markets and street vendors throughout Central Asia offer energy-dense products high in saturated and trans fats, refined carbohydrates and sugar, and sodium – including *samosa*, *piroshky*, *chebureki*, *shawarma*, hot dogs, sweet pastries, and candy, as well as sugar-sweetened beverages.[15]

Globally, Central Asia is among the regions with the highest sodium intake,[16] which is a major contributor to diet-related noncommunicable diseases. An estimated one in four deaths in Turkmenistan and Uzbekistan is attributable to dietary risks (such as diets low in whole grains, fruits, or vegetables, and/or high in sodium, red and processed meat, and sugar-sweetened beverages) – twice the global level – as is one in five deaths in the other Central Asian countries. Similarly, nearly half of all deaths in Turkmenistan and Uzbekistan are attributable to metabolic risks often related to diet quality (such as high blood sugar, high blood pressure, and high body mass index), as are more than one in three deaths in the other Central Asian countries.[17]

MICRONUTRIENT DEFICIENCIES

Micronutrient deficiencies are a critical concern in Central Asia, with minor to no improvement achieved in the last decade. Anemia is present among 30 percent of all women (15-49 years) in the region, and affects 35.8 percent of women in the Kyrgyz Republic and 35.2 percent in Tajikistan.[18] Among pregnant women, this prevalence is even higher, with 34.0 percent having anemia in the region – again, this is highest in the Kyrgyz Republic (36.3 percent) and Tajikistan (38.6 percent), the latter bordering on "severe" prevalence (more than 40 percent). Similarly, between 20 and 40 percent of young children (6-59 months) in the region are affected by anemia, with the highest levels in Tajikistan (37.0 percent), the Kyrgyz Republic (33.4 percent), and Turkmenistan (33.1 percent).[19]

While most of the Central Asian population are able to meet their daily calorie intake needs, significant lack of dietary diversity and inadequate nutrient intake contribute to the rise in overweight and micronutrient deficiencies. Recent surveys using dietary recall, conducted in late summer, a time of the year when food availability and food security are typically at their best, show that 87-89 percent of women of reproductive age consume diets that meet minimum dietary diversity across Central Asian countries.[20] However, during other times of the year – especially winter – and in vulnerable areas, diet quality is significantly lower and may also differ by gender (see Box 1). Cereals, mainly wheat products, are the traditional staples of Central Asians and account for nearly half of the calorie intake in most countries. Specifically, cereals account for 55.6 percent of calorie intake in Turkmenistan (50.7 percent from wheat), 48.4 percent in Tajikistan (44.2 percent from wheat), 45.7 percent in the Kyrgyz Republic (36.1 percent from wheat), and 44.2 percent in Uzbekistan (40.9 percent from wheat).[21] The fortification of wheat flour, typically with iron and folate, is mandatory in all countries (see Chapter 6); Tajikistan was the last to sign a national fortification law, in 2019.[22] However, effective measures to ensure implementation of these laws have yet to be enacted.

KEY CHALLENGES

The key obstacles to improving diet quality and nutrition in Central Asia include socioeconomic challenges, the high cost of a healthy diet, inadequate nutrition knowledge, unhealthy consumption habits, and domestic and regional policies (such as constraints on farm decision-making, trade restrictions, and poor enforcement of flour fortification and salt iodization), which all hamper a shift to production and consumption of more nutritious foods. The improvements in nutritional outcomes witnessed in past decades were mainly due to a significant reduction in poverty, yet poverty rates remain relatively high in the region. Energy-dense, less nutritious foods are widely available and affordable, while nutritious foods are often more expensive and unaffordable for low-income households.

AFFORDABILITY OF HEALTHY DIETS. Overall, 24.4 percent of Central Asian people are unable to afford a healthy diet, which is considerably higher than in Eastern Europe (2.5 percent) and West Asia (9 percent), but significantly lower than in Southeast (54.9 percent) and South Asia (72.2 percent). Among countries in the region, there are stark differences in the affordability of a healthy diet. According to the latest estimates (2021), 2.3 percent of the population is unable to afford a healthy diet in Kazakhstan, while 58.2 percent of the population in the Kyrgyz Republic and 44.3 percent in Tajikistan cannot afford a healthy diet. This amounts to a total of 8.7 million people who cannot afford a healthy diet in just these three countries.[23] The total number of people unable to afford a healthy diet in Central Asia is likely significantly higher, given that data are lacking from both Turkmenistan and Uzbekistan, which report some of the highest levels of moderate and severe food insecurity in the region.[24]

PRICE SHOCKS. Poor households are the most vulnerable to food price shocks. Prices for staple foods (wheat flour and derived products) increased sharply in Central Asian countries that import food (the Kyrgyz Republic, Tajikistan, and Uzbekistan) when Kazakhstan and the Russian Federation responded to the COVID-19 pandemic by restricting wheat exports. While the Russia-Ukraine war has not directly disrupted food trade between Russia and Central Asia, it has negatively affected the region's trade with Ukraine and raised food prices by increasing uncertainty in agrifood markets. Increases in staple food prices in the past three to five years have reduced consumers' purchasing power and made healthy diets even less affordable.[25,26]

BEHAVIORAL FACTORS AND GENDER. Social and behavioral factors also present significant barriers to improving nutrition in the region. Basic nutritional knowledge is often inadequate. For example, recent evidence from Tajikistan found significant misconceptions about what constitutes a health-promoting diet and appropriate IYCF practices.[27] In addition, levels of physical activity are low, and recent increases in welfare have come with a more sedentary lifestyle.

Culturally and socially driven gender roles likewise have notable effects on nutrition and health. Women are disproportionately exposed to multiple burdens of malnutrition as a result of gender inequality and their limited decision-making power, among other factors.[28] For example, gendered differences in dietary knowledge and practices were apparent in a study conducted in rural Tajikistan.[29] Such differences were also found in the IFPRI study in the Khatlon Region of Tajikistan, which showed that men consume more diverse diets than women (Box 1). Moreover, gender norms and roles can also present notable barriers to women's participation in physical activity. The largest gender gaps in physical activity are seen in Tajikistan, where 38.7 percent of women were insufficiently physically active compared with 19.9 percent of men in 2016; and Uzbekistan, where 24.4 percent of women and 13.3 percent of men are considered insufficiently physically active.[30]

POLICY RESPONSES

Several policy interventions have potential to transform food systems in the region for better nutrition and diet quality. These include improving policy responses to crises; enhancing trade openness and diversity in trading partners;[31] implementing flour fortification; and promoting crop diversity, school meal programs, and policies to improve the food environment (see Chapter 5), among others.

AGRICULTURAL DIVERSIFICATION. In the past, regional agriculture following the central planning mandates focused singularly on specific products: the Kyrgyz Republic specialized in livestock, Tajikistan and Uzbekistan in cotton, and Kazakhstan in wheat. In the past two decades, national governments have facilitated agricultural diversification by focusing more on high-value, nutrient-rich food crops. For example, in the 2010s, the Uzbek government shifted its policy toward promoting horticultural crops and received large loans from international donors such as the World Bank and Asian Development Bank to promote this policy. As a result, by 2022, more than 21 percent of agricultural land was allocated to horticultural crops, representing a nearly 8 percentage point increase compared with 2010.[32] A similar increase occurred in Tajikistan.[33] Recent evidence from Tajikistan suggests that promoting nutrition-sensitive agricultural diversification (see Chapters 3 and 6) is a viable strategy to improve nutrition and diet quality in Central Asia. Strong linkages have been observed between dietary diversity and diversity in food production by smallholders, especially when market access is limited.[34] Further promotion of crop diversity by allowing farmers more freedom to farm and improving access to innovative horticultural technologies is necessary to enhance diet quality and diversity in the region.

SCHOOL MEAL PROGRAMS. School meal programs can improve food security and nutrition (see Chapter 3). While these programs are present in all Central Asian countries, some countries have national school feeding policies (Kazakhstan), while others rely largely on donor-supported programs (the Kyrgyz Republic and Tajikistan). In Tajikistan, the World Food Programme (WFP) supports a school feeding program for primary school children that reaches more than half of the country's schools and nearly a quarter of its school children. WFP also supports a similar program in the Kyrgyz Republic. In Kazakhstan, the government's national school feeding program aims to further improve nutritional outcomes through nutrition education. In 2022, Uzbekistan's government began to provide free meals to primary school students in two regions and subsequently expanded the program to all primary schools. While there is no credible evidence of the impact of these programs on children's welfare and nutrition in the region, evidence from Armenia, a neighboring country with similar socioeconomic conditions and a comparable school meal program, shows that such programs have a modest impact on poverty.[35] Thus, better assessment of these programs in terms of their impact on nutritional outcomes is necessary as countries consider ways to enhance their design.

POLICIES TO IMPROVE FOOD ENVIRONMENTS. Assessing existing food environments is necessary to identify strategies and policies to promote healthy food environments in the region. The evidence suggests that countries in the region face significant problems related to food safety and sanitary and phytosanitary (SPS) standards. Outdated legislation, poor laboratory capacity, and poor coordination between border controls create vulnerability to transboundary pests and diseases, and constrain the potential of Central Asian countries to expand agricultural food trade.[36] Thus, aligning food safety systems and SPS standards with international standards will help boost food trade within the region and ensure food is available and affordable. Developing food-based dietary guidelines, promoting food labeling, and including nutrition information and caloric content on food product packages and restaurant menus will also contribute to healthy food environments in the region.

NUTRITION AND SOCIAL BEHAVIOR CHANGE COMMUNICATION. Behavior change campaigns are needed to improve basic nutritional knowledge, promote more diverse diets and consumption of whole grains, limit intake of processed food, reduce the use of oil and salt in both traditional and more newly introduced foods, and emphasize the importance of physical activity (see Chapters 3 and 5). These campaigns can prompt individual-level action and contribute to the critically needed efforts at the policy level to reduce malnutrition. Targeting this communication to both men and women, with attention to cultural factors such as gender-related norms and traditional roles, will be key in achieving improvements among men and women alike, across different age ranges. In addition, regulations on marketing ultra-processed foods and sugar-sweetened beverages to children could promote the establishment of healthy eating patterns during childhood and adolescence that reduce micronutrient deficiencies and mitigate increases in overweight and obesity.

DATA AND ANALYTICS. Central Asian countries currently lack comprehensive data on nutrition and dietary practices at the household and community levels. This lack of information, especially the absence of age- and gender-disaggregated data, poses a significant challenge in understanding disparities and inequalities of different demographic groups, including men and women, as well as children and adults. Moreover, none of the region's countries have national food-based dietary guidelines (see Chapter 3), though these are currently being developed in Tajikistan and Kyrgyzstan. Development of food-based dietary guidelines can lay the foundation for national food, nutrition, and health policies and programs. There is also a pressing need for enhanced data analysis capabilities and assessment in Central Asian countries. Investments in collecting age- and gender-disaggregated survey data and building analytical research capacity are essential to gain a deeper understanding of how to develop effective policy solutions to transform food systems for better nutrition and diet quality.

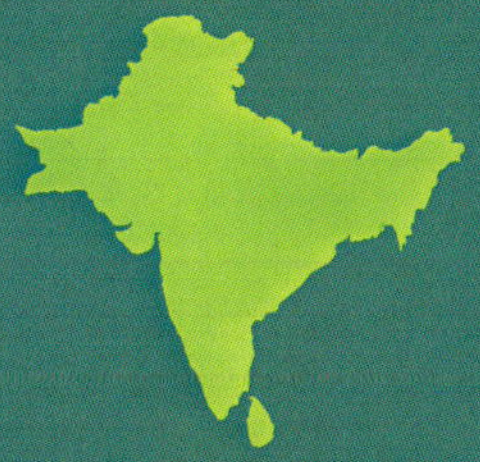

SOUTH ASIA

AVINASH KISHORE

Avinash Kishore is a senior research fellow, Development Strategies and Governance Unit, International Food Policy Research Institute, New Delhi.

Malnutrition rates are high across South Asia, and poor diet quality is a major contributor to this problem throughout the region. Cereals and starchy roots account for a large share of total calories consumed, and the consumption of calorie-dense foods, such as fried snacks, is high and increasing,[1] while the consumption of vegetables and other micronutrient-rich foods is low (Figure 1).[2] As a result, high levels of undernutrition (stunting and wasting) and micronutrient deficiencies persist even as the prevalence of overweight, obesity, and related noncommunicable diseases (NCDs) is rising (Table 1).

DRIVERS OF POOR DIET QUALITY

The factors underlying poor diets are well known – they include affordability constraints, behavioral and cultural preferences, agriculture and food policies, and food environments that favor rice, wheat, sugar, and calorie-dense foods.

FIGURE 1 Share of population consuming all five recommended food groups, salty or fried snacks, and no vegetables or fruits, 2021-2022

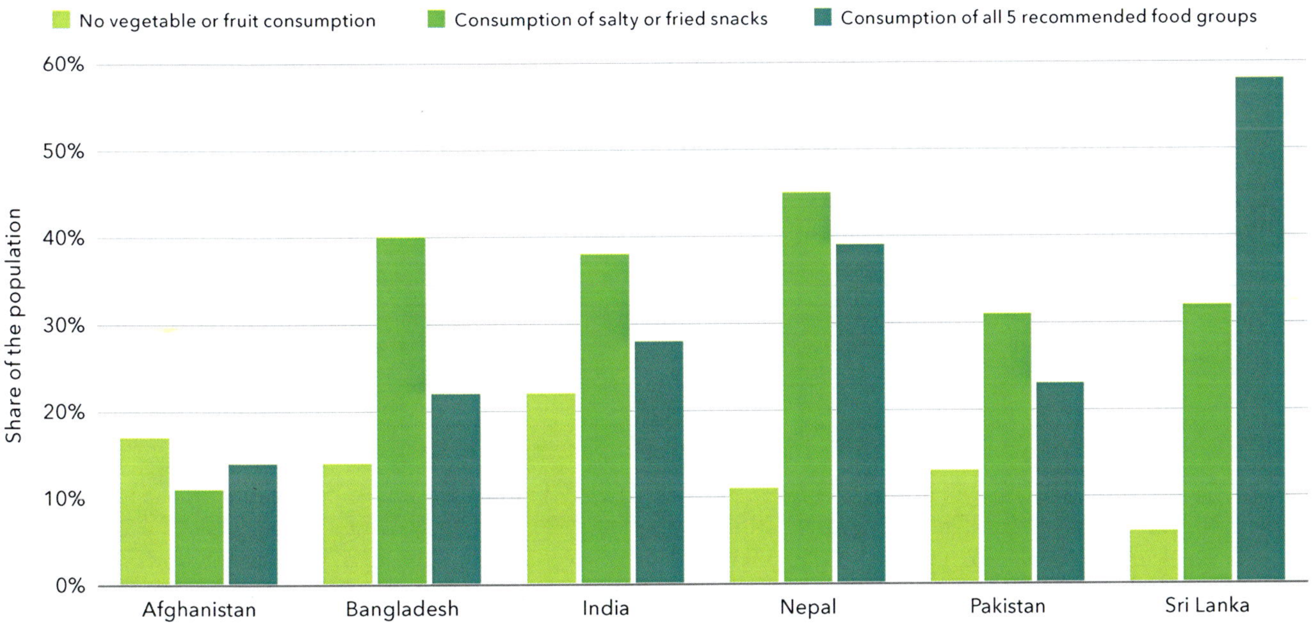

Source: Based on data from the Global Diet Quality Project, accessed January 2024. https://www.dietquality.org/indicators

Note: All five recommended food groups includes (1) at least one starchy staple food; (2) at least one vegetable; (3) at least one fruit; (4) at least one pulse, nut, or seed; and (5) at least one animal-source food.

TABLE 1 Prevalence of malnutrition and noncommunicable diseases in the six most populous countries of South Asia

Country	Prevalence of undernourishment (%)		Prevalence of stunting in children under 5 years (%)		Prevalence of overweight in adults (%)		Prevalence of raised blood pressure in adults (%)		Prevalence of diabetes in adults (%)	
	2011	2021	2011	2016–2019	2006	2016	2011	2015	2011	2014
Afghanistan	19.7	30.1	40.4 (2013)	38.2 (2018)	14.4	18.1	30.3	30.6	11.1	11.9
Bangladesh	16.1	11.2	41.3	28.0 (2019)	12.9	17.1	25.2	24.7	9.2	9.8
India	15.4	16.6	38.7 (2012)	34.7 (2017)	12.9	16.4	25.7	25.7	8.5	8.7
Nepal	9.1	5.4	40.1	31.5 (2019)	13.8	17.6	29.1	29.6	10.0	10.6
Pakistan	14.9	18.5	43.6	37.6 (2018)	17.0	20.6	30.2	30.4	11.6	12.4
Sri Lanka	14.0	5.3	14.6 (2012)	17.3 (2016)	14.8	18.6	21.9	22.3	6.9	7.4

Source: Based on data from the Food Systems Dashboard, accessed January 2024. www.foodsystemsdashboard.org/indicators

Note: "Prevalence of undernourishment" is the percentage of the population whose habitual food consumption is insufficient to provide the dietary energy levels required to maintain a normal active and healthy life. For data on the prevalence of stunting, numbers in parentheses indicate the year data were collected.

POOR AFFORDABILITY. South Asia is among the world's poorest regions. More than 10 percent of the population (nearly 200 million people) live in extreme poverty (at or below $2.15/capita/day), and 44 percent (814 million) live below the poverty line for lower-middle-income countries ($3.65/day).[3] Nearly half of the more than 2 billion people worldwide who cannot afford a healthy diet reside in South Asia,[4] with the cost of the EAT-Lancet reference diet exceeding the daily incomes of more than 600 million people in the region (38.4 percent of the total population),[5] and too expensive for 75 percent of the population (see Chapter 4).[6] Even the least-cost nutrient-adequate diets are unaffordable for a third of all households in South Asia.[7]

RELATIVE PRICES. Micronutrient-rich foods are expensive in South Asia, while cereals, fats and oils, sugar, and sugary and salty snacks are relatively cheap (see Chapter 4). The cost premium – that is, the additional cost, for the least-cost nutrient-adequate diet above the least-cost source of calorie adequacy – is larger in South Asia than in any other region.[8] For example, dark green leafy vegetables and vitamin A-rich fruits and vegetables cost 8 to 22 times more per calorie than starchy staples and twice as much per calorie as sugary and salty snacks. In addition, calories from fats and oils and sugar cost even less than those from staples in India and other South Asian countries.[9]

CEREAL-CENTRIC AGRICULTURE AND FOOD POLICIES. As in many other parts of the developing world, agriculture and food policies across South Asia continue to focus on keeping starchy staples affordable, rather than on the diverse diets needed for lifelong health.[10] The need for balanced diets rich in micronutrients is widely recognized but largely ignored in allocation of resources. For example, rice, wheat, and sugarcane growers are entitled to price guarantees in India. Similarly, rice farmers in Sri Lanka have preferential access to subsidized fertilizers. This bias also extends to public investments in agricultural R&D, which have prioritized enhancing the productivity of rice and wheat, while neglecting coarse grains and pulses.[11] These cereal-centric policies have led to low crop diversity across South Asia, with more than two-thirds of the region's arable land under cereals, and thus have contributed to poor nutritional outcomes.

ROLE OF SOCIAL SAFETY NET PROGRAMS. South Asian countries implement some of the world's largest food-based social safety net programs to support poor households, pregnant women, new mothers, and young children (see Chapters 3 and 4). Many of these programs subsidize rice and/or wheat for target households. For example, Bangladesh's Food Friendly Program (Khaddo Bandhob Karmasuchi) provides 30 kg of highly subsidized rice to the country's poorest households during the lean seasons between harvests (March–April and September–November). India's public distribution system (PDS) provides up to 25 kg of free rice and/or wheat every month to two-thirds of the country's poorest households. While the PDS may reduce hunger, it has not improved access to balanced diets for the targeted households (Box 1).

One study found that access to the PDS has no effect on consumption of micronutrient rich food[12]; rather, the PDS skews household consumption toward cereals, thus reducing consumption of items like fruits and milk. In addition, households with access to the PDS have reported replacing nutritionally richer coarse cereals with subsidized rice and wheat.[13] However, other studies suggest that subsidized rice and wheat act as income transfers and have a positive impact on consumption of all food groups.[14]

Switching from in-kind transfers to direct cash transfers for food subsidies could reduce the cost of this support for governments and eliminate the distortions affecting household choices.[15] However, in societies with high levels of poverty, poorly developed credit and factor and product markets, and widespread inequality, cash may not ensure the same food security that food transfers provide for households.[16] Moreover, households have been found to prefer food over cash in regions where the PDS is functioning well.[17]

BEHAVIORAL AND CULTURAL PREFERENCES. In addition to prices, incomes, and government policies, non-economic cultural factors, including vegetarianism and unusually late introduction of solid foods to infants, also have a strong influence on diets in South Asia.[18] Moreover, even the wealthiest households (in the top decile of monthly per capita consumption expenditure) consume less than the recommended quantity of vegetables and spend a large share of their food budgets on processed and ultra-processed foods.[19]

BOX 1 INDIA'S PUBLIC DISTRIBUTION SYSTEM AND DIVERSIFYING DIETS

There is an increasing demand in India to diversify the public distribution system (PDS) food basket by adding pulses, coarse cereals, and other nutrient-rich foods to make it more nutrition-sensitive. The state government of Karnataka in India has begun distributing 2 kg of subsidized finger millets per family per month through the PDS, and the governments of Madhya Pradesh, Maharashtra, Haryana, and Odisha are also introducing millets, including finger millets, in the PDS. Pulses have been added to the basket of subsidized goods sold through the PDS in states including Andhra Pradesh, Himachal Pradesh, Tamil Nadu, and Telangana.

However, adding subsidized pulses to the PDS basket led to only a small increase in household pulse consumption and almost negligible net nutritional impact, largely because the increase in consumption of PDS-subsidized pulses was offset by decreases in pulses purchased from the market.[a] The quantity of subsidized pulses or coarse cereals provided would have to increase dramatically to have any real impact on total consumption and nutrition. Small transfers of 2 kg per family per month are not enough to improve diet quality.

Expanding the PDS to include a sufficient amount of pulses and coarse cereals requires building a public procurement system and setting remunerative minimum support prices (MSP) for these crops, as is done for rice and wheat. Historically, MSPs for millets and pulses have generally been low compared to their market prices.[b] To encourage millet cultivation and its inclusion in the PDS, India's government has created an entity under the National Food Security Mission, but its impact remains to be seen.

EMERGING TRENDS IN SOUTH ASIAN DIETS

Consumption of calorie-dense and processed foods (chocolates and sugar confectioneries, salty snacks, beverages, ready-made and convenience foods, and breakfast cereals) is increasing in India and other countries of South Asia. After cereals and milk, snacks and prepared foods make up the largest share of Indian food budgets. Our analysis of data from a large nationally representative panel of households shows that India's total annual household expenditure on paid meals consumed away from home increased from Rs. 619 billion (US$8.8 billion) in 2015 to Rs. 820 billion (US$11.6 billion) in 2019 in real terms, an increase of about US$3 billion.[20] Similarly, the share of packaged (highly processed and calorie-dense) foods in household food budgets nearly doubled during this period, from 6.5 to 12 percent. Wealthier households spend a greater share of their food budgets on processed foods (Figure 2). A recent World Health Organization report also finds that sales of highly processed foods increased at an annual rate of 13.4 percent between 2011 and 2021.[21] It is not clear, however, whether increasing expenditure on prepared and ultra-processed foods is crowding out the consumption of healthier foods such as fruits and vegetables.

THE WAY FORWARD

To support a shift toward better nutrition and healthier diets, South Asian governments must correct the historical bias in their agriculture and food policies and allocate more resources to promote production and consumption of non-staple foods. "Crop-neutral" policies would allow farmers to respond to market signals,[22] including demand for more diverse diets (see Chapter 6), and the resulting diversification in domestic food production could also reduce poverty in the region.[23]

Rice and wheat subsidies are popular in many parts of India, but switching to direct cash transfers for food subsidies is worth trying in areas where grain markets are well developed and where consumers have easy access to banking services.[24] Cash transfers would reduce the cost to the government of food

FIGURE 2 Share of urban household food budgets spent on processed foods and purchased meals, by per capita consumption expenditure, India

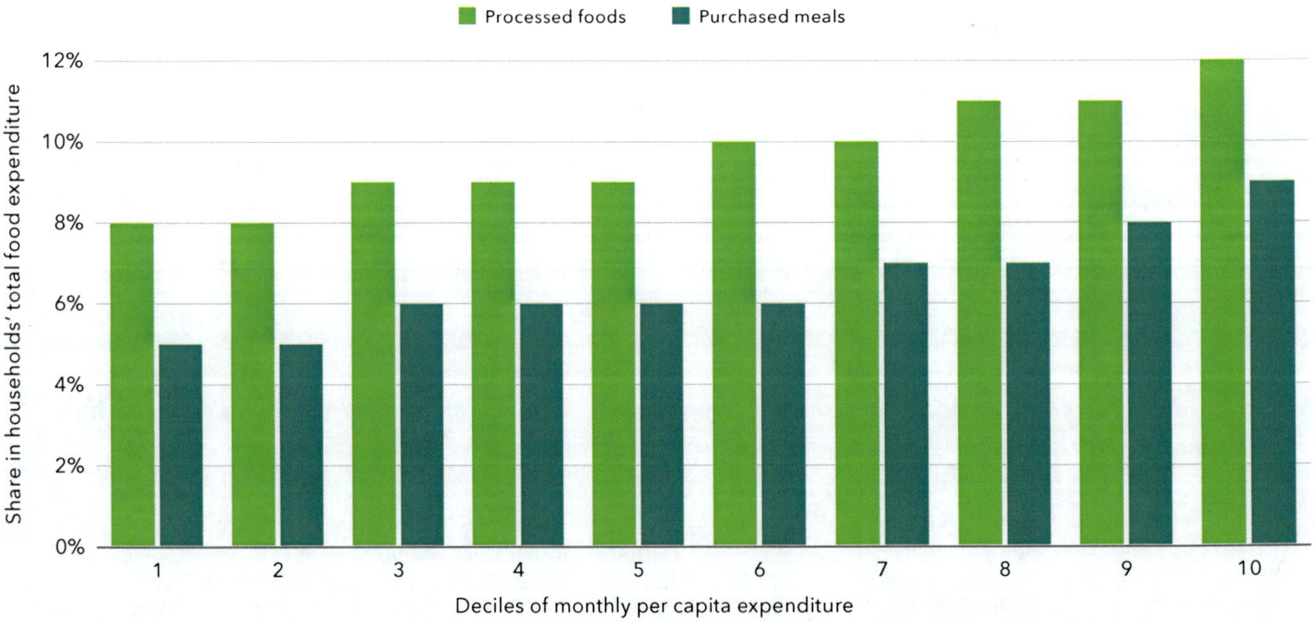

Source: Based on data from the Centre for Monitoring Indian Economy's Consumer Pyramids Household Surveys, www.cmie.com

subsidies, reduce distortions in food production and consumption, and afford consumers more choices. When combined with nutritional behavior change and communication training (see Chapter 3), cash transfers have also been shown to have a significant positive impact on children's nutritional status.[25]

Tax rates are not aligned with the nutritional content of foods in South Asia. Higher taxes on foods high in fat, sugar, and salt could help to slow the rapid increase in consumption of these foods (see Chapter 5). Many countries in Asia, including India, the Philippines, Saudi Arabia, Sri Lanka, and Thailand, have imposed corrective taxes on sugar-sweetened beverages, with some impact on lowering the average sugar content of the taxed items.[26]

Effective front-of-package labeling that provides consumers with easy-to-understand nutrition information can promote healthy food choices and incentivize reformulation by manufacturers (see Chapter 5). This form of nutrition labeling is strongly recommended by international health agencies. Color-coded labeling of sugar-sweetened beverages along with media campaigns to raise awareness in Sri Lanka has led to reduction in the sugar content of beverages and a drop in sales of carbonated drinks.[27] However, efforts to implement similar, accessible front-of-package labeling is facing stiff resistance from the food industry (see Chapters 3 and 8).[28]

In countries like India, 90 percent of food enterprises are small, informal, and outside the regulatory and tax net.[29] The predominance of these in the region may limit the impact of taxes and regulations on food quality and may even divert demand to informal food enterprises. To address this gap, taxes and other regulations should be combined with awareness campaigns to improve nutrition literacy. Effective food labeling and corrective taxes on foods high in fat, sugar, and salt, combined with nutrition literacy, may reduce the supply and consumption of unhealthy foods.

Over the past decade, efforts to improve nutrition knowledge and awareness in South Asia have included several large-scale social and behavior change initiatives (see Chapter 3). These have included efforts conducted through frontline health workers and community platforms, for example, the National Nutrition Mission and women's group programs in India, frontline health worker programs in Nepal and Bangladesh, and more. Evidence of the impact of these programs on dietary diversity is quite robust, but evidence on improving other aspects of healthy diets, such as reducing the consumption of ultra-processed foods, is very limited. New policies and programs targeting all components of a sustainable healthy diet will be essential across South Asia, especially considering the persistence of multiple forms of malnutrition and the increasing burden of NCDs.

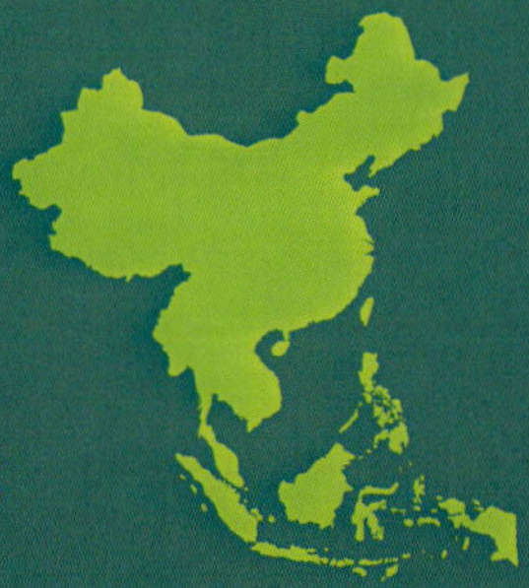

EAST AND SOUTHEAST ASIA

PHUONG HONG NGUYEN, KEVIN Z. CHEN, AND JODY HARRIS

Phuong Hong Nguyen is a senior research fellow, Nutrition, Diets, and Health Unit, International Food Policy Research Institute (IFPRI), Hanoi, Viet Nam. **Kevin Z. Chen** is a senior research fellow, Development Strategies and Governance Unit, IFPRI, Beijing, and Qiushi chair professor, Zhejiang University, Hangzhou. **Jody Harris** is a research fellow, Institute of Development Studies, United Kingdom, and adjunct professor, Institute of Nutrition, Mahidol University, Thailand.

The food systems of East and Southeast Asia (ESEA) are shaped by a unique interplay between the major role of traditional smallholders in food production, widespread informal employment in food systems, and the region's high level of urbanization, as well as impacts of regional trade on food supply, all of which affect diets and nutrition. The double burden of malnutrition – hunger and micronutrient deficiencies, plus overweight and obesity – is evident across the region, driven by inadequate diets and the food systems that underpin them. The region is also highly diverse, both across countries (ranging from the smallest to the largest economies in the world) and within countries (home to some of the richest urbanites and some of the most marginalized rural and urban communities). This section describes the dietary trends in the region, highlights key food system drivers of the double burden, and suggests policy options to mitigate the challenges and build on successful experiences.

DIET AND NUTRITION TRENDS AND ISSUES

Regional diets have historically been predominantly rice-based and characterized by seasonal scarcity, particularly of fruits and vegetables. Many ESEA countries also have strong food cultures (the cuisine, ingredients, cooking methods, and attitudes about the production, preparation, consumption, and sharing of food). While calorie availability has improved across the region as a result of the Green Revolution and economic and trade reforms, both food insecurity and lack of dietary diversity remain persistent problems.[1] The ongoing nutrition transition from traditional to modern diets, which emerged in the region in the early 1990s, has led to increased consumption of ultra-processed foods and animal-source foods and a decline in heavily staple-based fresh and local foods.[2] Over the past three decades (1990–2017), inadequate diets (either nutrient-poor, staple-based diets in food insecure areas or diets high in ultra-processed foods, particularly in urban areas) have been responsible for 30 percent of all adult deaths and 21 percent of illness in East Asia and 22 percent of deaths and 17 percent of illness in Southeast Asia.[3]

While hunger, micronutrient deficiencies, and overnutrition coexist within the same countries and sometimes the same households, there are notable differences in diets and nutrition outcomes across countries. These differences reflect wide variations in food insecurity and access to healthy diets that disproportionately affect marginalized communities or populations. Nearly a quarter of the ESEA population experiences at least moderate food insecurity (limited access to adequate and nutritious food), ranging from less than 5 percent in Singapore and Japan to more than 30 percent in Cambodia, the Philippines, Thailand, and Lao PDR.[4] Diets do not meet recommendations for healthy and sustainable diets on average in the region (Figure 1, panel A),[5] with average intake of fruits, vegetables, legumes, nuts, and whole grains below recommended levels and intake of red meat above the recommended level. There is high consumption of sodium

FIGURE 1 Diets in East and Southeast Asia

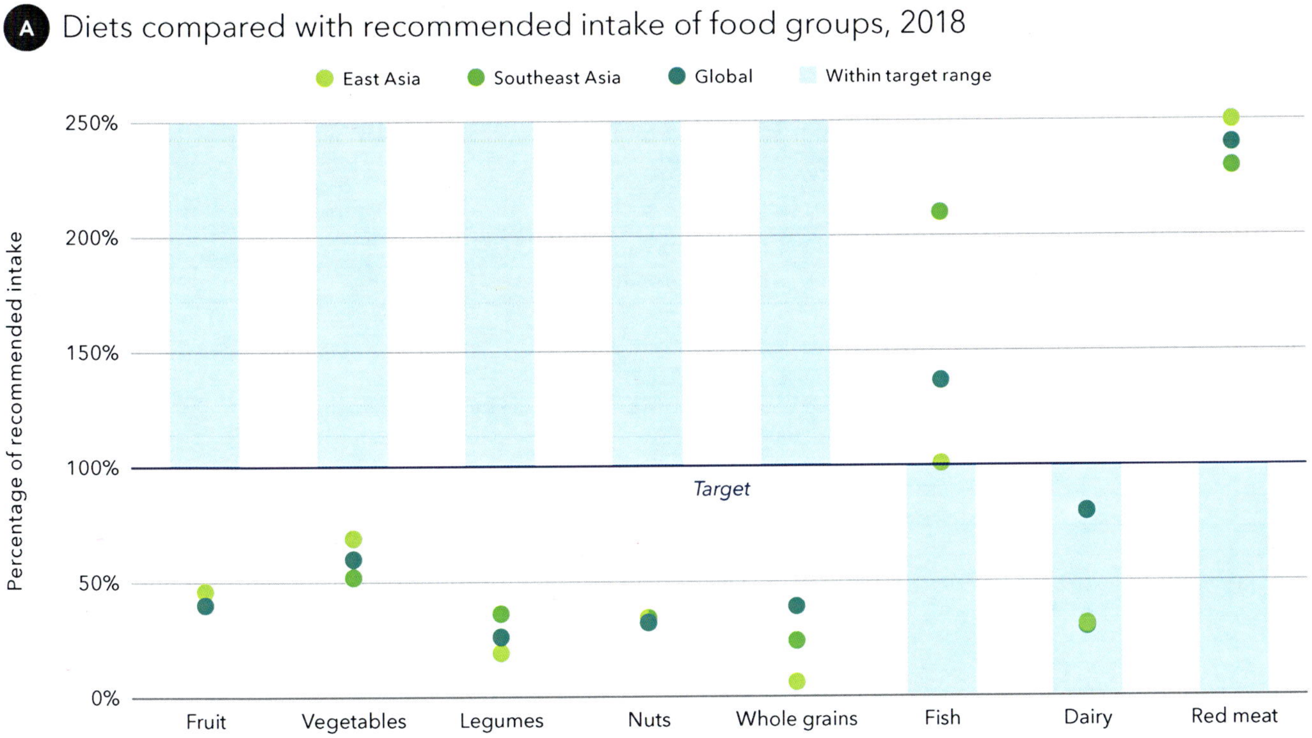

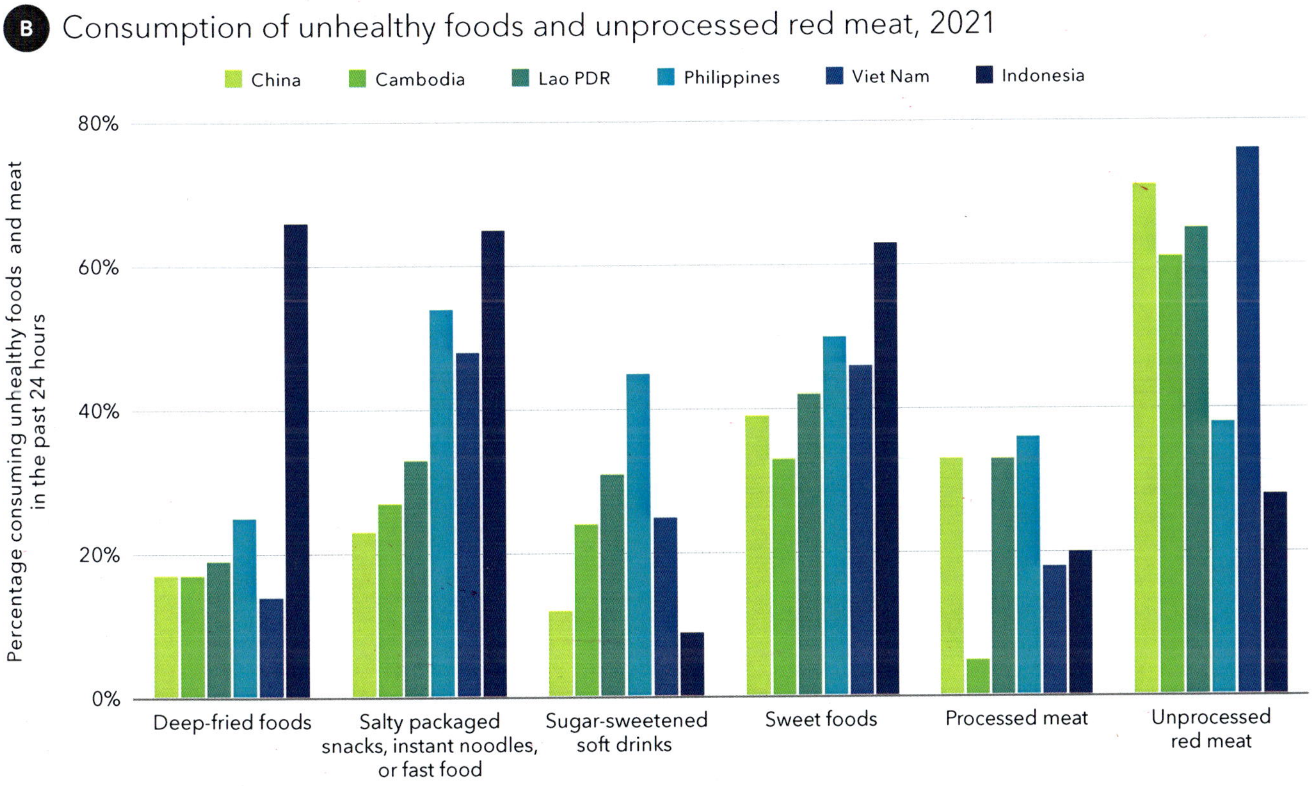

Source: Panel A: Adapted from Development Initiatives, *2021 Global Nutrition Report: The State of Global Nutrition* (Bristol, UK: 2021); Panel B: Adapted from GBD 2017 Diet Collaborators, "Health Effects of Dietary Risks in 195 Countries, 1990-2017: A Systematic Analysis for the Global Burden of Disease Study 2017," *Lancet* 393, 10184 (2019): 1958-1972; data from Global Diet Quality Project, "Global Diet Quality Project," accessed November 2023. https://www.dietquality.org/

(through salt, salty snacks, and traditional condiments)[6] and of unhealthy and ultra-processed foods (high in sugar, fat, or salt and with ultra-high levels of processing or additives) across the region (Figure 1, panel B), though consumption of the latter is notably higher in some countries and populations than others.[7]

Poor diets lead to multiple micronutrient deficiencies. Nineteen percent of women in East Asia and 28 percent in Southeast Asia have anemia, and an estimated half of all children in the region have at least one micronutrient deficiency.[8] At the same time, the nutrition transition[9] is driving an increase in overweight and obesity across the region, though with large variations related to national food system characteristics and food cultures. Almost 58 percent of adults in Malaysia and around 20 percent in Viet Nam are overweight or obese,[10] and related noncommunicable diseases (NCDs) are significant. About 8 percent of adults in ESEA have diabetes, and high blood pressure affects 21 percent of adults in East Asia and 23 percent in Southeast Asia.[11]

FOOD SYSTEM DRIVERS AND CHALLENGES

Several food system drivers play a role in shaping diets in ESEA, including regional trade, the critical but stagnant role of smallholder farming, rapid urbanization, climate change and biodiversity loss, the nutrition transition, and food cultures. All of these, along with uncertain livelihoods and incomes, also have implications for affordability of healthy diets.

FIGURE 2 Availability of fruits and vegetables in East and Southeast Asia

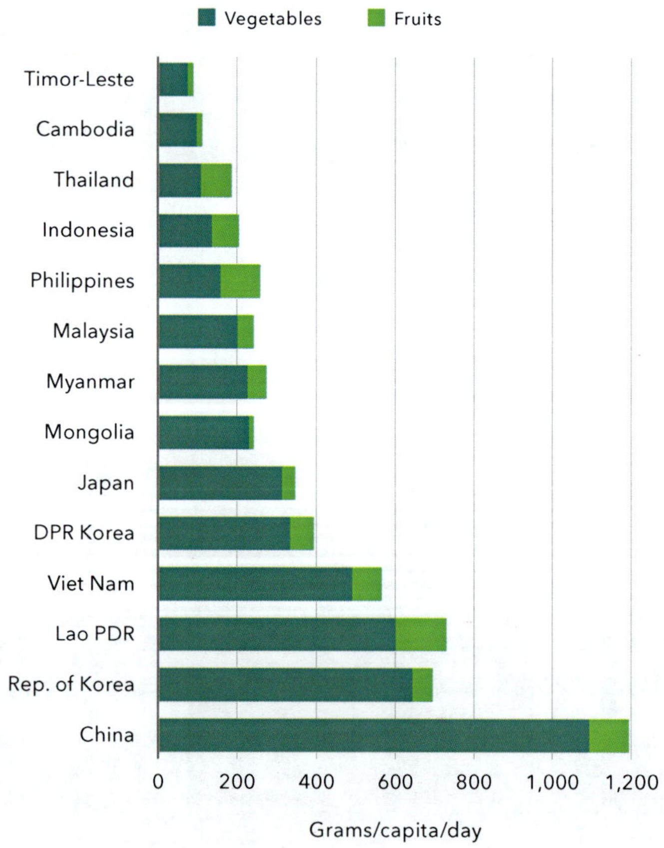

Source: Based on data from the Food Systems Dashboard, accessed February 2024. www.foodsystemsdashboard.org

Note: Recommendation is 400 grams of fruits and vegetables a day. Amount available is calculated as the sum of production, imports, and net stocks minus exports, food manufacturing, feed, seed, waste, and other uses.

TRADE. While ESEA contributes significantly to current global rice and aquatic food production and export,[12] many countries within the region (including some of the largest) are net importers of food.[13] The diversity in national food trade profiles – ranging from import dependence to export orientation to self-sufficiency goals for particular foods – poses a challenge for coherent regional trade policy that considers nutrition alongside economic goals. This diversity is desirable particularly for evening out availability of nutrient-dense perishable foods such as fruits and vegetables, but important regional trade policies rarely consider nutrition and health issues, and in some cases, these policies are contrary to national public health policy goals.[14] Figure 2 shows the differences in fruit and vegetable availability across ESEA countries, which reflect limited regional trade.

FOOD SYSTEM EMPLOYMENT. In many countries, the share of agricultural employment, particularly among the working poor, remains high, and smallholder farmers are among those most likely to experience poor diets and malnutrition.[15] Although the region is home to some of the world's largest agribusinesses, smallholder and peasant systems involve 450 million smallholders and produce 80 percent of the region's food, often under poor working conditions and with uncertain land tenure.[16] Employment in agriculture, and in food systems in general, is largely informal, with informal livelihoods accounting for an estimated 37 percent of agricultural employment in Thailand and as much as 90 percent in Cambodia (with the caveat that informal employment data are difficult to standardize across countries).[17] The range and informality of agricultural and food system work in ESEA have implications for designing food system policies that support livelihoods while improving the availability of nutritious foods for consumers.

URBANIZATION. Urbanization is the most important demographic trend and a key driver of food system change in ESEA in recent years, but with mixed impacts. ESEA is the world's most rapidly urbanizing region, with an average annual urbanization rate of 3 percent.[18] More than 60 percent of ESEA's population and over 70 percent of East Asia's population[19] now live in urban areas, though urban populations still account for as little as one-third in some Southeast Asian countries. Of the region's urban population, approximately 40 percent live in informal settlements, while cities are also home to the region's wealthiest people.[20] Urbanization has driven increased demand for ultra-processed foods, which are often cheaper and more convenient but less healthy options for busy or poor urban workers (see Chapters 4 and 5). Urban markets enable more targeted transportation and logistical networks, contributing to market concentration (which reduces food choices for purchasers and market choices for producers), the proliferation of supermarkets and convenience stores, and increased sales of prepared foods and sugar-sweetened beverages from global and Asian firms.[21] These sales have accelerated recently because of increased use of delivery apps, largely for unhealthy foods.[22]

CLIMATE CHANGE AND BIODIVERSITY LOSS. Climate change and biodiversity loss can have complex and interconnected effects on diets, affecting food availability, diversity, dietary patterns, and nutritional quality.[23] Climate change affects crop yields and nutrient levels in plant-based foods, particularly cereals and legumes, due to increased carbon dioxide levels. Loss of genetic diversity limits the ability to breed resilient crops and reduces the variety of crops and livestock for a healthy diet. Rising temperatures lead to higher levels of heavy metals in crops and disrupt ecosystems by reducing beneficial organisms like pollinators and pest-control regulators. In addition, shifts in agricultural practices in response to climate change, such as changes in crop selection or farming techniques, may influence the types of foods that are produced and consumed.

FOOD CULTURES AND FOOD SAFETY. Strong traditional food cultures in the region have tempered the nutrition transition to some extent, and traditional foods remain a preferred element of many daily diets. However, while traditional diets may offer diversity and freshness, they are not always synonymous with healthy eating because they often contain large amounts of sugar or salt or rely heavily on low-nutrient starchy foods.[24] Asian food consumption is also characterized by informal food distribution, such as wet markets and food stalls, and by out-of-home eating. These sales outlets provide opportunities for accessing fresh foods as well as unhealthy snacks, but they lack robust food safety standards, which can drive consumers away from fresh foods (see Chapter 3).

AFFORDABILITY. Most importantly, healthy diets remain out of reach for a substantial population across all of Asia. An estimated 1.9 billion people in Asia could not afford a healthy diet in 2021[25] (see Chapter 4), with recent data showing that the proportion varies widely across the region (Figure 3). Less than 5 percent of the population in the Republic of Korea, Japan, and Malaysia faced affordability issues, whereas more than 50 percent in Indonesia, Lao PDR, Mongolia, Myanmar, and the Philippines struggled to afford nutritious food. The cost of a nutritionally adequate diet in ESEA averages about US$1.51 per person, per day, with nutrient-rich foods such as fish, vegetables, and legumes accounting for much of the cost.[26] In 2022, between 1 percent (Thailand, Malaysia) and 33 percent (Indonesia) of the Southeast Asian population lived

FIGURE 3 Share of population who cannot afford a healthy diet, 2017–2020

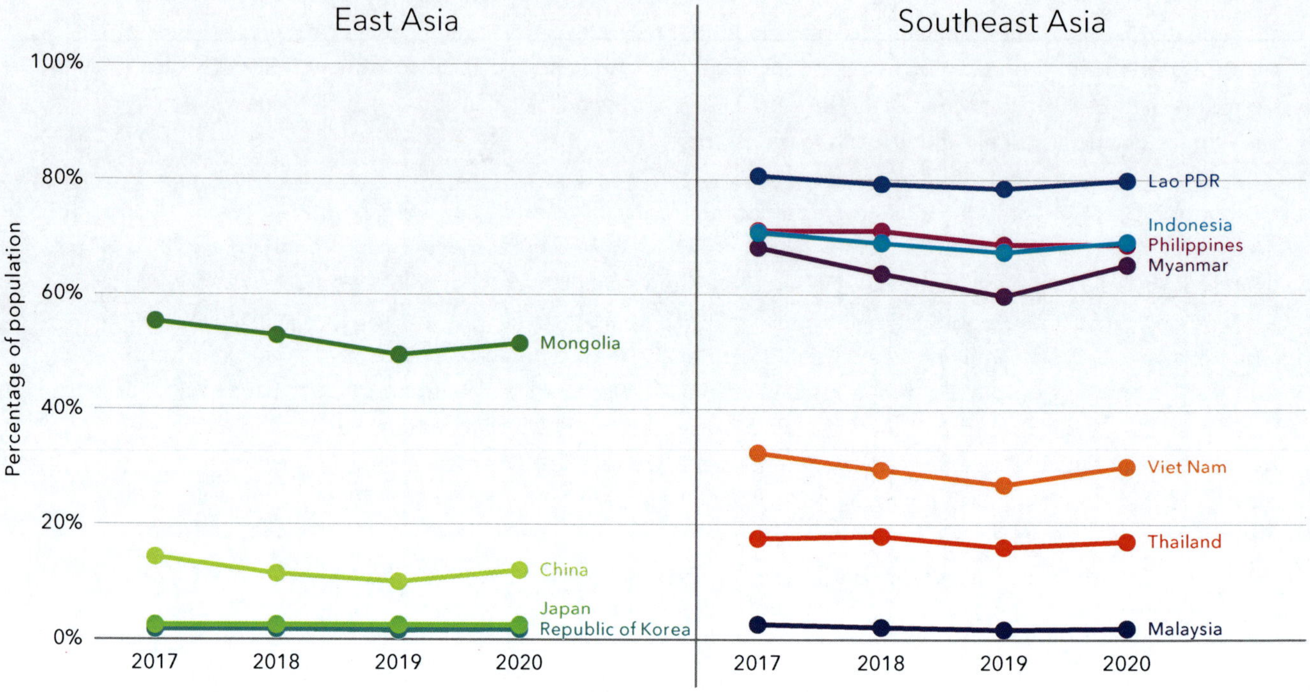

Source: Data from Food Systems Dashboard, accessed November 2023. www.foodsystemsdashboard.org

on less than US$3.65 per day (a key cut-off for poverty), representing millions of people and underscoring the challenge of food affordability in some countries.[27] In addition, shocks such as the COVID-19 pandemic have disproportionately affected ESEA because of the strong lockdown policies adopted and the large share of informal-sector workers in food systems, with the greatest impacts on marginalized populations, who faced both high food prices and lost livelihoods.[28]

Box 1 describes how some of these issues play out in two very different country contexts – China and Cambodia – and lead to different diet and nutrition outcomes, as well as distinct policy priorities. Other countries in the region fall somewhere between these two extremes.

OPTIONS FOR ACTION

Urbanization, income growth, and environmental changes in ESEA are occurring at a rapid pace, positioning the region both as an early-warning context for global shifts and as a potential model for policy responses that may be applicable elsewhere.

Food system surveys across the region consistently highlight several common food system challenges, most notably poor food standards; lack of consideration of diets and health in trade; and rising demand for healthier food, especially among wealthier and urbanizing populations,[29] as well as the insecure and risky livelihoods that continue to affect rural food producers. To address these issues, policies must consider the needs and preferences of diverse populations facing various food system issues; support the agency of the most marginalized producers and consumers; and strengthen regional cooperation to make diverse, healthy food available and accessible for all. Food systems, however, are often a blind spot for policymakers in ESEA and elsewhere. Sectoral policies in agriculture, economy, health, and other areas are often siloed, and decision-makers fail to consider their interconnections or combined effect on the diets and health of citizens. In addition, disaggregated data on different socioeconomic groups remain limited in many contexts.[30]

BOX 1 CASE STUDIES

Cambodia

Cambodia is among the world's smallest economies and remains largely rural. Its food system depends largely on traditional smallholder farmers, who are the major food producers and who focus predominantly on staple crops, seeking their own food security amid significant food imports. Some urban areas are expanding, along with modern fresh food and convenience retail chains. Agriculture contributes about 22 percent of gross domestic product (GDP) and employs a third of working-age adults (of whom 39 percent are women), but productivity growth in the sector is low.[a]

Diets in Cambodia are largely based on rice, roots, and tubers, which provide 69 percent of dietary energy.[b] Compared with the Southeast Asian average, Cambodian diets are low in fruits, vegetables, legumes, nuts, whole grains, and dairy, though they are relatively high in meat, fish, and sugar-sweetened beverages. Food and beverages account for 46 percent of average household expenditures (57 percent for the poorest), while a nutrient-adequate diet would cost 74 percent of an average household's income.[c] The most marginalized groups within Cambodia's food system – including Indigenous peoples, landless and tenant smallholder farmers, informal food system workers, and daily wage earners – are most affected by inadequate employment opportunities, limited land rights, and poor food security and nutrition outcomes.[d]

Beyond low incomes and a largely rural population, Cambodia's food system drivers include a high level of market liberalization, efforts to increase regional trade, and a relatively rich endowment of natural resources such as land and water. In contexts like this, policymakers are advised to address calorie and nutrient shortfalls through greater support to farmers and more diverse farming systems. Policymakers should also prioritize nutrition and health in regional food trade deals; food safety regulation (on-farm and in the retail sector); and steps to limit consumption of ultra-processed foods, such as taxes and regulation.[e]

China

China, one of the world's largest economies, has a complex food system geared both to feeding its huge population and to regional and global exports, and has made tremendous progress in reducing hunger in recent decades. However, current Chinese diets are characterized not only by an overconsumption of cereals and meat, accompanied by an insufficient intake of vegetables and fruits, but also by the heavy use of cooking oil and salt.[f] Average daily meat consumption reached 191 grams in 2023, approximately 2.6 times the amount recommended by the national dietary guidelines (the Chinese Food Guide Pagoda), and the average daily fat-to-energy ratio of food consumed is 34.6 percent, which exceeds the recommended limit of 30 percent.[g]

This dietary imbalance creates both health and environmental problems. In particular, overweight and obesity, along with major, chronic diet-related diseases, are becoming more prevalent. At the same time, the environmental burden of food consumption is growing, with CO_2 emissions expected to rise from 1.18 billion tons in 2020 to 1.28 billion tons by 2030.[h] Shifting Chinese dietary patterns toward a sustainable healthy diet is widely recognized as key to addressing these challenges. A complete shift in the current diet toward the national guidelines could avoid at least 1.15 million deaths and 425,000 premature deaths in China by 2030[i] and reduce CO_2 emissions by 146 million tons.[j]

China's government has initiated public campaigns to promote healthy diets, and more policy support is under consideration. Already, increased spending on agricultural research and development has increased the production of nutrition-enriched foods and facilitated access to healthier foods. Targeted interventions, such as the Nutrition Improvement Program, are promoting healthy diets for China's poorer regions. Chinese experts also recommend a strategic shift in investment and trade that emphasizes a nutrition-centric food supply both domestically and internationally.[k] In addition, social protection programs for low-income individuals could enhance their purchasing power and improve diet quality.[l]

Several policy responses can address these challenges:

- Promote engagement of nutrition and health representatives in trade negotiations, and inform trade negotiators of the food system implications of trade agreements.[31]

- Support small and marginalized food producers and promote diversified systems.[32] Initiatives for farmers can include better labor standards, inclusive rural development, and responsible investment in food and agriculture that supports farmers' livelihoods and diversified food production.[33] Diversified farming systems that move away from the existing rice-centric system can provide healthier food choices and also greater resilience to shocks such as COVID-19.[34] Given regional diversity, countries will need to address the particular barriers to better farm livelihoods that are relevant for their food systems, such as land tenure, access to extension for crops other than rice, and farmers' empowerment in engagement with buyers and contractors.

- Regulate food retail to limit sale of unhealthy foods and promote healthy foods, for example, through taxes and less preferential trade deals on ultra-processed foods and sugar-sweetened beverages[35] and through provision of healthy meals in public institutions (schools, hospitals) as well as in private sector workplaces.[36]

- Improve food safety through stronger implementation and enforcement of existing Association of Southeast Asian Nations (ASEAN) and national food safety policies, while protecting the livelihoods of informal food system workers.[37]

- Leverage strong traditional food cultures for healthier diets through (1) locally tailored dietary messaging to enhance nutrition literacy[38] and (2) locally adapted and environmentally sustainable food-based dietary guidelines that focus on local and regional production and trade, such as those recently released by China.[39]

- Strengthen social protection systems to (1) explicitly consider the ability to afford a healthy diet alongside other household expenditures and (2) connect the most nutritionally vulnerable groups to additional support services.

- Enhance data collection, particularly disaggregated by geography and population with an equity lens, for informed decision-making.

Raising the priority given to food and diets through advocacy and information sharing is crucial. Greater intraregional cooperation, such as within ASEAN, will be necessary to tackle issues of trade regulation and harmonization.[40] In addition, granting more autonomy to provinces or cities through careful decentralization can facilitate the creation of grounded, agile, and context-specific solutions.[41] All policies should consider equity and ensure that marginalized groups are not left behind.[42] Given the region's double burden of malnutrition, double-duty or multi-duty food system policies that address undernutrition and micronutrient deficiencies together with overnutrition need to be considered, as well as the synergies and trade-offs that these entail, including for the environment and sustainability.[43] Recommendations are available to help countries prioritize policy solutions that consider food systems, equity, and nutrition based on their particular context.[44] Ultimately, a proactive approach to food policy that is both integrative (considering synergies, trade-offs, and spillovers from multiple sectors) and inclusive (attentive to the welfare of the most marginalized stakeholders in food systems) is vital for healthy diets and the well-being of all in the region.

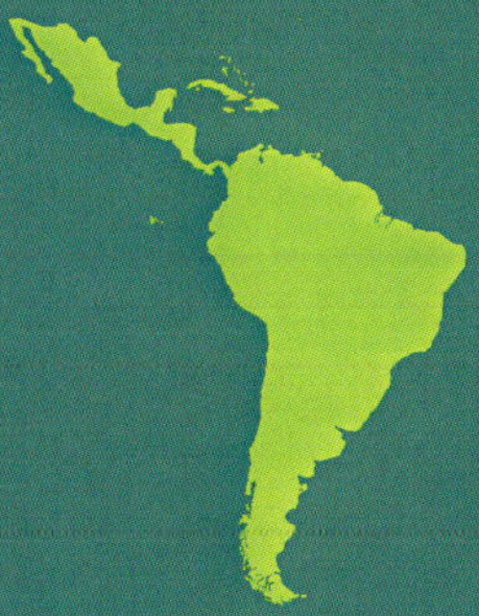

LATIN AMERICA AND THE CARIBBEAN

EUGENIO DÍAZ-BONILLA AND VALERIA PIÑEIRO

Eugenio Díaz-Bonilla is a visiting senior research fellow, Director General's Office, International Food Policy Research Institute (IFPRI), and special advisor, Inter-American Institute for Cooperation in Agriculture. **Valeria Piñeiro** is acting head, Latin America and the Caribbean, and senior research coordinator, Development Strategies and Governance Unit, IFPRI.

The nutrition transition in Latin America and the Caribbean (LAC) is well advanced compared with other developing regions, with high rates of urbanization and relatively higher incomes leading to an epidemic of obesity alongside persistent undernutrition and micronutrient deficiencies – known as the double burden of malnutrition. The great diversity of the region's countries – in terms of economic size and income levels – is reflected in the range and types of nutritional challenges they face.

Figure 1 compares four global indicators[1] with the averages in the LAC region: the prevalence of hunger (or undernourishment, the indicator used for Sustainable Development Goal 2.1.1); wasting (low weight-for-height) and stunting (low height-for-age) in children under five years of age; and poverty rates at the US$2.15 purchasing power parity (PPP) level, which indicates extreme poverty in the LAC region.

All four indicators in LAC are below the world averages. After showing some improvement from the early 2000s until about 2015, however, these indicators stagnated over the past decade as a result of several negative developments, most notably the end of the upward commodity cycle that had fueled growth in the region. In 2020, the COVID-19 pandemic and related responses led to an increase in all four indicators, and the subsequent shocks related to Russia's invasion of Ukraine and to climate challenges in different subregions within LAC have kept these levels relatively high. The most recent data show some improvement, but levels have not yet fallen to pre-COVID-19 numbers.[2] However, there are substantial differences across countries, such as the case of Haiti, where undernutrition and poverty rates are high.[3]

Dietary diversity and consumption of nutrient-rich foods, including fruits and vegetables, legumes, nuts, and animal-source foods (in moderation), contribute to health and are crucial to preventing maternal and child undernutrition and micronutrient deficiencies. For many people, however, healthy diets are unaffordable (see Chapter 4). Figure 2 compares the share of global and LAC

FIGURE 1 Indicators of hunger, undernutrition, and poverty, global and LAC, 2020–2022

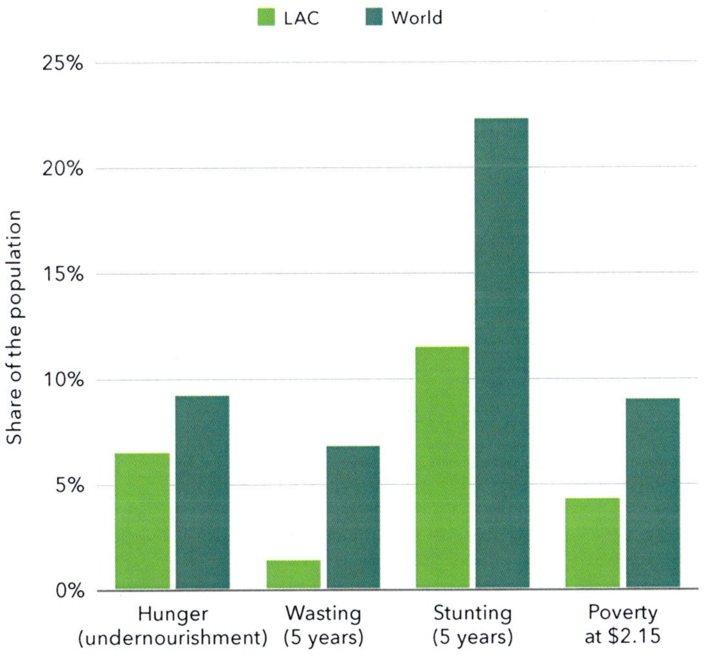

Source: Data on prevalence of hunger (undernourishment), wasting, and stunting in children from FAOSTAT; data on poverty from the World Bank's World Development Indicators, both accessed January 2024.

FIGURE 2 Share of global and LAC populations unable to afford a healthy diet, 2017–2021

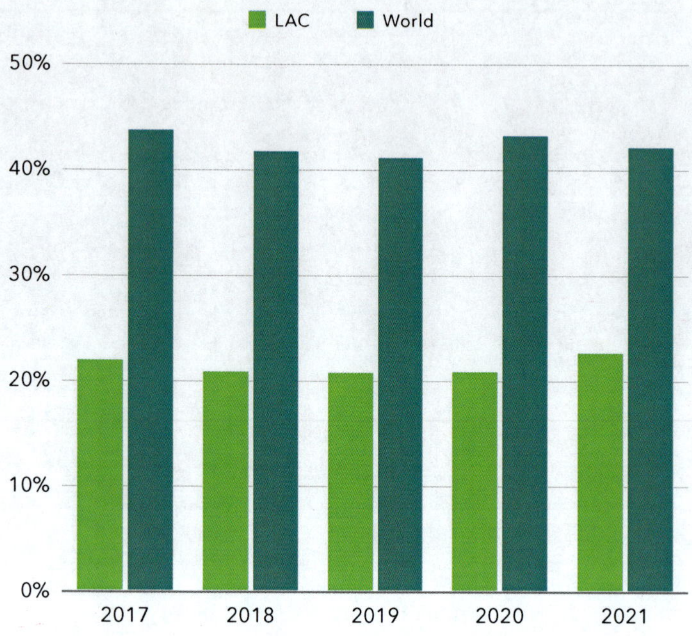

Source: Data from FAOSTAT, accessed January 2024.

populations who could not afford a healthy diet in recent years. While the LAC rate is well below the global average, at less than 23 percent in 2021, it is still high, and in several LAC countries it is much higher. Five countries (Belize, Haiti, Honduras, Jamaica, and Suriname) show levels above the world rate of more than 40 percent.[4]

Limited availability of the diverse foods needed for a healthy diet contributes to micronutrient deficiencies in the region. Figure 3 maps the number of major food groups for which national production is insufficient, with darker shades representing less diversity in production. In general, production is more diversified in LAC, with the exception of a few countries such as Venezuela, than in most of the developing world. However, low levels of intraregional trade mean that the region's population does not enjoy the full advantages of this diversity.

Obesity and overweight rates are higher in LAC than in other global regions. While obesity has been increasing globally, 24 percent of the adult

FIGURE 3 Number of food groups with insufficient national production

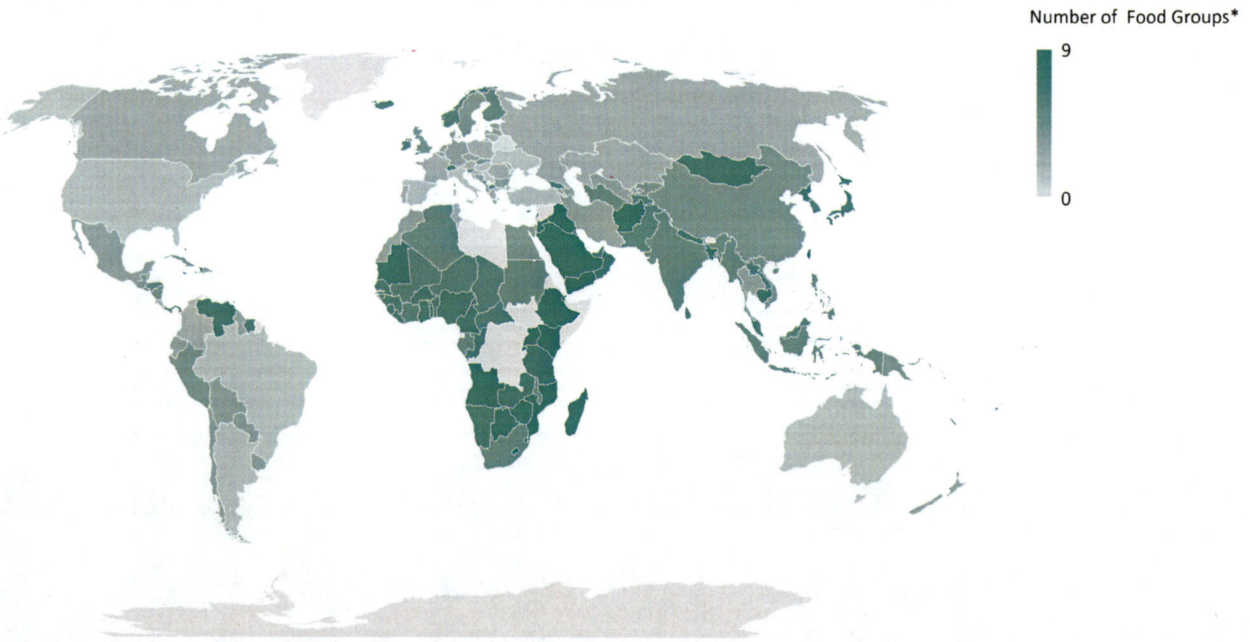

Source: D. Laborde Debucquet, V. Piñeiro, and J. Swinnen, "Tomorrow's Agri-food System: The Connections between Trade, Food Security, and Nutrition for a Sustainable Diet," in *Routledge Handbook of Sustainable Diets*, eds. K. Kevany and P. Prosperi (Routledge: 2022). Reproduced with permission of Informa UK Limited through PLSclear.

Note: The nine food groups are animal products (excluding dairy), milk, starches, legumes and beans, nuts and seeds, fruits, vegetables, vegetable oils, and sugar. This classification is more general than the one proposed by the EAT-Lancet report, allowing a degree of flexibility for substitution of foods at the national level. Numbers are adjusted for food loss and waste.

population in LAC was considered obese, compared with 13 percent worldwide, as of 2016. In addition, almost 8 percent of children under five years of age in LAC were considered overweight, compared with 5.5 percent globally. As a result, more people are suffering from obesity (110 million in 2016) in LAC than from hunger (43 million in 2022, using the prevalence of undernourishment).[5] Within LAC, obesity is most common in Argentina, Chile, Mexico, Uruguay, and some English-speaking Caribbean countries (all with a prevalence of about 28 percent or higher), while undernutrition is a larger problem in Haiti, Venezuela, and several countries in Central America.

WHAT CAN BE DONE?

The LAC region must address the double burden of malnutrition, including the associated economic and social costs, while also tackling the issues of accessibility and affordability of healthy diets. The region's heterogeneity affects the national extent of these problems, and each country will need to identify the set of policy solutions that best fits their particular context. Most will require a combination of demand- and supply-side responses, discussed in this section.

DEFINING THE PROBLEM

Public policy decisions must take a comprehensive view of the multiple malnutrition problems facing LAC countries. National programs for improving nutrition must start by defining the set of targets to address: undernutrition, micronutrient deficiencies, and/or obesity; access to and affordability of diverse and healthy diets; or a combination of these. Policies and programs must also clearly identify the groups of people affected and establish quantitative objectives for improved nutrition and the time frame for achieving them. This type of analysis will require broader and more frequent collection of basic information, which is lacking in many LAC countries. In particular, data on dietary diversity and anthropometric measures are needed, and should be standardized and collected uniformly in schools and health centers.

DEMAND-SIDE SOLUTIONS

SOCIAL SAFETY NETS. Undernutrition and lack of economic access to healthy and diverse diets are largely caused by poverty and inequality.[6] Of the 30 countries with the worst inequality indicators globally, approximately half are in the LAC region. LAC was a pioneer in the use of conditional cash transfers as a social safety net to combat poverty and inequality, and most LAC countries now have some variety of cash transfer program. But, given persistent problems of malnutrition and the high cost of nutritious diets, LAC countries need to expand program coverage and redesign their existing social protection programs, including the use of double- or multi-duty actions (Chapters 2 and 3).[7] With some estimates suggesting that up to half of the money for social safety nets goes to the non-poor, targeting must be improved.[8] Program design and operation also need to be expanded to include components for productivity, nutrition, and the environment; to better integrate emergency programs with more permanent ones to create shock-responsive safety nets;[9] and to improve other operational aspects, such as developing detailed registries of beneficiaries. School meal programs are among the region's most important social protection programs (see Chapter 3). Given their effectiveness, school-based programs should be expanded and made more nutrition sensitive. In some countries, including Brazil, school feeding interventions have been linked to food procurement programs that work with small farmers, thus adding regional economic multiplier effects.

INCREASING DEMAND FOR HEALTHY FOODS. The nutrition transition in LAC is closely related to the increased availability of cheap diets heavy in calories but lacking in necessary nutrients, as well as to more sedentary lives and marketing of ultra-processed foods high in sugar, fat, and salt. The problem has been exacerbated by poverty and the impact of COVID-19, which led to the consumption of cheaper, less healthy diets as healthier options became more expensive.[10] While access to healthy diets can be addressed to some extent through social protection programs, combating obesity and micronutrient deficiencies will require additional policy tools.

Most prominently, interventions are needed to increase demand for healthy foods, reduce demand for ultra-processed foods and sugar-sweetened beverages, and make food environments more conducive to healthy food choices (see Chapters 3 and 5). These include the use of taxes and/or the elimination of subsidies for less nutritious food products; subsidies and support for the production of healthy foods to increase availability and lower costs (see Chapter 6); and subsidies to help vulnerable populations access healthy diets.

The LAC region has been a leader in addressing the growing consumption of ultra-processed foods through stricter regulations for labeling and information requirements to inform consumers' food choices (see Chapter 5), including on the types and amounts of some potentially unhealthy ingredients. For example, Chile has established a system of front-of-package labeling using black hexagons (acting as stop signs) to inform consumers about excess calories, salt, sugar, and fats. Evidence so far has shown that consumer awareness increased in Chile, and inclusion of those products in school lunches decreased, but behavior changes have been less pronounced (see Chapter 5 for a longer discussion).[11] Adoption of taxes on sugar-sweetened beverages in several LAC countries also shows potential for reducing consumption (see Chapters 5 and 8).[12] These policies also need to consider gender and nutrition, the roles played by men and women in food systems, and the different impacts they experience. For example, obesity in LAC affects far more women (28 percent as of 2016) than men (20 percent).

In addition to these policies focused on food systems, other approaches may be needed to control obesity, such as infrastructure for sports and exercise, alternative transportation methods, or behavioral nudges to avoid sedentary lifestyles.

SUPPLY-SIDE SOLUTIONS

PRODUCTION OF HEALTHY AND DIVERSIFIED PRODUCTS. Making healthy diets more accessible and affordable will require increasing the production and diversity of healthy food in the region, which will help to stabilize and even reduce prices for consumers. Greater investments in agricultural R&D are needed for fruits, vegetables, legumes, and nuts (see Chapters 4 and 6). Promotion of local "orphan" crops that have been marginalized and underutilized would also help, as the example of the recent expansion of quinoa in Bolivia and Peru has shown.[13] Support to family farms and home gardens to diversify their production and link them to short supply chains could both increase household incomes and increase the local affordability of healthy diets (see Chapter 3).[14] Public procurement schemes also need to consider gender aspects: for instance, Brazil's Food Acquisition Program, created in 2003, added a requirement in 2011 that a minimum of 40 percent of its suppliers be women.

THE ROLE OF TRADE. Diversity in production and availability of healthy foods for consumption differ in large part due to the key role of trade (see Chapter 4).[15] A global study using data for 151 countries has found a positive correlation between trade openness and key indicators of dietary health, such as dietary energy supply, diversity, and overall quality.[16] Moreover, adherence to science-based standards and regulations in food trade can further bolster food safety measures, ensuring the integrity of traded food products. By facilitating year-round access to a diverse range of food products, trade benefits countries with distinct seasonal conditions, serving as a crucial mechanism for mitigating variability and volatility in food supply. This suggests that differentiated strategies are needed to address nutritional deficiencies related to the limited availability and affordability of nutritious foods. For instance, while low-income nations may prioritize diversifying domestic production, middle- and high-income countries could leverage their economic resources to access a wider array of nutritional options through international markets. Strengthening intraregional trade in LAC, which is relatively low compared with other regions, could also contribute to more diversified and affordable diets.[17]

In sum, LAC faces the complex challenge of identifying the most effective policies and standards associated with developing efficient and balanced national food systems that can meet the growing demand for food while ensuring environmental sustainability, food safety, nutritional quality, and economic and social sustainability. Clearly defining objectives, strengthening social protection programs, addressing the drivers of obesity and overweight, and increasing the availability and affordability of nutritious foods, including through trade, will all contribute to more sustainable healthy diets in the region, while maintaining and expanding the crucial role LAC plays in global food security and nutrition.

Notes

GLOSSARY

1 T. Beal, C.D. Gardner, M. Herrero, L.L. Iannotti, L. Merbold, S. Nordhagen, and A. Mottet, "Friend or Foe? The Role of Animal-Source Foods in Healthy and Environmentally Sustainable Diets," *The Journal of Nutrition* 153, 2 (2023): 409-425.

2 World Health Organization (WHO), "Malnutrition," March 1, 2024, 2024. https://www.who.int/news-room/fact-sheets/detail/malnutrition

3 WHO, *The Double Burden of Malnutrition: Policy Brief*, fact sheet (Geneva: 2017).

4 C. Hawkes, M.T. Ruel, L. Salm, B. Sinclair, and F. Branca, "Double-Duty Actions: Seizing Programme and Policy Opportunities to Address Malnutrition in All Its Forms," *Lancet* 395, 10218 (2020): 142-155.

5 WHO, "Malnutrition," March 1, 2024, update. https://www.who.int/news-room/fact-sheets/detail/malnutrition

6 C.A. Monteiro, G. Cannon, R.B. Levy, et al., "Ultra-Processed Foods: What They Are and How to Identify Them," *Public Health Nutrition* 22, 5 (2019): 936-941.

7 Food and Agriculture Organization of the United Nations and WHO, *Sustainable Healthy Diets–Guiding Principles* (Rome: 2019).

CHAPTER 1

1 Global Diet Quality Project, *Measuring What the World Eats: Insights from a New Approach* (Geneva: GAIN; Boston, MA: Harvard T.H. Chan School of Public Health, Department of Global Health and Population, 2022).

2 M. Crippa, E. Solazzo, D. Guizzardi, F. Monforti-Ferrario, F.N. Tubiello, and A. Leip. "Food Systems are Responsible for a Third of Global Anthropogenic GHG Emissions." *Nature Food* 2, 3 (2021): 198-209.

3 Food and Agriculture Organization of the United Nations (FAO) and World Health Organization (WHO), *Sustainable Healthy Diets - Guiding Principles* (Rome: FAO and WHO, 2019).

4 High Level Panel of Experts on Food Security and Nutrition of the Committee on World Food Security (HLPE), *Food Security and Nutrition: Building a Global Narrative Towards 2030* (Rome: 2020).

5 FAO and WHO, *Sustainable Healthy Diets - Guiding Principles* (Rome: FAO, 2019).

6 FAO, Food-Based Dietary Guidelines, www.fao.org/nutrition/education/food-based-dietary-guidelines

7 A. Webb Girard, E. Waugh, S. Sawyer, L. Golding, and U. Ramakrishnan, "A Scoping Review of Social-Behaviour Change Techniques Applied in Complementary Feeding Interventions," *Maternal & Child Nutrition* 16, 1 (2020): e12882.

8 S.S. Kim, P.H. Nguyen, L.M. Tran, S. Alayon, P. Menon, and E.A. Frongillo, "Different Combinations of Behavior Change Interventions and Frequencies of Interpersonal Contacts Are Associated with Infant and Young Child Feeding Practices in Bangladesh, Ethiopia, and Vietnam," *Current Developments in Nutrition* 4, 2 (2020): nzz140.

9 A. Ahmed, F. Coleman, J. Ghostlaw, et al., "Increasing Production Diversity and Diet Quality: Evidence from Bangladesh," *American Journal of Agricultural Economics*, in print, 2023. https://doi.org/10.1111/ajae.12427

10 D.K. Olney, A. Gelli, N. Kumar, H. Alderman, A. Go, and A. Raza, "Social Assistance Programme Impacts on Women's and Children's Diets and Nutritional Status," *Maternal & Child Nutrition* 18, 4 (2022): e13378.

11 D.D. Headey, K. Hirvonen, and H. Alderman, "Estimating the Cost and Affordability of Healthy Diets: How Much Do Methods Matter?" IFPRI Discussion Paper 2179, IFPRI, Washington, DC, 2023.

12 See calculations in Chapter 5 and K. Hirvonen, Y. Bai, D.D. Headey, and W.A. Masters, "Affordability of the EAT-Lancet Reference Diet: A Global Analysis," *Lancet Global Health* 8, 1 (2020): e59-e66; D.D. Headey, K. Hirvonen, and H. Alderman, "Estimating the Cost and Affordability of Healthy Diets: How Much Do Methods Matter?" IFPRI Discussion Paper 2179, IFPRI, Washington, DC, 2023.

13 O. Ecker, H. Alderman, A.R. Comstock, D.D. Headey, K. Mahrt, and A. Pradesha, "Mitigating Poverty and Undernutrition through Social Protection: A Simulation Analysis of the COVID-19 Pandemic in Bangladesh and Myanmar," *Applied Economic Perspectives and Policy* 45, 4 (2023): 2034-2055.

14 A. Ahmed, J. Hoddinott, and S. Roy, "Food Transfers, Cash Transfers, Behavior Change Communication and Child Nutrition: Evidence from Bangladesh," IFPRI Discussion Paper 1868, IFPRI, Washington, DC, 2019; E.M. Maffioli, D.D. Headey, I. Lambrecht, T.Z. Oo, and N.T. Zaw, "A Prepandemic Nutrition-Sensitive Social Protection Program Has Sustained Benefits for Food Security and Diet Diversity in Myanmar during a Severe Economic Crisis," *The Journal of Nutrition* 153, 4 (2023): 1052-1062.

15 A. Alcorta, A. Porta, A. Tárrega, M.D. Alvarez, and M.P. Vaquero, "Foods for Plant-Based Diets: Challenges and Innovations," *Foods* 10, 2 (2021): 293; T. Beal, F. Ortenzi, and J. Fanzo, "Estimated Micronutrient Shortfalls of the EAT-Lancet Planetary Health Diet," *Lancet Planetary Health* 7, 3 (2023): e233-e237.

16 FAO, International Fund for Agricultural Development (IFAD), UNICEF, World Food Programme (WFP), and WHO, *The State of Food Security and Nutrition in the World 2020* (Rome: FAO, 2020).

17 P.L. Pingali, "Green Revolution: Impacts, Limits, and the Path Ahead," *Proceedings of the National Academy of Sciences* 109, 31 (2012): 12302-12308.

18 A.Z. Alem, Y. Yeshaw, A.M. Liyew, et al., "Double Burden of Malnutrition and Its Associated Factors among Women in Low and Middle Income Countries: Findings from 52 Nationally Representative Data," *BMC Public Health* 23, 1 (2023): 1479.

19 E.C. Keats, LM. Neufeld, G.S. Garrett, M.N.N. Mbuya, and Z.A. Bhutta, "Improved Micronutrient Status and Health Outcomes in Low- and Middle-Income Countries Following Large-Scale Fortification: Evidence from a Systematic Review and Meta-Analysis," *American Journal of Clinical Nutrition* 109, 6 (2019): 1696-1708.

20 A. Mottet, C. de Haan, A. Falcucci, G. Tempio, C. Opio, and P. Gerber, "Livestock: On Our Plates or Eating at Our Table? A New Analysis of the Feed/Food Debate," *Global Food Security* 14 (2017): 1-8.

21 WHO, *Red and Processed Meat in the Context of Health and the Environment: Many Shades of Red and Green*, Information Brief (Geneva: 2023); IARC Working Group on the Evaluation of Carcinogenic Risks to Humans, *Red Meat and Processed Meat - IARC Monographs on the Evaluation of Carcinogenic Risks to Humans* (Lyon, France: IARC, 2018).

22 Pan American Health Organization (PAHO) and WHO, *Guiding Principles for Complementary Feeding of the Breastfed Child* (Washington, DC: 2003).

23 FAO and Intergovernmental Technical Panel on Soils (ITPS), *Status of the World's Soil Resources (SWSR) - Main Report* (Rome: 2015); N. Ramankutty, Z. Mehrabi, K. Waha, L. Jarvis, C. Kremen, M. Herrero, and L.H. Rieseberg, "Trends in Global Agricultural Land Use: Implications for Environmental Health and Food Security," *Annual Review of Plant Biology* 69 (2018): 789-815.

24 J.A. Painter, R.M. Hoekstra, T. Ayers, R.V. Tauxe, C.R. Braden, F.J. Angulo, and P.M. Griffin, "Attribution of Foodborne Illnesses, Hospitalizations, and Deaths to Food Commodities by Using Outbreak Data, United States, 1998-2008," *Emerging Infectious Diseases* 19, 3 (2013): 407-415.

25 J. Fanzo, L. Haddad, K.R. Schneider, et al., "Viewpoint: Rigorous Monitoring Is Necessary to Guide Food System Transformation in the Countdown to the 2030 Global Goals," *Food Policy* 104 (2021): 102163; K.R. Schneider, J. Fanzo, L. Haddad, et al., "The State of Food Systems Worldwide in the Countdown to 2030," *Nature Food* 4, 12 (2023): 1090-1110.

26 J.K. Hanson and R. Sigman, "Leviathan's Latent Dimensions: Measuring State Capacity for Comparative Political Research," *Journal of Politics* 83, 4 (2021): 1495-1510; P. Evans, *Embedded Autonomy: States and Industrial Transformation* (Princeton, NJ: Princeton University Press, 1995); A. Kohli, *State-Directed Development: Political Power and Industrialization in the Global Periphery* (New York: Cambridge University Press, 2004).

27 D. Pomeranz and J. Vila-Belda, "Taking State-Capacity Research to the Field: Insights from Collaborations with Tax Authorities," *Annual Review of Economics* 11, 1 (2019): 755-781; J. Weigel, "The Participation Dividend of Taxation: How Citizens in Congo Engage More with the State When It Tries to Tax Them," *Quarterly Journal of Economics* 134, 4 (2020): 1849-1903.

28 A. Buyse, "Squeezing Civic Space: Restrictions on Civil Society Organizations and the Linkages with Human Rights," *The International Journal of Human Rights* 22, 8 (2018): 966-988; D. Resnick and S. Deshpande, "Illiberal Democracy and Nutrition Advocacy," *Development Policy Review* 41, 6 (2023): e12726.

29 M. Gautam, D. Laborde, A. Mamun, W. Martin, V. Piñeiro, and R. Vos, *Repurposing Agricultural Policies and Support: Options to Transform Agriculture and Food Systems for Better Health of People, Economies and the Planet*, Technical Report (Washington, DC: World Bank and IFPRI, 2022).

30 C. Zorbas, D. Resnick, E. Jones, et al., "From Promises to Action: Analyzing Global Commitments on Food Security and Diets Since 2015," IFPRI Discussion Paper 2238, IFPRI, Washington, DC, 2024.

31 L.M. Neufeld, S. Nordhagen, J.L. Leroy, et al., "Food Systems Interventions for Nutrition: Lessons from 6 Program Evaluations in Africa and South Asia," *The Journal of Nutrition*, April 4, 2024, online preprint.

BOX 1

a Food and Agriculture Organization of the United Nations (FAO), "Hunger and Food Insecurity," accessed April 1, 2024. www.fao.org/hunger/en/

b Our World in Data, Micronutrient Deficiency, accessed April 1, 2024. https://ourworldindata.org/micronutrient-deficiency

c FAO, International Fund for Agricultural Development (IFAD), UNICEF, World Food Programme (WFP), and World Health Organization (WHO), *The State of Food Security and Nutrition in the World 2020* (Rome: FAO, 2020).

d WHO, "Obesity and Overweight," accessed April 1, 2024. www.who.int/en/news-room/fact-sheets/detail/obesity-and-overweight

e F. Branca, A. Lartey, S. Oenema, et al., "Transforming the Food System to Fight Non-communicable Diseases," *BMJ* 364 (2019): l296.

f GBD 2017 Causes of Death Collaborators, "Global, Regional, and National Age-Sex-Specific Mortality for 282 Causes of Death in 195 Countries and Territories, 1980-2017: A Systematic Analysis for the Global Burden of Disease Study 2017," *Lancet Global Health Metrics* 392, 10159 (2018): 1736-1788.

g GBD 2017 Diet Collaborators, "Health Effects of Dietary Risks in 195 Countries, 1990-12017: A Systematic Analysis for the Global Burden of Disease Study 2017," *Lancet* 393, 10184 (2019): 1958-1972.

BOX 2

a Food and Agriculture Organization of the United Nations, "Hunger and Food Insecurity," accessed April 1 2024. www.fao.org/hunger/en/; Our World in Data, Micronutrient Deficiency, accessed April 1, 2024. https://ourworldindata.org/micronutrient-deficiency

b L. Depenbusch, P. Schreinemachers, S. Brown, and R. Roothaert, "Impact and Distributional Effects of a Home Garden and Nutrition Intervention in Cambodia," *Food Security* 14 (2022): 865-881; D.K. Olney, A. Gelli, N. Kumar, H. Alderman, A. Go, and A. Raza, "Social Assistance Programme Impacts on Women's and Children's Diets and Nutritional Status," *Maternal & Child Nutrition* 18, 4 (2022): e13378; A.C. Palmer, K. Healy, M.A. Barffour, et al., "Provitamin A Carotenoid-Biofortified Maize Consumption Increases Pupillary Responsiveness among Zambian Children in a Randomized Controlled Trial," *The Journal of Nutrition* 146, 12 (2016): 2551-2558; C. Hotz, C. Loechl, A. Lubowa, et al., "Introduction of B-carotene-rich Orange Sweet Potato in Rural Uganda Resulted in Increased Vitamin A Intakes among Children and Women and Improved Vitamin A Status among Children," *The Journal of Nutrition* 142, 10 (2012): 1871-1880; J.W. Low, M. Arimond, N. Osman, B. Cunguara, F. Zano, and D. Tschirley, "A Food-Based Approach Introducing Orange-Fleshed Sweet Potatoes Increased Vitamin A Intake and Serum Retinol Concentrations in Young Children in Rural Mozambique," *The Journal of Nutrition* 137, 5 (2007): 1320-1327; P.J. Van Jaarsveld, M. Faber, S.A. Tanumihardjo, P. Nestel, C.J. Lombard, and A.J.S. Benadé, "B-carotene-rich Orange-Fleshed Sweet Potato Improves the Vitamin A Status of Primary School Children Assessed with the Modified-Relative-Dose-Response Test," *The American Journal of Clinical Nutrition* 81, 5 (2005): 1080-1087; R. Engle-Stone, M. Nankap, A.O. Ndjebayi, et al., "Iron, Zinc, Folate, and Vitamin B-12 Status Increased among Women and Children in Yaoundé and Douala, Cameroon, 1 Year after Introducing Fortified Wheat Flour," *The Journal of Nutrition* 147, 7 (2017): 1426-1436; F. Rohner, M. Leyvraz, A.G. Konan, et al., "The Potential of Food Fortification to Add Micronutrients in Young Children and Women of Reproductive Age: Findings from a Cross-Sectional Survey in Abidjan, Côte d'Ivoire," *PLoS ONE* 11, 7 (2016): e0158552; D.K. Olney, L. Bliznashka, A. Pedehombga, A. Dillon, M.T. Ruel, and J. Heckert, "A 2-Year Integrated Agriculture and Nutrition Program Targeted to Mothers of Young Children in Burkina Faso Reduces Underweight among Mothers and Increases Their Empowerment: A Cluster-Randomized Controlled Trial," *The Journal of Nutrition* 146 (2016): 1109-1117.

BOX 3

a C.A. Monteiro, G. Cannon, R.B. Levy, et al., "Ultra-processed Foods: What They Are and How to Identify Them," *Public Health Nutrition* 22, 5 (2019): 936-941.

BOX 4

a See IFPRI's work on trade, export restrictions, and food price impacts during the COVID-19 pandemic (https://www.ifpri.org/covid-19) and related to the Russia-Ukraine War (https://www.ifpri.org/spotlight/food-prices-war-ukraine).

b J. Glauber, D. Laborde, A. Mamun, E. Olivetti, and V. Piñero, "MC12: How to Make the WTO Relevant in the Middle of a Food Price Crisis," IFPRI Blog, June 11, 2022.

c Food and Agriculture Organization of the United Nations (FAO), International Fund for Agricultural Development, UNICEF, World Food Programme, The State of Food Security and Nutrition in the World 2023: Urbanization, Agrifood Systems Transformation and Healthy Diets Across the Rural-Urban Continuum (Rome: FAO, 2023).

CHAPTER 2

1 S. Gillespie and J. Harris, "How Nutrition Improves: Half a Century of Understanding and Responding to the Problem of Malnutrition," in *Nourishing Millions: Stories of Change in Nutrition*, eds. S. Gillespie, J. Hodge, S. Yosef, and R. Pandya-Lorch, 1-13 (Washington, DC: IFPRI, 2016).

2 United Nations (UN), "The Food Systems Summit," New York, September 23, 2021.

3 High Level Panel of Experts (HLPE), *Food Security and Nutrition: Building a Global Narrative Towards 2030*, A report by the High Level Panel of Experts on Food Security and Nutrition of the Committee on World Food Security (Rome: FAO, 2020).

4 UN-Nutrition, "The Coalition on Action for Healthy Diets from Sustainable Food Systems for Children and All," accessed March 25, 2024. https://www.unnutrition.org/coalition-action-healthy-diets-sustainable-food-systems-children-and-all-hdsfs

5 H.E. Bouis and R.M. Welch, "Biofortification: A Sustainable Agricultural Strategy for Reducing Micronutrient Malnutrition in the Global South," *Crop Science* 50 (2010): S20-S32.

6 Council for Agricultural Science and Technology (CAST), "Food Biofortification: Reaping the Benefits of Science to Overcome Hidden Hunger," CAST Issue Paper No. 69, CAST, Ames, Iowa, 2020.

7 M.T. Ruel, *Can Food-Based Strategies Help Reduce Vitamin A and Iron Deficiencies? A Review of Recent Evidence* (Washington, DC: IFPRI, 2001); P.R. Berti, J. Krasevec, and S. FitzGerald, "A Review of the Effectiveness of Agriculture Interventions in Improving Nutrition Outcomes," *Public Health Nutrition* 7, 5 (2004): 599-609; C. Hawkes and M.T. Ruel, *From Agriculture to Nutrition: Pathways, Synergies and Outcomes*, Agricultural and Rural Development Note No. 40 (Washington, DC: World Bank 2007); E. Masset, L. Haddad, A. Cornelius, and J. Isaza-Castro, "Effectiveness of Agricultural Interventions that Aim to Improve Nutritional Status of Children: Systematic Review," *BMJ* 344 (2012): d8222; A. Webb-Girard, J.L. Self, C. McAuliffe, and O. Olude, "The Effects of Household Food Production Strategies on the Health and Nutrition Outcomes of Women and Young Children: A Systematic Review," *Paediatric and Perinatal Epidemiology* 26, S1 (2012): 205-222; M.T. Ruel and H. Alderman, "Nutrition-Sensitive Interventions and Programmes: How Can They Help to Accelerate Progress in Improving Maternal and Child Nutrition?" *Lancet* 382, 9891 (2013): 536-551; J. Leroy and E. Frongillo, "Can Interventions to Promote Animal Production Ameliorate Undernutrition?" *The Journal of Nutrition* 137, 10 (2007): 2311-2316; J.L. Leroy, M. Ruel, E. Verhofstadt, and D.K. Olney, "The Micronutrient Impact of Multisectoral Programs Focusing on Nutrition: Examples from Conditional Cash Transfer, Microcredit with Education, and Agricultural Programs," paper presented at the *Micronutrient Forum*, 2008.

8 M.T. Ruel, A.R. Quisumbing, and M. Balagamwala, "Nutrition-Sensitive Agriculture: What Have We Learned So Far?" *Global Food Security* 17 (2018): 128-153; A. Margolies, C.G. Kemp, E.M. Choo, C. Levin, D. Olney, N. Kumar, A. Go, H. Alderman, and A. Gelli, "Nutrition-Sensitive Agriculture Programs Increase Dietary Diversity in Children Under 5 Years: A Review and Meta-Analysis," *Journal of Global Health* 12 (2022): 08001; I.K. Sharma, S. Di Prima, D. Essink, and J.E.W. Broerse, "Nutrition-Sensitive Agriculture: A Systematic Review of Impact Pathways to Nutrition Outcomes," *Advances in Nutrition* 12, 1 (2021): 251-275.

9 M.T. Ruel, A.R. Quisumbing, and M. Balagamwala, "Nutrition-Sensitive Agriculture: What Have We Learned So Far?" *Global Food Security* 17 (2018): 128-153; I.K. Sharma, S. Di Prima, D. Essink, and J.E.W. Broerse, "Nutrition-Sensitive Agriculture: A Systematic Review of Impact Pathways to Nutrition Outcomes," *Advances in Nutrition* 12, 1 (2021): 251-275.

10 C. Hawkes, J. Harris, and S. Gillespie, "Changing Diets: Urbanization and the Nutrition Transition," in *2017 Global Food Policy Report*, Chapter 4, 34-41 (Washington, DC: IFPRI, 2017).

11 C. Hawkes, J. Harris, and S. Gillespie, "Changing Diets: Urbanization and the Nutrition Transition," in *2017 Global Food Policy Report*, Chapter 4, 34-41 (Washington, DC: IFPRI, 2017); B.M. Popkin, C. Corvalan, and L.M. Grummer-Strawn, "Dynamics of the Double Burden of Malnutrition and the Changing Nutrition Reality," *Lancet* 395, 10217 (2020): 65-74; P. Baker, P. Machado, T. Santos, et al., "Ultra-Processed Foods and the Nutrition Transition: Global, Regional and National Trends, Food Systems Transformations and Political Economy Drivers," *Obesity Reviews* 21, 12 (2020): e13126; G. Pagliai, M. Dinu, M.P. Madarena, M. Bonaccio, L. Iacoviello, and F. Sofi, "Consumption of Ultra-processed Foods and Health Status: A Systematic Review and Meta-analysis," *British Journal of Nutrition* 125, 3 (2021): 308-318; M.T. Ruel, J.L. Leroy, O. Ecker, M.A. Hernandez, D. Resnick, and J. Thurlow, "Urban Food Systems and Diets, Nutrition and Health of the Poor: Challenges, Opportunities, and Research Gaps," in *Handbook on Urban Food Security in the Global South*, eds. J. Crush, B. Frayne, and G. Hawsom, Chapter 19, 380-396. (Cheltenham, UK: Edward Elgar Publishing, 2020).

12 P. Baker, P. Machado, T. Santos, et al., "Ultra-processed Foods and the Nutrition Transition: Global, Regional and National Trends, Food Systems Transformations and Political Economy Drivers," *Obesity Reviews* 21, 12 (2020): e13126; G. Pagliai, M. Dinu, M.P. Madarena, M. Bonaccio, L. Iacoviello, and F. Sofi, "Consumption of Ultra-processed Foods and Health Status: A Systematic Review and Meta-analysis," *British Journal of Nutrition* 125, 3 (2021): 308-318.

13 I.D. Brouwer, M.J. van Liere, A. de Brauw, et al., "Reverse Thinking: Taking a Healthy Diet Perspective Towards Food Systems Transformations," *Food Security* 13 (2021): 1497-1523.

14 S.D. Nguyen, "Improving Vietnamese Diets: Balancing Multiple Sustainability Domains," PhD thesis, Wageningen University, Netherlands, 2024.

15 World Health Organization (WHO), *WHO Guideline for Complementary Feeding of Infants and Young Children 6-23 Months of Age* (Geneva: 2023); WHO, *Guideline: Implementing Effective Actions for Improving*

Adolescent Nutrition (Geneva: 2018). WHO, *A Healthy Diet Sustainably Produced*, Information Sheet (Geneva: 2018).

16 T.C. Wallace, R.L. Bailey, J.B. Blumberg, et al., "Fruits, Vegetables, and Health: A Comprehensive Narrative, Umbrella Review of the Science and Recommendations for Enhanced Public Policy to Improve Intake," *Critical Reviews in Food Science Nutrition* 60, 13 (2020): 2174-2211; GBD 2017 Diet Collaborators, "Health Effects of Dietary Risks in 195 Countries, 1990-2017: A Systematic Analysis for the Global Burden of Disease Study 2017," *Lancet* 393, 10184 (2019): 1958-1972.

17 A. Kalmpourtzidou, A. Eilander, and E.F. Talsma, "Global Vegetable Intake and Supply Compared to Recommendations: A Systematic Review," *Nutrients* 12, 6 (2020): 1558.

18 D.D. Headey, O. Ecker, A.R. Comstock, and M.T. Ruel, "Poverty, Price and Preference Barriers to Improving Diets in Sub-Saharan Africa," *Global Food Security* 36 (2023): 100664.

19 A. Muhammad, A. D'Souza, B. Meade, R. Micha, and D. Mozaffarian, "How Income and Food Prices Influence Global Dietary Intakes by Age and Sex: Evidence from 164 Countries," *BMJ Global Health* 2, 3 (2017): e000184.

20 W. Willett, J. Rockström, B. Loken, et al., "Food in the Anthropocene: The EAT-Lancet Commission on Healthy Diets from Sustainable Food Systems," *Lancet* 393, 10170 (2019): 447-492.

21 P. Baker, P. Machado, T. Santos, et al., "Ultra-processed Foods and the Nutrition Transition: Global, Regional and National Trends, Food Systems Transformations and Political Economy Drivers," *Obesity Reviews* 21, 12 (2020): e13126; G. Pagliai, M. Dinu, M.P. Madarena, M. Bonaccio, L. Iacoviello, and F. Sofi, "Consumption of Ultra-processed Foods and Health Status: A Systematic Review and Meta-analysis," *British Journal of Nutrition* 125, 3 (2021): 308-318; M.A. Lane, E. Gamage, S. Du, et al., "Ultra-processed Food Exposure and Adverse Health Outcomes: Umbrella Review of Epidemiological Meta-analyses," *BMJ* 384 (2024): e077310.

22 M.J. Gibney, C.G. Forde, D. Mullally, and E.R. Gibney, "Ultra-processed Foods in Human Health: A Critical Appraisal," *The American Journal of Clinical Nutrition* 106, 3 (2017): 717-724.

23 Food and Agriculture Organization of the United Nations (FAO), *Food Systems-Based Dietary Guidelines: An Overview* (Rome: 2024).

24 M.T. Ruel and J. Fanzo, "Nutrition and Climate Change: Shifting to Sustainable Healthy Diets," in *2022 Global Food Policy Report: Climate Change and Food Systems*, 72-81 (Washington, DC: IFPRI, 2022); J. Fanzo, C. Davis, R. McLaren, and J. Choufani, "The Effect of Climate Change across Food Systems: Implications for Nutrition Outcomes," *Global Food Security* 18 (2018): 12-19.

25 V. Owino, C. Kumwenda, B. Ekesa, M.E. Parker, L. Ewoldt, N. Roos, W.T. Lee, and D. Tome, "The Impact of Climate Change on Food Systems, Diet Quality, Nutrition, and Health Outcomes: A Narrative Review," *Frontiers in Climate* 4 (2022): 941842.

26 E.O. Verger, M. Savy, Y. Martin-Prével, et al., *Healthy Diet Metrics: A Suitability Assessment of Indicators for Global and National Monitoring Purposes* (Rome: FAO and WHO, 2023).

27 Intake, *The Intake4Earth App: An Invitation to Collect Data on the Environmental Impact of Diets* (Washington, DC: Intake, 2022).

28 WHO, "Healthy Diets Monitoring Initiative (HDMI)," accessed March 25, 2024. https://www.who.int/groups/who-unicef-technical-expert-advisory-group-on-nutrition-monitoring/healthy-diets-monitoring-initiative

29 FAO, "FAO/WHO GIFT | Global Individual Food Consumption Data Tool," accessed March 25, 2024. https://www.fao.org/gift-individual-food-consumption/en/

30 Intake, "What We Do," accessed March 25, 2024. https://www.intake.org/what-we-do

31 Food Systems Dashboard, "Food Systems Dashboard," accessed March 25, 2024. www.foodsystemsdashboard.org

32 K.R. Schneider, J. Fanzo, L. Haddad, et al., "The State of Food Systems Worldwide in the Countdown to 2030," *Nature Food* 4 (2023): 1090-1110.

33 IFPRI, "Foresight and Policy Modeling (FPM)," accessed March 24, 2025. https://www.ifpri.org/unit/foresight-and-policy-modeling-fpm

34 An example of work on assessing the key drivers of food choices using mixed methods can be found on Drivers of Food Choice. https://driversoffoodchoice.org/

35 M. Herrero, M. Hugas, U. Lele, A. Wirakartakusumah, and M. Torero, "A Shift to Healthy and Sustainable Consumption Patterns," in *Science and Innovations for Food Systems Transformation*, eds. J. von Braun, K. Afsana, L.O. Fresco, and M.H.A. Hassan, 59-85 (Cham, Switzerland: Springer Cham, 2023).

BOX 1

a D.E. Medek, J. Schwartz, and S.S. Myers, "Estimated Effects of Future Atmospheric CO_2 Concentrations on Protein Intake and the Risk of Protein Deficiency by Country and Region," *Environmental Health Perspectives* 125, 8 (2017): 087002; S.S. Myers, M.R. Smith, S. Guth, C.D. Golden, B. Vaitla, N.D. Mueller, A.D. Dangour, and P. Huybers, "Climate Change and Global Food Systems: Potential Impacts on Food Security and Undernutrition," *Annual Review of Public Health* 38 (2017): 259-277.

b R.H. Beach, T.B. Sulser, A. Crimmins, et al., "Combining the Effects of Increased Atmospheric Carbon Dioxide on Protein, Iron, and Zinc Availability and Projected Climate Change on Global Diets: A Modelling Study," *Lancet Planet Health* 3, 7 (2019): e307-e317.

c R.D. Semba, S. Askari, S. Gibson, M.W. Bloem, and K. Kraemer, "The Potential Impact of Climate Change on the Micronutrient-Rich Food Supply," *Advances in Nutrition* 13, 1 (2022): 80-100.

d J. Fanzo, C. Davis, R. McLaren, and J. Choufani, "The Effect of Climate Change across Food Systems: Implications for Nutrition Outcomes," *Global Food Security* 18 (2018): 12-19.

CHAPTER 3

1 Food and Agriculture Organization of the United Nations (FAO) and World Health Organization (WHO), *Sustainable Healthy Diets: Guiding Principles* (Rome: FAO, 2021).

2 L.J. Haddad, C. Hawkes, E. Achadi, et al., *Global Nutrition Report 2015: Actions and Accountability to Advance Nutrition and Sustainable Development* (Washington, DC: IFPRI, 2015).

3 FAO and WHO, *Sustainable Healthy Diets: Guiding Principles* (Rome: FAO, 2019).

4 FAO and WHO, *Sustainable Healthy Diets: Guiding Principles* (Rome: FAO, 2019).

5 H. Ritchie, P. Rosado, and M. Roser, "Food Prices," Our World in Data, published online 2023. https://ourworldindata.org/food-prices

6 Global Diet Quality Project, *Measuring What the World Eats: Insights from a New Approach* (Geneva: GAIN; Boston, MA: Harvard T.H. Chan School of Public Health, Department of Global Health and Population, 2022).

7 T. Beal and F. Ortenzi, "Priority Micronutrient Density in Foods," *Frontiers in Nutrition* 9 (2022): 806566.

8 L.I. Reyes, S.V. Constantinides, S. Bhandari, et al., "Actions in Global Nutrition Initiatives to Promote Sustainable Healthy Diets," *Global Food Security* 31 (2021): 100585; International Food Policy Research Institute (IFPRI), *2022 Global Food Policy Report: Climate Change and Food Systems* (Washington, DC: 2022).

9 C.E. Blake, E.A. Frongillo, A.M. Warren, S.V. Constantinides, K.K. Rampalli, and S. Bhandari, "Elaborating the Science of Food Choice for Rapidly Changing Food Systems in Low- and Middle-Income Countries," *Global Food Security* 28 (2021): 100503.

10 C.E. Blake, E.A. Frongillo, A.M. Warren, S.V. Constantinides, K.K. Rampalli, and S. Bhandari, "Elaborating the Science of Food Choice for Rapidly Changing Food Systems in Low- and Middle-Income Countries," *Global Food Security* 28 (2021): 100503.

11 U.S. Department of Agriculture, Economic Research Service, "Food Demand Analysis," accessed March 2024. https://ers.usda.gov/topics/food-choices-health/food-consumption-demand/food-demand-analysis

12 High Level Panel of Experts on Food Security and Nutrition of the Committee on World Food Security (HLPE), *Food Security and Nutrition: Building a Global Narrative Towards 2030* (Rome: 2020).

13 M. Boncyk, S. Isanovic, S. Samin, et al., *Development of a Methods Repository for Food Choice Behaviors and Drivers at the Household- and Individual-Levels*, TAFSSA Research Note 1 (Washington, DC: IFPRI, 2023).

14 S. Isanovic, S.V. Constantinides, E.A. Frongillo, et al., "How Perspectives on Food Safety of Vendors and Consumers Translate into Food-Choice Behaviors in 6 African and Asian Countries," *Current Developments in Nutrition* 7, 1 (2023): 100015.

15 C.E. Blake, E.C. Monterrosa, K.K. Rampalli, et al., "Basic Human Values Drive Food Choice Decision-Making in Different Food Environments of Kenya and Tanzania," *Appetite* 188, 1 (2023): 106620; S.D. Drew, C.E. Blake, L.I. Reyes, W. Gonzalez, and E.C. Monterrosa, "Attributes of Parenting Identities and Food Practices among Parents in Nairobi, Kenya," *Appetite* 180, 1 (2023): 106370.

16 E. Kenney, K.K. Rampalli, S. Samin, et al., "How Livelihood Change Affects Food Choice Behaviors in Low- and Middle-Income Countries: A Scoping Review," *Advances in Nutrition* 15, 5 (2024): 100203.

17 K. van der Gaast, E. van Leeuwen, and S. Wertheim-Heck, "Food Systems in Transition: Conceptualizing Sustainable Food Entrepreneu rship," *International Journal of Agricultural Sustainability* 20, 5 (2022): 705-721.

18 FAO and WHO, *Sustainable Healthy Diets: Guiding Principles* (Rome: FAO, 2019).

19 FAO and WHO, *Sustainable Healthy Diets: Guiding Principles* (Rome: FAO, 2019).

20 FAO, "Food-Based Dietary Guidelines," accessed March 2024. https://fao.org/nutrition/education/food-based-dietary-guidelines

21 Sri Lanka, Ministry of Health, Nutrition Division, *Food-Based Dietary Guidelines for Sri Lankans: Practitioner's Handbook* (2021).

22 FAO, "Food-Based Dietary Guidelines," accessed March 2024. https://fao.org/nutrition/education/food-based-dietary-guidelines

23 M. Springmann, L. Spajic, M.A. Clark, et al., "The Healthiness and Sustainability of National and Global Food Based Dietary Guidelines: Modelling Study," *BMJ* 370 (2020): m2322.

24 M. Springmann, L. Spajic, M.A. Clark, et al., "The Healthiness and Sustainability of National and Global Food Based Dietary Guidelines: Modelling Study," *BMJ* 370 (2020): m2322.

25 M. Springmann, L. Spajic, M.A. Clark, et al., "The Healthiness and Sustainability of National and Global Food Based Dietary Guidelines: Modelling Study," *BMJ* 370 (2020): m2322.

26 A. Webb Girard, E. Waugh, S. Sawyer, L. Golding, and U. Ramakrishnan, "A Scoping Review of Social-Behaviour Change Techniques Applied in Complementary Feeding Interventions," *Maternal & Child Nutrition* 16, 1 (2020): p.e12882.

27 S. Kachwaha, S.S. Kim, J.K. Das, S. Rasheed, S.M. Gavaravarapu, P. Pandey Rana, and P. Menon, "Behavior Change Interventions to Address Unhealthy Food Consumption: A Scoping Review," *Current Developments in Nutrition* 8, 3 (2024): 102104.

28 Pan American Health Organization, *Guiding Principles for Complementary Feeding of the Breastfed Child* (Washington, DC: 2003).

29 Z.S. Lassi, F. Rind, O. Irfan, R. Hadi, J.K. Das, and Z.A. Bhutta, "Impact of Infant and Young Child Feeding (IYCF) Nutrition Interventions on Breastfeeding Practices, Growth and Mortality in Low- and Middle-Income Countries: Systematic Review," *Nutrients* 12, 3 (2020): 722; R.K. Hodder, F.G. Stacey, R.J. Wyse, et al., "Interventions for Increasing Fruit and Vegetable Consumption in Children Aged Five Years and Under," *Cochrane Database of Systematic Reviews* 9, 9 (2020): CD008552.

30 E.J. Vargas-Garcia, C.E.L. Evans, A. Prestwich, B.J. Sykes-Muskett, J. Hooson, and J.E. Cade, "Interventions to Reduce Consumption of Sugar-Sweetened Beverages or Increase Water Intake: Evidence from a Systematic Review and Meta-Analysis," *Obesity Reviews* 18, 11 (2017): 1350-1363.

31 S.S. Kim, P.H. Nguyen, L.M. Tran, S. Alayon, P. Menon, and E.A. Frongillo, "Different Combinations of Behavior Change Interventions and Frequencies of Interpersonal Contacts Are Associated with Infant and Young Child Feeding Practices in Bangladesh, Ethiopia, and Vietnam," *Current Developments in Nutrition* 4, 2 (2020): nzz140.

32 FAO, International Fund for Agricultural Development, UNICEF, World Food Programme, and WHO, *The State of Food Security and Nutrition in the World 2022: Repurposing Food and Agricultural Policies to Make Healthy Diets More Affordable* (Rome: FAO, 2022).

33 World Bank, *Food Prices for Nutrition DataHub: Global Statistics on the Cost and Affordability of Healthy Diets* (Washington, DC: 2023).

34 A. Ahmed, F. Coleman, J. Ghostlaw, et al., "Increasing Production Diversity and Diet Quality: Evidence from Bangladesh," *American Journal of Agricultural Economics*, in print, 2023.

35 L. Depenbusch, P. Schreinemachers, S. Brown, and R. Roothaert, "Impact and Distributional Effects of a Home Garden and Nutrition Intervention in Cambodia," *Food Security* 14 (2022): 865-881.

36 A. Margolies, C.G. Kemp, E.M. Choo, et al., "Nutrition-Sensitive Agriculture Programs Increase Dietary Diversity in Children under 5 Years: A Review and Meta-Analysis," *Journal of Global Health* 12 (2022): 08001; M.T. Ruel, A.R. Quisumbing, and M. Balagamwala, "Nutrition-Sensitive Agriculture: What Have We Learned So Far?" *Global Food Security* 17 (2018): 128-153.

37 A. Margolies, C.G. Kemp, E.M. Choo, et al., "Nutrition-Sensitive Agriculture Programs Increase Dietary Diversity in Children under 5 Years: A Review and Meta-Analysis," *Journal of Global Health* 12 (2022): 08001.

38 S. Kadiyala, H. Harris-Fry, R. Pradhan, et al., "Effect of Nutrition-Sensitive Agriculture Interventions with Participatory Videos and Women's Group Meetings on Maternal and Child Nutritional Outcomes in Rural Odisha,

India (UPAVAN trial): A Four-Arm, Observer-Blind, Cluster-Randomised Controlled Trial," *Lancet Planetary Health* 5, 5 (2021): e263-e276.

39 G.S. Marquis, E.K. Colecraft, R. Kanlisi, B.A. Aidam, A. Atuobi-Yeboah, C. Pino, and R. Aryeetey, "An Agriculture-Nutrition Intervention Improved Children's Diet and Growth in a Randomized Trial in Ghana," *Maternal & Child Nutrition* 14, Suppl 3 (2018): e12677; A. Gelli, A. Margolies, M. Santacroce, et al., "Using a Community-Based Early Childhood Development Center as a Platform to Promote Production and Consumption Diversity Increases Children's Dietary Intake and Reduces Stunting in Malawi: A Cluster-Randomized Trial," *The Journal of Nutrition* 148, 10 (2018): 1587-1597; A.F. Darrouzet-Nardi, L.C. Miller, N. Joshi, S. Mahato, M. Lohani, and B.L. Rogers, "Child Dietary Quality in Rural Nepal: Effectiveness of a Community-Level Development Intervention," *Food Policy* 61 (2016): 185-197.

40 M. Hidrobo, J. Hoddinott, N. Kumar, and M. Olivier, "Social Protection, Food Security, and Asset Formation," *World Development* 101 (2018): 88-103.

41 D.K. Olney, A. Gelli, N. Kumar, H. Alderman, A. Go, and A. Raza, "Social Assistance Programme Impacts on Women's and Children's Diets and Nutritional Status," *Maternal & Child Nutrition* 18, 4 (2022): e13378.

42 D.K. Olney, A. Gelli, N. Kumar, H. Alderman, A. Go, and A. Raza, "Social Assistance Programme Impacts on Women's and Children's Diets and Nutritional Status," *Maternal & Child Nutrition* 18, 4 (2022): e13378.

43 D.K. Olney, A. Gelli, N. Kumar, H. Alderman, A. Go, and A. Raza, "Social Assistance Programme Impacts on Women's and Children's Diets and Nutritional Status," *Maternal & Child Nutrition* 18, 4 (2022): e13378.

44 J. Manley, Y. Balarajan, S. Malm, et al., "Cash Transfers and Child Nutritional Outcomes: A Systematic Review and Meta-Analysis," *BMJ Global Health* 5, 12 (2020): e003621.

45 D.K. Olney, A. Gelli, N. Kumar, H. Alderman, A. Go, and A. Raza, "Social Assistance Programme Impacts on Women's and Children's Diets and Nutritional Status," *Maternal & Child Nutrition* 18, 4 (2022): e13378.

46 Global Child Nutrition Foundation, *School Meal Programs Around the World: Results from the 2021 Global Survey of School Meal Programs©* (2022).

47 S. Chakrabarti, S.P. Scott, H. Alderman, P. Menon, and D.O. Gilligan, "Intergenerational Nutrition Benefits of India's National School Feeding Program," *Nature Communications* 12, 1 (2021): 4248.

48 WHO, "How School Systems Can Improve Health and Wellbeing," Topic Brief: Mental Health (May 3, 2023); J.J. Metcalfe, B. Ellison, N. Hamdi, R. Richardson, and M.P. Prescott, "A Systematic Review of School Meal Nudge Interventions to Improve Youth Food Behaviors," *International Journal of Behavioral Nutrition and Physical Activity* 17, 1 (2020): 1-9.

49 K.M. O'Brien, C. Barnes, S. Yoong, et al, "School-Based Nutrition Interventions in Children Aged 6 to 18 Years: An Umbrella Review of Systematic Reviews," *Nutrients* 13, 11 (2021): 4113.

50 H. Alderman, D. Bundy, and A. Gelli, "School Meals Are Evolving. Has the Evidence Kept Up?" *World Bank Research Observer*, in print, 2023.

BOX 1

a C.E. Blake, E.A. Frongillo, A.M. Warren, S.V. Constantinides, K.K. Rampalli, and S. Bhandari, "Elaborating the Science of Food Choice for Rapidly Changing Food Systems in Low- and Middle-Income Countries," *Global Food Security* 28 (2021): 100503.

b U.S. Department of Agriculture, Economic Research Service, "Food Consumption & Demand," accessed March 2024. https://www.ers.usda.gov/topics/food-choices-health/food-consumption-demand/

BOX 2

a N. Akseer, H. Tasic, O. Adeyemi, and R. Heidkamp, "Concordance and Determinants of Mothers' and Children's Diets in Nigeria: An In-Depth Study of the 2018 Demographic and Health Survey," *BMJ Open* 13, 7 (2023): e070876.

b V.L. Flax, A. Ipadeola, C.H. Schnefke, et al., "Complementary Feeding Social and Behavior Change Communication for Fathers and Mothers Improves Children's Consumption of Fish and Eggs and Minimum Meal Frequency in Kaduna State, Nigeria," *Current Developments in Nutrition* 6, 5 (2022): nzac075.

c P. Menon, P.H. Nguyen, K.K. Saha, et al., "Combining Intensive Counseling by Frontline Workers with a Nationwide Mass Media Campaign Has Large Differential Impacts on Complementary Feeding Practices but Not on Child Growth: Results of a Cluster-Randomized Program Evaluation in Bangladesh," *The Journal of Nutrition* 146, 10 (2016): 2075-2084.

d M. Saaka, K. Wemah, F. Kizito, and I. Hoeschle-Zeledon, "Effect of Nutrition Behaviour Change Communication Delivered through Radio on Mothers' Nutritional Knowledge, Child Feeding Practices and Growth," *Journal of Nutritional Science* 10 (2021): e44.

e C. Abiyu and T. Belachew, "Effect of Complementary Feeding Behavior Change Communication Delivered through Community-Level Actors on Dietary Adequacy of Infants in Rural Communities of West Gojjam Zone, Northwest Ethiopia: A Cluster-Randomized Controlled Trial," *PLoS ONE* 15, 9 (2020): e0238355.

f L.Z. Katenga-Kaunda, P.R. Kamudoni, G. Holmboe-Ottesen, H.E. Fjeld, I. Mdala, Z. Shim and P.O. Iversen, "Enhancing Nutrition Knowledge and Dietary Diversity among Rural Pregnant Women in Malawi: A Randomized Controlled Trial," *BMC Pregnancy and Childbirth* 21 (2021): 644.

BOX 3

a A.M. Pries, N. Sharma, A. Upadhyay, A.M. Rehman, S. Filteau, and E.L. Ferguson, "Energy Intake from Unhealthy Snack Food/Beverage among 12-23-Month-Old Children in Urban Nepal," *Maternal & Child Nutrition* 15 (2019): e12775.

b S.M. Frank, J. Webster, B. McKenzie, et al., "Consumption of Fruits and Vegetables among Individuals 15 Years and Older in 28 Low- and Middle-Income Countries," *The Journal of Nutrition* 149, 7 (2019): 1252-1259.

c P. Schreinemachers, R.M. Shrestha, B. Gole, D.R. Bhattarai, P.L. Ghimire, B.P. Subedi, T. Brück, G. Baliki, I.P. Gautam, and C.E. Blake, "Drivers of Food Choice among Children and Caregivers in Post-Earthquake Nepal," *Ecology of Food and Nutrition* 60, 6 (2021): 826-846.

d P. Schreinemachers, R.M. Shrestha, B. Gole, et al., "Drivers of Food Choice among Children and Caregivers in Post-Earthquake Nepal," *Ecology of Food and Nutrition* 60, 6 (2021): 826-846.

BOX 4

a N. Kumar, K. Raghunathan, A. Arrieta, A. Jilani, and S. Pandey, "The Power of the Collective Empowers Women: Evidence from Self-Help Groups in India," *World Development* 146 (2021): 105579; S. Desai, M. Misra, A. Das, R.J. Singh, M. Sehgal, L. Gram, N. Kumar, and A. Prost,"Community Interventions with Women's Groups to Improve Women's and Children's Health in India: A Mixed-Methods Systematic Review of Effects, Enablers and Barriers," *BMJ Global Health* 5, 12 (2020): e003304.

b N. Kumar, S. Scott, P. Menon, et al., "Pathways from Women's Group-Based Programs to Nutrition Change in South Asia: A Conceptual Framework and Literature Review," *Global Food Security* 17 (2018): 172-185.

CHAPTER 4

1 F. Dizon and A. Herforth, "The Cost of Nutritious Food in South Asia," World Bank Policy Research Working Paper No. 8557, World Bank, Washington, DC, 2018; K. Mahrt, D. Mather, A. Herforth, and D.D. Headey, "Household Dietary Patterns and the Cost of a Nutritious Diet in Myanmar," IFPRI Discussion Paper 1854, IFPRI, Washington, DC, 2019; F. Dizon, A. Herforth, and Z. Wang, "The Cost of a Nutritious Diet in Afghanistan, Bangladesh, Pakistan, and Sri Lanka," *Global Food Security* 21 (2019): 38-51.

2 K. Hirvonen, Y. Bai, D.D. Headey, and W.A. Masters, "Affordability of the EAT-Lancet Reference Diet: A Global Analysis," *Lancet Global Health* 8, 1 (2020): e59-e66.

3 Food and Agriculture Organization of the United Nations (FAO), International Fund for Agricultural Development (IFAD), UNICEF, World Food Programme (WFP), and World Health Organization (WHO), *The State of Food Security and Nutrition in the World (SOFI): 2020* (Rome: FAO, 2020).

4 D.D. Headey, K. Hirvonen, and H. Alderman, "Estimating the Cost and Affordability of Healthy Diets: How Much Do Methods Matter?" IFPRI Discussion Paper 2179, IFPRI, Washington, DC, 2023.

5 W. Willett, J. Rockström, B. Loken, et al., "Food in the Anthropocene: The EAT-Lancet Commission on Healthy Diets from Sustainable Food Systems," *Lancet* 393, 10170 (2019): 447-492.

6 Note that, technically speaking, the diet cost is formulated for a 30-year-old non-pregnant and non-lactating woman. This has been found to be a relatively representative demographic for the population at large, although calorie requirements are substantially lower for young children, especially.

7 This is just the cost of cash required, under the assumption of perfect targeting and without any regard to administrative costs; a very hypothetical number, but nevertheless illustrative.

8 This is somewhat below the 3 billion estimate reported in the SOFI reports using the same underlying price and income/expenditure data but a different definition of a healthy diet. However, the regional composition of results is similar.

9 This refers to the latest round of India's national Household Consumption Expenditure Survey. More recent data on household consumption expenditure is being collected through the Centre for Monitoring the Indian Economy's Consumer Pyramids Household Survey (CMIE CPHS), but this dataset has been criticized for its severe underrepresentation of the poor.

10 Seasonal fluctuations in healthy diet costs are also important, partly due to income fluctuations and especially to huge fluctuations in vegetable and fruit prices in particular; K. Raghunathan, D.D. Headey, and A. Herforth, "Affordability of Nutritious Diets in Rural India," *Food Policy* 99 (2020): 101982; Y. Bai, E.N. Naumova, and W.A. Masters, "Seasonality of Diet Costs Reveals Food System Performance in East Africa," *Science Advances* 6, 49 (2020): eabc2162.

11 D.D. Headey, K. Hirvonen, and H. Alderman, "Estimating the Cost and Affordability of Healthy Diets: How Much Do Methods Matter?" IFPRI Discussion Paper 2179, IFPRI, Washington, DC, 2023.

12 O. Ecker, H. Alderman, A.R. Comstock, D.D. Headey, K. Mahrt, and A. Pradesha, "Mitigating Poverty and Undernutrition through Social Protection: A Simulation Analysis of the COVID-19 Pandemic in Bangladesh and Myanmar," *Applied Economic Perspectives and Policy* 45, 4 (2023): 2034-2055.

13 A. Ahmed, J. Hoddinott, and S. Roy, "Food Transfers, Cash Transfers, Behavior Change Communication and Child Nutrition: Evidence from Bangladesh," IFPRI Discussion Paper 1868, IFPRI, Washington, DC, 2019; E.M. Maffioli, D.D. Headey, I. Lambrecht, T.Z. Oo, and N.T. Zaw, "A Prepandemic Nutrition-Sensitive Social Protection Program Has Sustained Benefits for Food Security and Diet Diversity in Myanmar during a Severe Economic Crisis," *The Journal of Nutrition* 153, 4 (2023): 1052-1062.

14 For example, Pakistan's Benazir Nashonuma Program Supplementary Nutritious Food to vulnerable mothers and children under 2 years of age.

15 H. Alderman, U. Gentilini, and R. Yemtsov, *The 1.5 Billion People Question: Food, Vouchers, or Cash Transfers?* (Washington, DC: World Bank, 2017).

16 World Bank, *The State of Social Safety Nets 2018* (Washington, DC: 2018).

17 To estimate this, we use a very simple cross-country regression, which shows that countries that spend more on social protection tend to have faster poverty reduction, even after controlling for their economic growth rate.

18 FAO, IFAD, UNICEF, WFP, and WHO, *The State of Food Security and Nutrition in the World (SOFI): 2022* (Rome: FAO, 2022).

19 P.L. Pingali, "Green Revolution: Impacts, Limits, and the Path Ahead," *Proceedings of the National Academy of Sciences* 109, 31 (2012): 12302-12308.

20 IFPRI's RIAPA models are a prime example of a tool specifically designed to assess investment-specific synergies and tradeoffs across different welfare objectives. www.ifpri.org/project/riapa-model

21 S.S. Morris, K. Beesabathuni, and D.D. Headey, "An Egg for Everyone: Pathways to Universal Access to One of Nature's Most Nutritious Foods," *Maternal & Child Nutrition* 14, S3 (2018): e12679.

22 J.M. Scott, B. Belton, K. Mahrt, S.H. Thilsted, and J.R. Bogard, "Food Systems Transformation, Animal-Source Foods Consumption, Inequality, and Nutrition in Myanmar," *Food Security* 15 (2023): 1345-1364.

23 While Figure 3 shows a bivariate association, we also estimated the association between EAT-Lancet diet costs and the transport and infrastructure logistics index in multivariate regressions that controlled for GDP per capita, agricultural productivity, and climate conditions.

24 For example, India's baseline score is 3.12, so its simulated improvement in the logistics index is 3.75-3.12 = 0.63, rather than a full unit increase.

25 FAO, FAOSTAT database, accessed February 24, 2024. www.fao.org/faostat/en/

26 S. Smitasiri and S. Chotiboriboon, "Experience with Programs to Increase Animal Source Food Intake in Thailand," *The Journal of Nutrition* 133, 11 (2003): 4000S-4005S.

27 J. Yothasamut, L. Camfield, and M. Pfeil, "Practices and Values Regarding Milk Consumption among Pre-schoolers in Bangkok," *International Journal of Qualitative Studies on Health and Well-Being* 13, 1 (2018): 1461515.

28 D.D. Headey, F. Bachewe, Q. Marshall, K. Raghunathan, and K. Mahrt, "Food Prices and the Wages of the Poor: A Cost-effective Addition to High-frequency Food Security Monitoring," *Food Policy* 125 (2024): 102630.

29 S. Gourlay, T. Kilic, A. Martuscelli, P. Wollburg, and A. Zezza, "Viewpoint: High-Frequency Phone Surveys on COVID-19: Good Practices, Open Questions," *Food Policy* 105 (2021): 102153; D.D. Headey and C.B. Barrett, "Opinion: Measuring Development Resilience in the World's Poorest Countries," *Proceedings of the National Academy of Sciences* 112, 37 (2015): 11423-11425.

CHAPTER 5

1 C. Turner, A. Aggarwal, H. Walls, et al., "Concepts and Critical Perspectives for Food Environment Research: A Global Framework with Implications for Action in Low- and Middle-Income Countries," *Global Food Security* 18 (2018): 93-101.

2 S. Ahmed, "Missing Wild and Cultivated Environments in Food Environment Measures," *ANH Academy Blogs*, August 30, 2017.

3 C.E. Blake, E.A. Frongillo, M. Warren Andrea, S.V. Constantinides, K.K. Rampalli, and S. Bhandari, "Elaborating the Science of Food Choice for Rapidly Changing Food Systems in Low- and Middle-Income Countries," *Global Food Security* 28 (2021): 100503.

4 Global Panel on Agriculture and Food Systems for Nutrition (GloPAN), *Improving Nutrition through Enhanced Food Environments* (London: 2017); C.B. Barrett, T. Reardon, J. Swinnen, and D. Zilberman, "Agri-food Value Chain Revolutions in Low- and Middle-Income Countries," *Journal of Economic Literature* 60, 4 (2022): 1316-1377.

5 Food and Agriculture Organization of the United Nations (FAO), International Fund for Agricultural Development (IFAD), UNICEF, World Food Programme (WFP), and World Health Organization (WHO), *The State of Food Security and Nutrition in the World 2023: Urbanization, Agrifood Systems Transformation and Healthy Diets Across the Rural-Urban Continuum* (Rome: FAO, 2023).

6 T. Reardon, D. Tschirley, M. Dolislager, J. Snyder, C. Hu, and S. White, *Urbanization, Diet Change, and Transformation of Food Supply Chains in Asia* (Michigan State University, Global Center for Food Systems Innovation: 2014).

7 S. Shapouri and S. Rosen, "Global Diet Composition: Factors Behind the Changes and Implications of the New Trends," in *Food Security Assessment 2007*, 28-37 (Washington, DC: USDA, 2007).

8 C.M. Sauer, T. Reardon, D. Tschirley, et al., "Consumption of Processed Food & Food Away from Home in Big Cities, Small Towns, and Rural Areas of Tanzania," *Agricultural Economics* 52, 5 (2021): 749-770.

9 J.M. Harris and R. Shiptsova, "Consumer Demand for Convenience Foods: Demographics and Expenditures," *Journal of Food Distribution Research* 38, 3 (2007): 1-15; T. Reardon, D. Tschirley, L.S.O. Liverpool-Tasie, et al., "The Processed Food Revolution in African Food Systems and the Double Burden of Malnutrition," *Global Food Security* 28 (2021): 100466.

10 C.A. Monteiro, G. Cannon, R.B. Levy, et al., "Ultra-Processed Foods: What They Are and How to Identify Them," *Public Health Nutrition* 22, 5 (2019): 936-941.

11 FAO, IFAD, UNICEF, WFP, and WHO, *The State of Food Security and Nutrition in the World 2023: Urbanization, Agrifood Systems Transformation and Healthy Diets Across the Rural-Urban Continuum* (Rome: FAO, 2023).

12 T. Reardon, D. Tschirley, L.S.O. Liverpool-Tasie, et al., "The Processed Food Revolution in African Food Systems and the Double Burden of Malnutrition," *Global Food Security* 28 (2021): 100466.

13 M.I. Gómez and K.D. Ricketts, "Food Value Chain Transformations in Developing Countries: Selected Hypotheses on Nutritional Implications," *Food Policy* 42 (2013): 139-150.

14 M. Berger and B. van Helvoirt, "Ensuring Food Secure Cities: Retail Modernization and Policy Implications in Nairobi, Kenya," *Food Policy* 79 (2018): 12-22; Global Alliance for Improved Nutrition (GAIN), *Informal Food Retail in Urban Areas* (Geneva: 2020).

15 J. Battersby and V. Watson, "Addressing Food Security in African Cities," *Nature Sustainability* 1, 4 (2018): 153-155.

16 FAO, *The State of Food and Agriculture 2019. Moving Forward on Food Loss and Waste Reduction* (Rome: 2019).

17 C. Muyanja, L. Nayiga, N. Brenda, and G. Nasinyama, "Practices, Knowledge and Risk Factors of Street Food Vendors in Uganda," *Food Control* 22, 10 (2011): 1551-1558.

18 D. Resnick, "Governance: Informal Food Markets in Africa's Cities," in *Global Food Policy Report 2017*, 50-57 (Washington, DC: IFPRI, 2017).

19 J.E. Carins and S.R. Rundle-Thiele, "Eating for the Better: A Social Marketing Review (2000-2012)," *Public Health Nutrition* 17, 7 (2014): 1628-1639; A. Finlay, E. Robinson, A. Jones, et al., "A Scoping Review of Outdoor Food Marketing: Exposure, Power and Impacts on Eating Behaviour and Health," *BMC Public Health* 22, 1 (2022): 1431; B. Kelly, S. Vandevijvere, S.H. Ng, et al., "Global Benchmarking of Children's Exposure to Television Advertising of Unhealthy Foods and Beverages across 22 Countries," *Obesity Reviews* 20, S2 (2019): 116-128.

20 E.J. Boyland, S. Nolan, B. Kelly, C. Tudur-Smith, A. Jones, J.C.G. Halford, and E. Robinson, "Advertising as a Cue to Consume: A Systematic Review and Meta-analysis of the Effects of Acute Exposure to Unhealthy Food and Nonalcoholic Beverage Advertising on Intake in Children and Adults," *American Journal of Clinical Nutrition*, 103, 2 (2016) 519-533; WHO, *Food Marketing Exposure and Power and Their Associations with Food-Related Attitudes, Beliefs and Behaviours: A Narrative Review* (Geneva: 2022).

21 E. Boyland, L. McGale, M. Maden, J. Hounsome, A. Boland, and A. Jones, "Systematic Review of the Effect of Policies to Restrict the Marketing of Foods and Non-alcoholic Beverages to which Children are Exposed," *Obesity Reviews* 23, 8 (2022): e13447; A.J. Kucharczuk, T.L. Oliver, and E.B. Dowdell, "Social Media's Influence on Adolescents' Food Choices: A Mixed Studies Systematic Literature Review," *Appetite* 168 (2022): 105765.

22 WHO, *Food Marketing Exposure and Power and Their Associations with Food-Related Attitudes, Beliefs and Behaviours: A Narrative Review* (Geneva: 2022).

23 S.I. Granheim, A.L. Løvhaug, L. Terragni, L.E. Torheim, and M. Thurston, "Mapping the Digital Food Environment: A Systematic Scoping Review," *Obesity Reviews* 23, 1 (2022): e13356.

24 K. Brar and L.M. Minaker, "Geographic Reach and Nutritional Quality of Foods Available from Mobile Online Food Delivery Service Applications: Novel Opportunities for Retail Food Environment Surveillance," *BMC Public Health* 21, 1 (2021): 458; P.M. Horta, J. de Paula Matos Souza, L.L. Rocha, and L.L. Mendes, "Digital Food Environment of a Brazilian Metropolis: Food Availability and Marketing Strategies Used by Delivery Apps," *Public Health Nutrition* 24, 3 (2021): 544-548.

25 WHO, *Food Marketing Exposure and Power and Their Associations with Food-Related Attitudes, Beliefs and Behaviours: A Narrative Review* (Geneva: 2022).

26 L.M. Neufeld, E.B. Andrade, A. Ballonoff Suleiman, et al., "Food Choice in Transition: Adolescent Autonomy, Agency, and the Food Environment," *Lancet* 399, 10320 (2022): 185-197.

27 A.J. Kucharczuk, T.L. Oliver, and E.B. Dowdell, "Social Media's Influence on Adolescents' Food Choices: A Mixed Studies Systematic Literature Review," *Appetite* 168 (2022): 105765.

28 F. Folkvord and R.C.J. Hermans, "Food Marketing in an Obesogenic Environment: A Narrative Overview of the Potential of Healthy Food Promotion to Children and Adults," *Current Addiction Reports* 7, 4 (2020): 431-436.

29 Market Development Facility, *What's for Breakfast? The COVID-19 Crisis and Rising Food Prices, A Year On* (Suva, Fiji: 2021).

30 S. Alonso, M.D. Angel, E. Muunda, E. Kilonzi, G. Palloni, D. Grace, and J.L. Leroy, "Consumer Demand for Milk and the Informal Dairy Sector Amidst COVID-19 in Nairobi, Kenya," *Current Developments in Nutrition* 7, 4 (2023): 100058.

31 H.-J. Brinkman, S. de Pee, I. Sanogo, L. Subran, and M.W. Bloem, "High Food Prices and the Global Financial Crisis Have Reduced Access to Nutritious Food and Worsened Nutritional Status and Health," *The Journal of Nutrition* 140, 1 (2010): 153S-161S; World Bank, *Food Security and COVID-19*, Brief (Washington, DC: 2021).

32 C. Corvalan, M. Reyes, M.L. Garmendia, and R. Uauy, "Structural Responses to the Obesity and Non-communicable Diseases Epidemic: Update on the Chilean Law of Food Labelling and Advertising," *Obesity Reviews* 20, 3 (2019): 367-374; A. Jones, B. Neal, B. Reeve, C. Ni Mhurchu, and A.M. Thow, "Front-of-Pack Nutrition Labelling to Promote Healthier Diets: Current Practice and Opportunities to Strengthen Regulation Worldwide," *BMJ Global Health* 4, 6 (2019): e001882.

33 C.A. Roberto, S.W. Ng, M. Ganderats-Fuentes, D. Hammond, S. Barquera, A. Jauregui, and L.S. Taillie, "The Influence of Front-of-Package Nutrition Labeling on Consumer Behavior and Product Reformulation," *Annual Review of Nutrition* 41, 1 (2021): 529-550.

34 A. Contreras-Manzano, C.M. White, C. Nieto, et al., "Self-Reported Decreases in the Purchases of Selected Unhealthy Foods Resulting from the Implementation of Warning Labels in Mexican Youth and Adult Population," medRxiv Pre-print, 2023; L.S. Taillie, M. Reyes, M.A. Colchero, B. Popkin, and C. Corvalan, "An Evaluation of Chile's Law of Food Labeling and Advertising on Sugar-Sweetened Beverage Purchases from 2015 to 2017: A Before-and-After Study," *PLoS Medicine* 17, 2 (2020): e1003015.

35 M. Reyes, L.S. Taillie, B. Popkin, R. Kanter, S. Vandevijvere, and C. Corvalan, "Changes in the Amount of Nutrient of Packaged Foods and Beverages after the Initial Implementation of the Chilean Law of Food Labelling and Advertising: A Nonexperimental Prospective Study," *PLoS Medicine* 17, 7 (2020): e1003220.

36 G. Fretes, C. Corvalán, M. Reyes, L.S. Taillie, C.D. Economos, N.L.W. Wilson, and S.B. Cash, "Changes in Children's and Adolescents' Dietary Intake after the Implementation of Chile's Law of Food Labeling, Advertising and Sales in Schools: A Longitudinal Study," *International Journal of Behavioral Nutrition and Physical Activity* 20, 1 (2023): 40; C. Massri, S. Sutherland, C. Kallestal, and S. Pena, "Impact of the Food-Labeling and Advertising Law Banning Competitive Food and Beverages in Chilean Public Schools, 2014-2016," *American Journal of Public Health* 109, 9 (2019): 1249-1254.

37 E. Sidaner, D. Balaban, and L. Burlandy, "The Brazilian School Feeding Programme: An Example of an Integrated Programme in Support of Food and Nutrition Security," *Public Health Nutrition* 16, 6 (2013): 989-994.

38 WHO, "WHO Recommends Stronger Policies to Protect Children from the Harmful Impact of Food Marketing," *WHO Departmental News*, July 3, 2023.

39 E. Boyland, L. McGale, M. Maden, J. Hounsome, A. Boland, and A. Jones, "Systematic Review of the Effect of Policies to Restrict the Marketing of Foods and Non-alcoholic Beverages to which Children are Exposed," *Obesity Reviews* 23, 8 (2022): e13447; L.S. Taillie, E. Busey, F. Mediano Stoltze, and F.R. Dillman Carpentier, "Governmental Policies to Reduce Unhealthy Food Marketing to Children," *Nutrition Reviews* 77, 11 (2019): 787-816.

40 C. Corvalan, M. Reyes, M.L. Garmendia, and R. Uauy, "Structural Responses to the Obesity and Non-communicable Diseases Epidemic: Update on the Chilean Law of Food Labelling and Advertising," *Obesity Reviews* 20, 3 (2019): 367-374; Diario Oficial de la Federación, "Decreto por el Que Se Reforman, Adicionan y Derogan Diversas Disposiciones del Reglamento de Control Sanitario de Productos y Servicios y del Reglamento de la Ley General de Salud en Materia de Publicidad," *Diario Oficial de la Federación*, September 8, 2023; Diario Oficial del Bicentenario - El Peruano, *Aprueban Manual de Advertencias Publicitarias en el Marco de lo Establecido en la Ley N° 30021, Ley de Promoción de la Alimentación Saludable para Niños, Niñas y Adolescentes, y Su Reglamento Aprobado por Decreto Supremo N° 017-2017-SA*, Decreto Supremo - N° 012-2018 - SA (2018).

41 B. Kelly, K. Backholer, E. Boyland, M.P. Kent, M.A. Bragg, T. Karupaiah, and S. Ng, "Contemporary Approaches for Monitoring Food Marketing to Children to Progress Policy Actions," *Current Nutrition Reports* 12, 1 (2023): 14-25.

42 G. Sacks and E.S.Y. Looi, "The Advertising Policies of Major Social Media Platforms Overlook the Imperative to Restrict the Exposure of Children and Adolescents to the Promotion of Unhealthy Foods and Beverages," *International Journal of Environmental Research and Public Health* 17, 11 (2020): 4172.

43 Global Food Research Program, "Taxes on Unhealthy Foods and Beverages," updated November 6, 2023. https://www.globalfoodresearchprogram.org/resource/taxes-on-unhealthy-foods-and-beverages/

44 T. Andreyeva, K. Marple, S. Marinello, T.E. Moore, and L.M. Powell, "Outcomes Following Taxation of Sugar-Sweetened Beverages," *JAMA Network Open* 5, 6 (2022): e2215276; J.C. Caro, C. Corvalan, M. Reyes, A. Silva, B. Popkin, and L.S. Taillie, "Chile's 2014 Sugar-Sweetened Beverage Tax and Changes in Prices and Purchases of Sugar-Sweetened Beverages: An Observational Study in an Urban Environment," *PLoS Medicine* 15, 7 (2018): e1002597; J. Cawley, A.M. Thow, K. Wen, and D. Frisvold, "The Economics of Taxes on Sugar-Sweetened Beverages: A Review of the Effects on Prices, Sales, Cross-Border Shopping, and Consumption," *Annual Review of Nutrition* 39, 1 (2019): 317-338; M.A. Colchero, J. Rivera-Dommarco, B.M. Popkin, and S.W. Ng, "In Mexico, Evidence of Sustained Consumer Response Two Years after Implementing a Sugar-Sweetened Beverage Tax," *Health Affairs* 36, 3 (2017): 564-571; L.S. Taillie, J.S. Rivera, B.M. Popkin, and C. Batis, "Do High vs. Low Purchasers Respond Differently to a Nonessential Energy-Dense Food Tax? Two-Year Evaluation of Mexico's 8% Nonessential Food Tax," *Preventive Medicine* 105 (2017): S37-S42.

45 M.A. Colchero, J. Rivera-Dommarco, B.M. Popkin, and S.W. Ng, "In Mexico, Evidence of Sustained Consumer Response Two Years after Implementing a Sugar-Sweetened Beverage Tax," *Health Affairs* 36, 3 (2017): 564-571.

46 A. Afshin, J.L. Peñalvo, L. Del Gobbo, et al., "The Prospective Impact of Food Pricing on Improving Dietary Consumption: A Systematic Review and Meta-analysis," *PLoS One* 12, 3 (2017): e0172277.

47 E. Crosbie, F.S. Gomes, J. Olvera, S. Rincón-Gallardo Patiño, S. Hoeper, and A. Carriedo, "A Policy Study on Front-of-Pack Nutrition Labeling in the Americas: Emerging Developments and Outcomes," *Lancet Regional Health – Americas* 18 (2023): 100400; M. White and S.

Barquera, "Mexico Adopts Food Warning Labels, Why Now?" *Health Systems & Reform* 6, 1 (2020): e1752063; World Cancer Research Fund International, *Building Momentum: Lessons on Implementing a Robust Front-of-Pack Food Label* (London: 2019).

48 A. Carriedo, A.D. Koon, L.M. Encarnación, K. Lee, R. Smith, and H. Walls, "The Political Economy of Sugar-Sweetened Beverage Taxation in Latin America: Lessons from Mexico, Chile and Colombia," *Globalization and Health* 17, 1 (2021): 5.

49 G. Rivlin, *Rigged: Supermarket Shelves for Sale* (Washington, DC: Center for Science in the Public Interest, 2016).

50 S.C. Shaw, G. Ntani, J. Baird, and C.A. Vogel, "A Systematic Review of the Influences of Food Store Product Placement on Dietary-Related Outcomes," *Nutrition Reviews* 78, 12 (2020): 1030-1045.

51 G. Pastori, I.D. Brouwer, M. Siemonsma, et al., "Fruit and Vegetable Intake of Females Before, During and After Introduction of Three Bundled Food System Interventions in Urban Vietnam and Nigeria," *Current Developments in Nutrition* in press (2023): 102050.

52 GAIN, "Vegetables for All," accessed March 28, 2024. https://www.gainhealth.org/impact/countries/kenya

53 International Livestock Research Institute, "MoreMilk: Making the Most of Milk," accessed March 28, 2024. https://www.ilri.org/research/projects/moremilk-making-most-milk

CHAPTER 6

1 Food and Agriculture Organization of the United Nations (FAO) and World Health Organization (WHO), *International Symposium on Sustainable Food Systems for Healthy Diets and Improved Nutrition: Key Messages* (Rome: FAO, 2017); V. Miller, P. Webb, R. Micha, and D. Mozaffarian, "Defining Diet Quality: A Synthesis of Dietary Quality Metrics and Their Validity for the Double Burden of Malnutrition," *Lancet Planetary Health* 4, 8 (2020): e352-e370; P. Agyemang, E.M. Kwofie, and J.I. Baum, "Transitioning to Sustainable Healthy Diets: A Model-Based and Conceptual System Thinking Approach to Optimized Sustainable Diet Concepts in the United States," *Frontiers in Nutrition* 9 (2022): 874721; International Atomic Energy Agency (IAEA), "Diet Quality," accessed January 2024, https://www.iaea.org/topics/diet-quality

2 W. Willett, J. Rockström, B. Loken, et al., "Food in the Anthropocene: The EAT-Lancet Commission on Healthy Diets from Sustainable Food Systems," *Lancet* 393, 10170 (2019): 447-492.

3 A. Alcorta, A. Porta, A. Tárrega, M.D. Alvarez, and M.P. Vaquero, "Foods for Plant-Based Diets: Challenges and Innovations," *Foods* 10, 2 (2021): 293; T. Beal, F. Ortenzi, and J. Fanzo, "Estimated Micronutrient Shortfalls of the EAT-Lancet Planetary Health Diet," *Lancet Planetary Health* 7, 3 (2023): e233-e237.

4 V. Miller, P. Webb, F. Cudhea, et al., "Global Dietary Quality in 185 Countries from 1990 to 2018 Show Wide Differences by Nation, Age, Education, and Urbanicity," *Nature Food* 3 (2022): 694-702.

5 G.A. Stevens, T. Beal, M.N.N. Mbuya, et al., "Micronutrient Deficiencies among Preschool-Aged Children and Women of Reproductive Age Worldwide: A Pooled Analysis of Individual-Level Data from Population-Representative Surveys," *Lancet Global Health* 10, 11 (2022): e1590-e1599.

6 F. Branca, A. Lartey, S. Oenema, et al., "Transforming the Food System to Fight Non-communicable Diseases," *BMJ* 364 (2019): l296; GBD 2017 Causes of Death Collaborators, "Global, Regional, and National Age-Sex-Specific Mortality for 282 Causes of Death in 195 Countries and Territories, 1980-2017: A Systematic Analysis for the Global Burden of Disease Study 2017," *Lancet Global Health Metrics* 392, 10159 (2018): 1736-1788.

7 G.A. Stevens, T. Beal, M.N.N. Mbuya, et al., "Micronutrient Deficiencies among Preschool-Aged Children and Women of Reproductive Age Worldwide: A Pooled Analysis of Individual-Level Data from Population-Representative Surveys," *Lancet Global Health* 10, 11 (2022): e1590-e1599.

8 GBD 2017 Diet Collaborators, "Health Effects of Dietary Risks in 195 Countries, 1990-12017: A Systematic Analysis for the Global Burden of Disease Study 2017," *Lancet* 393, 10184 (2019): 1958-1972.

9 J. Fanzo, C. Davis, R. McLaren, and J. Choufani, "The Effect of Climate Change across Food Systems: Implications for Nutrition Outcomes," *Global Food Security* 18 (2018): 12-19; M.R. Smith and S.S. Myers, "Impact of Anthropogenic CO2 Emissions on Global Human Nutrition," *Nature Climate Change* 8 (2018): 834-839; L. Ziska, "Rising Carbon Dioxide and Global Nutrition: Evidence and Action Needed," *Plants* 11 (2022): 1000.

10 FAO, International Fund for Agricultural Development (IFAD), UNICEF, World Food Programme (WFP) and WHO, *The State of Food Security and Nutrition in the World 2020* (Rome: FAO, 2020).

11 J. Harris, M. van Zonneveld, E.G. Achigan-Dako, et al., "Fruit and Vegetable Biodiversity for Nutritionally Diverse Diets: Challenges, Opportunities, and Knowledge Gaps," *Global Food Security* 33 (2022): 100618.

12 D. Mason-D'Croz, J.R. Bogard, T.B. Sulser, N. Cenacchi, S. Dunston, M. Herrero, and K. Wiebe, "Gaps between Fruit and Vegetable Production, Demand, and Recommended Consumption at Global and National Levels: An Integrated Modelling Study," *Lancet Planetary Health* 3, 7 (2019): e318-e329.

13 L.C. Del Gobbo, S. Khatibzadeh, F. Imamura, R. Micha, P. Shi, M. Smith, S.S. Meyers, and D. Mozaffarian, "Assessing Global Dietary Habits: A Comparison of National Estimates from the FAO and the Global Dietary Database," *American Journal of Clinical Nutrition* 101, 5 (2015): 1038-1046.

14 B. Stadlmayr, U. Trübswasser, S. McMullin, et al., "Factors Affecting Fruit and Vegetable Consumption and Purchase Behavior of Adults in Sub-Saharan Africa: A Rapid Review," *Frontiers in Nutrition* 10 (2023): 1113013.

15 D. Grace, "Food Safety in Low and Middle Income Countries," *International Journal of Environmental Research and Public Health* 12, 9 (2015): 10490-10507.

16 For information on FRESH, see https://www.cgiar.org/initiative/fruit-and-vegetables-for-sustainable-healthy-diets-fresh/

17 V. Taleon, M.Z. Hasan, R. Jongstra, R. Wegmüller, and M.K. Bashar, "Effect of Parboiling Conditions on Zinc and Iron Retention in Biofortified and Non-biofortified Milled Rice," *Journal of the Science of Food and Agriculture* 102, 2 (2022): 514-522; S. Gallego-Castillo, V. Taleon, E.F. Talsma, A. Rosales-Nolasco, and N. Palacios-Rojas, "Effect of Maize Processing Methods on the Retention of Minerals, Phytic Acid and Amino Acids When Using High Kernel-Zinc Maize," *Current Research in Food Science* 4 (2021): 279-286.

18 A.Z. Alem, Y. Yeshaw, A.M. Liyew, et al., "Double Burden of Malnutrition and Its Associated Factors among Women in Low and Middle Income Countries: Findings from 52 Nationally Representative Data," *BMC Public Health* 23, 1 (2023): 1479.

19 A.Z. Alem, Y. Yeshaw, A.M. Liyew, et al., "Double Burden of Malnutrition and Its Associated Factors among Women in Low and Middle Income Countries: Findings from 52 Nationally Representative Data," *BMC Public Health* 23, 1 (2023): 1479.

20 K.O. Fuglie, and R.G. Echeverria, "The Economic Impact of CGIAR-Related Crop Technologies on Agricultural Productivity in Developing Countries, 1961-2020," *World Development* 176 (2024): 106523.

21 B. Born and M. Purcell, "Avoiding the Local Trap," *Journal of Planning Education and Research* 26, 2 (2006): 195-207.

22 B. Born and M. Purcell, "Avoiding the Local Trap," *Journal of Planning Education and Research* 26, 2 (2006): 195-207.

23 K. Hirvonen, Y. Bai, D.D. Headey, and W.A. Masters, "Affordability of the EAT-Lancet Reference Diet: A Global Analysis," *Lancet Global Health* 8, 1 (2020): e59-e66.

24 J. Harris, M. van Zonneveld, E.G. Achigan-Dako, et al., "Fruit and Vegetable Biodiversity for Nutritionally Diverse Diets: Challenges, Opportunities, and Knowledge Gaps," *Global Food Security* 33 (2022): 100618.

25 T. Borelli, D. Hunye, S. Padulosi, et al., "Local Solutions for Sustainable Food Systems: The Contribution of Orphan Crops and Wild Edible Species," *Agronomy* 10, 2 (2020): 231.

26 P. Schreinemachers, G. Grovermann, S. Praneetvatakul, et al., "How Much is Too Much? Quantifying Pesticide Overuse in Vegetable Production in Southeast Asia," *Journal of Cleaner Production* 244 (2020): 118738.

27 J. Harris, B. de Steenhuijsen Piters, S. McMullin, B. Bajwa, I. de Jager, and I.D. Brouwer, "Fruits and Vegetables for Healthy Diets: Priorities for Food System Research and Action," in *Science and Innovations for Food Systems Transformation*, eds. J. von Braun, K. Afsana, L.O. Fresco, and M. Hag Ali Hassan, 87-104 (Cham, Switzerland: Springer International Publishing, 2023).

28 F. Andreotti, D. Bazile, C. Biaggi, et al., "When Neglected Species Gain Global Interest: Lessons Learned from Quinoa's Boom and Bust for Teff and Minor Millet," *Global Food Security* 32 (2022): 100613.

29 J. Hufnagel, M. Reckling, and F. Ewert, "Diverse Approaches to Crop Diversification in Agricultural Research. A Review," *Agronomy for Sustainable Development* 40, (2020): 14.

30 A.D. Jones, "Critical Review of the Emerging Research Evidence on Agricultural Biodiversity, Diet Diversity, and Nutritional Status in Low- and Middle-Income Countries," *Nutrition Reviews* 75, 10 (2017): 769-782; K.T. Sibhatu, V.V. Krishna, and M. Qaim, "Production Diversity and Dietary Diversity in Smallholder Farm Households," *Proceedings of the National Academy of Sciences* 112, 34 (2015): 10657-10662.

31 L. Stefan, M. Hartmann, N. Engbersen, J. Six, and C. Schöb, "Positive Effects of Crop Diversity on Productivity Driven by Changes in Soil Microbial Composition," *Frontiers in Microbiology* 12 (2021): 660749.

32 S. Lopez-Ridaura, L. Barba-Escoto, C.A. Reyna-Ramirez, C. Sum, N. Palacios-Rojas, and B. Gerard, "Maize Intercropping in the Milpa System. Diversity, Extent and Importance for Nutritional Security in the Western Highlands of Guatemala," *Scientific Reports* 11 (2021): 3696.

33 K.T. Sibhatu, V.V. Krishna, and M. Qaim, "Production Diversity and Dietary Diversity in Smallholder Farm Households," *PNAS* 112, 34 (2015): 10657-10662.

34 A.D. Jones, "Critical Review of the Emerging Research Evidence on Agricultural Biodiversity, Diet Diversity, and Nutritional Status in Low- and Middle-Income Countries," *Nutrition Reviews* 75, 10 (2017): 769-782.

35 T. Mitra-Ganguli, W.H. Pfeiffer, and J. Walton, "The Global Regulatory Framework for the Commercialization of Nutrient Enriched Biofortified Foods," *Annals of the New York Academy of Sciences* 1517, 1 (2022): 154-166.

36 J.A. Pickett, C.M. Woodcock, C.A.O. Midega, and Z.R. Khan, "Push-Pull Farming Systems," *Current Opinion in Biotechnology* 26 (2014): 125-132; R.D. Harrison, C. Thierfelder, F. Baudron, P. Chinwada, C. Midega, U. Schaffner, and J. van den Berg, "Agro-ecological Options for Fall Armyworm (*Spodoptera frugiperda* JE Smith) Management: Providing Low-Cost, Smallholder Friendly Solutions to an Invasive Pest," *Journal of Environmental Management* 243 (2019): 318-330.

37 G. Velu, L. Crespo Herrera, C. Guzman, J. Huerta, T. Payne, and R.P. Singh, "Assessing Genetic Diversity to Breed Competitive Biofortified Wheat with Enhanced Grain Zn and Fe Concentrations, *Frontiers in Plant Science* 9 (2019): 413924.

38 A.C. Sánchez, H.N. Kamau, F. Grazioli, and S.K. Jones, "Financial Profitability of Diversified Farming Systems: A Global Meta-analysis," *Ecological Economics* 201, (2022): 107595; Y. Zhang, Y. Wu, J. Yan, and T. Peng, "How Does Rural Labor Migration Affect Crop Diversification for Adapting to Climate Change in the Hehuang Valley, Tibetan Plateau?" *Land Use Policy* 113, (2022): 105928.

39 H.E. Bouis, E. Birol, E. Boy, and B. Gannon, "Food Biofortification-Reaping the Benefits of Science to Overcome Hidden Hunger," *CAST* Issue Paper 69 (Ames, Iowa: CAST, 2020).

40 FAO, IFAD, UNICEF, WFP and WHO, *The State of Food Security and Nutrition in the World 2020*, Global Health Estimates Technical Paper (Rome: FAO, 2020).

41 WHO, *WHO Methods and Data Sources for Global Burden of Disease Estimates 2000-2019* (Geneva: 2020).

42 E. Birol and H.E. Bouis, "Role of Socio-economic Research in Developing, Delivering and Scaling New Crop Varieties: The Case of Staple Crop Biofortification," *Frontiers in Plant Science* 14 (2023): 1099496.

43 T. Mitra-Ganguli, W.H. Pfeiffer, and J. Walton, "The Global Regulatory Framework for the Commercialization of Nutrient Enriched Biofortified Foods," *Annals of the New York Academy of Sciences* 1517 (2022): 154-166.

44 N. Neufingerl and A. Eilander, "Nutrient Intake and Status in Adults Consuming Plant-Based Diets Compared to Meat-Eaters: A Systematic Review," *Nutrients* 14, 1 (2021): 29.

45 E.C. Keats, L.M. Neufeld, G.S. Garrett, M.N.N. Mbuya, and Z.A. Bhutta, "Improved Micronutrient Status and Health Outcomes in Low- and Middle-Income Countries Following Large-Scale Fortification: Evidence from a Systematic Review and Meta-analysis," *American Journal of Clinical Nutrition* 109, 6 (2019): 1696-1708.

46 J. Monroy-Gomez, C. Ferraboschi, K.G. van Zutphen, B. Gavin-Smith, D. Amanquah, and K. Kraemer, "Small and Medium Enterprises' Perspectives on Food Fortification Amid the Growing Burden of Malnutrition," *Nutrients* 14, 18 (2022): 3837.

47 J. Monroy-Gomez, C. Ferraboschi, K.G. van Zutphen, B. Gavin-Smith, D. Amanquah, and K. Kraemer, "Small and Medium Enterprises' Perspectives on Food Fortification Amid the Growing Burden of Malnutrition," *Nutrients* 14, 18 (2022): 3837.

48 A.A. Harb, A. Shechter, P.A. Koch, and M.-P. St-Onge, "Ultra-processed Foods and the Development of Obesity in Adults," *European Journal of Clinical Nutrition* 77, 6 (2023): 619-627.

BOX 1

a S. Sazawal, U. Dhingra, P. Dhingra, et al., "Efficacy of High Zinc Biofortified Wheat in Improvement of Micronutrient Status, and Prevention of Morbidity among Preschool Children and Women: A Double Masked, Randomized, Controlled Trial," *Nutrition Journal* 17 (2018): 86.

b L.M. Pompano, S.V. Luna, S.A. Udipi, P.S. Ghugre, E.M. Przybyszewski, and J. Haas, "Iron-Biofortified Pearl Millet Consumption Increases Physical Activity in Indian Adolescent Schoolchildren after a 6-Month Randomised Feeding Trial," *British Journal of Nutrition* 127, 7 (2021): 1018-1025; S.P. Scott, L.E. Murray-Kolb, M.J. Wenger, S.A. Udipi, P.S. Ghugre, E. Boy, and J.D. Haas, "Cognitive Performance in Indian School-Going Adolescents is Positively Affected by Consumption of Iron-Biofortified Pearl Millet: A 6-Month Randomized Controlled Efficacy Trial," *The Journal of Nutrition* 148, 9 (2018): 1462-1471; J.L. Finkelstein, M. Saurabh, S.A. Udipi, et al., "A Randomized Trial of Iron-Biofortified Pearl Millet in School Children in India," *The Journal of Nutrition* 145, 7 (2015): 1576-1581; L.E. Murray-Kolb, M.J. Wenger, S.P. Scott, M.G. Lung'aho, and J.D. Haas, "Consumption of Iron-Biofortified Beans Positively Affects Cognitive Performance in 18- to 27-Year-Old Rwandan Female College Students in an 18-Week Randomized Controlled Efficacy Trial," *The Journal of Nutrition* 147, 11 (2017): 2109-2117; M.J. Wenger, S.E. Rhoten, L.E. Murray-Kolb, S.P. Scott, E. Boy, J.-B. Gahutu, and J.D. Haas, "Changes in Iron Status are Related to Changes in Brain Activity and Behavior in Rwandan Female University Students: Results from a Randomized Controlled Efficacy Trial Involving Iron-Biofortified Beans," *The Journal of Nutrition* 149, 4 (2019): 687-697; S.V. Luna, L.M. Pompano, M. Lung'aho, J.-B. Gahutu, and J.D. Haas, "Increased Iron Status during a Feeding Trial of Iron-Biofortified Beans Increases Physical Work Efficiency in Rwandan Women," *The Journal of Nutrition* 150, 5 (2020): 1093-1099.

c P.J. van Jaarsveld, M. Faber, S.A. Tanumihardjo, P. Nestel, C.J. Lombard, and A.J. Spinnler Benadé, "Beta-carotene-Rich Orange-Fleshed Sweet Potato Improves the Vitamin A Status of Primary School Children Assessed with the Modified-Relative-Dose-Response Test," *American Journal of Clinical Nutrition* 81, 5 (2005): 1080-1087; B. Gannon, C. Kaliwile, S.A. Arscott, et al., "Biofortified Orange Maize is as Efficacious as a Vitamin A Supplement in Zambian Children Even in the Presence of High Liver Reserves of Vitamin A: A Community-Based, Randomized Placebo-Controlled Trial," *American Journal of Clinical Nutrition* 100, 6 (2014): 1541-1550; A.C. Palmer, K. Healy, M.A. Barffour, et al., "Provitamin A Carotenoid-Biofortified Maize Consumption Increases Pupillary Responsiveness among Zambian Children in a Randomized Controlled Trial," *The Journal of Nutrition* 146, 12 (2016): 2551-2558; E.F. Talsma, I.D. Brouwer, H. Verhoef, et al., "Biofortified Yellow Cassava and Vitamin A Status of Kenyan Children: A Randomized Controlled Trial," *American Journal of Clinical Nutrition* 103, 1 (2016): 258-267; I. Afolami, M.B. Mwangi, F. Samuel, et al., "Daily Consumption of Pro-vitamin A Biofortified (Yellow) Cassava Improves Serum Retinol Concentrations in Preschool Children in Nigeria: A Randomized Controlled Trial," *American Journal of Clinical Nutrition* 113, 1 (2020): 221-231; C. Hotz, C. Lechl, A. de Brauw, Pet al., "A Large-Scale Intervention to Introduce Orange Sweet Potato in Rural Mozambique Increases Vitamin A Intakes among Children and Women," *British Journal of Nutrition* 108, 1 (2012): 163-176; C. Hotz, C. Loechle, A. Lubowa, et al., "Introduction of Beta-carotene-rich Orange Sweet Potato in Rural Uganda Resulted in Increased Vitamin A Intakes among Children and Women and Improved vitamin A Status among Children," *The Journal of Nutrition* 142, 10 (2012): 1871-1880.

d S.L. Huey, S. Venkatramanan, S.A. Udipi, et al., "Acceptability of Iron-and Zinc-Biofortified Pearl Millet (ICTP-8203)-Based Complementary Foods among Children in an Urban Slum of Mumbai, India," *Frontiers in Nutrition* 4 (2017): 39; S.L. Huey, A. Bhargava, V.M. Friesen, et al., "Sensory Acceptability of Biofortified Foods and Food Products: A Systematic Review," Nutrition Reviews (2023): nuad100.

e E. Birol and H.E. Bouis, "Role of Socio-economic Research in Developing, Delivering and Scaling New Crop Varieties: The Case of Staple Crop Biofortification," *Frontiers in Plant Science* 14 (2023): 1099496.

CHAPTER 7

1 B.M. Popkin, C. Corvalan, and L.M. Grummer-Strawn, "Dynamics of the Double Burden of Malnutrition and the Changing Nutrition Reality," *Lancet* 395, 10217 (2020): 65-74; S.J. Vermeulen, T. Park, C.K. Khoury, and C. Béné, "Changing Diets and the Transformation of the Global Food System," *Annals of the New York Academy of Sciences* 1478, 1 (2020): 3-17; Global Panel on Agriculture and Food Systems for Nutrition (GLOPAN), *Urban Diets and Nutrition: Trends, Challenges and Opportunities for Policy Action* (London: 2017).

2 V. Miller, J. Reedy, F. Cudhea, et al., "Global, Regional, and National Consumption of Animal-Source Foods Between 1990 and 2018: Findings from the Global Dietary Database," *Lancet Planetary Health* 6, 3 (2022): e243-256.

3 N. Alexandratos and J. Bruinsma, "World Agriculture Towards 2030/2050: The 2012 Revision," ESA Working Paper No. 12-03, Food and Agriculture Organization of the United Nations (FAO), Rome, 2012.

4 A. Mottet, C. de Haan, A. Falcucci, G. Tempio, C. Opio, and P. Gerber, "Livestock: On Our Plates or Eating at Our Table? A New Analysis of the Feed/Food Debate," *Global Food Security* 14 (201): 1-8.

5 World Health Organization (WHO), *Red and Processed Meat in the Context of Health and the Environment: Many Shades of Red and Green*, Information Brief (Geneva: 2023); IARC Working Group on the Evaluation of Carcinogenic Risks to Humans, *Red Meat and Processed Meat: IARC Monographs on the Evaluation of Carcinogenic Risks to Humans* (Lyon, France: IARC, 2018).

6 FAO and WHO, *Sustainable Healthy Diets: Guiding Principles* (Rome: 2019).

7 Vitamin B12 is also found in some algae.

8 S.P. Murphy and L.H. Allen, "Nutritional Importance of Animal Source Foods," *The Journal of Nutrition* 133, 11 (2003): 3932S-3935S.

9 D. Swanson, R. Block, and S.A. Mousa, "Omega-3 Fatty Acids EPA and DHA: Health Benefits Throughout Life," *Advances in Nutrition* 3, 1 (2012): 1-7.

10 G. Wu, "Important Roles of Dietary Taurine, Creatine, Carnosine, Anserine and 4-Hydroxyproline in Human Nutrition and Health," *Amino Acids* 52 (2020): 329-360.

11 L.H. Allen and N. Ahluwalia, *Improving Iron Status through Diet: The Application of Knowledge Concerning Dietary Iron Bioavailability in Human Populations* (Arlington, VA: OMNI Project, 1997).

12 K.G. Dewey and K.H. Brown, "Update on Technical Issues Concerning Complementary Feeding of Young Children in Developing Countries and Implications for Intervention Programs," *Food and Nutrition Bulletin* 24, 1 (2003): 5-28.

13 T. Beal, C.D. Gardner, M. Herrero, L.L. Iannotti, L. Merbold, S. Nordhagen, and A. Mottet, "Friend or Foe? The Role of Animal-Source Foods in Healthy and Environmentally Sustainable Diets," *The Journal of Nutrition* 153, 2 (2023): 409-425.

14 K.G. Dewey and K.H. Brown, "Update on Technical Issues Concerning Complementary Feeding of Young Children in Developing Countries and Implications for Intervention Programs," *Food and Nutrition Bulletin* 24, 1 (2003): 5-28.

15 Pan American Health Organization (PAHO) and WHO, *Guiding Principles for Complementary Feeding of the Breastfed Child* (Washington, DC: 2003).

16 FAO, *Contribution of Terrestrial Animal Source Food to Healthy Diets for Improved Nutrition and Health Outcomes: An Evidence and Policy Overview on the State of Knowledge and Gaps* (Rome: 2023).

17 H. Asare, A. Rosi, M. Faber, C.M. Smuts, and C. Ricci, "Animal-Source Foods as a Suitable Complementary Food for Improved Physical Growth in 6 to 24-Month-Old Children in Low- and Middle-Income Countries: A Systematic Review and Meta-analysis of Randomised Controlled Trials," *British Journal of Nutrition* 128, 12 (2022): 2453-2463.

18 FAO, *Contribution of Terrestrial Animal Source Food to Healthy Diets for Improved Nutrition and Health Outcomes: An Evidence and Policy Overview on the State of Knowledge and Gaps* (Rome: 2023); L. Lu, P. Xun, Y. Wan, K. He, and W. Cai, "Long-Term Association Between Dairy Consumption and Risk of Childhood Obesity: A Systematic Review and Meta-analysis of Prospective Cohort Studies," *European Journal of Clinical Nutrition* 70 (2016): 414-423.

19 FAO, *Contribution of Terrestrial Animal Source Food to Healthy Diets for Improved Nutrition and Health Outcomes: An Evidence and Policy Overview on the State of Knowledge and Gaps* (Rome: 2023).

20 FAO, *Contribution of Terrestrial Animal Source Food to Healthy Diets for Improved Nutrition and Health Outcomes: An Evidence and Policy Overview on the State of Knowledge and Gaps* (Rome: 2023).

21 GBD 2017 Causes of Death Collaborators, "Global, Regional, and National Age-Sex-Specific Mortality for 282 Causes of Death in 195 Countries and Territories, 1980-2017: A Systematic Analysis for the Global Burden of Disease Study 2017," *Lancet Global Health Metrics* 392, 10159 (2018): 1736-1788.

22 IARC Working Group on the Evaluation of Carcinogenic Risks to Humans, *Red Meat and Processed Meat: IARC Monographs on the Evaluation of Carcinogenic Risks to Humans* (Lyon, France: 2018).

23 WHO, *Red and Processed Meat in the Context of Health and the Environment: Many Shades of Red and Green*, Information Brief (Geneva: 2023).

24 Y. Ma, F.J. He, Q. Sun Q, et al., "24-Hour Urinary Sodium and Potassium Excretion and Cardiovascular Risk," *New England Journal of Medicine* 386 (2022): 252-263.

25 IARC Working Group on the Evaluation of Carcinogenic Risks to Humans, *Red Meat and Processed Meat: IARC Monographs on the Evaluation of Carcinogenic Risks to Humans* (Lyon, France: 2018).

26 WHO, *Red and Processed Meat in the Context of Health and the Environment: Many Shades of Red and Green*, Information Brief (Geneva: 2023).

27 WHO, *Red and Processed Meat in the Context of Health and the Environment: Many Shades of Red and Green*, Information Brief (Geneva: 2023); T. Beal, C.D. Gardner, M. Herrero, L.L. Iannotti, L. Merbold, S. Nordhagen, and A. Mottet, "Friend or Foe? The Role of Animal-Source Foods in Healthy and Environmentally Sustainable Diets," *The Journal of Nutrition* 153, 2 (2023): 409-425.

28 R. Rubin, "Backlash Over Meat Dietary Recommendations Raises Questions About Corporate Ties to Nutrition Scientists," *JAMA* 323, 5 (2020): 401-404.

29 WHO, *Saturated Fatty Acid and Trans-fatty Acid Intake for Adults and Children: WHO Guideline* (Geneva: 2023).

30 A.H. Havelaar, M.D. Kirk, P.R. Torgerson, et al., "World Health Organization Global Estimates and Regional Comparisons of the Burden of Foodborne Disease in 2010," *PLoS Medicine* 12, 12 (2015): e1001923.

31 S.A. Richard, R.E. Black, R.H. et al., "Catch-Up Growth Occurs after Diarrhea in Early Childhood," *The Journal of Nutrition* 144, 6 (2014): 965-971.

32 S.A. Richard, R.E. Black, R.H. et al., "Catch-Up Growth Occurs after Diarrhea in Early Childhood," *The Journal of Nutrition* 144, 6 (2014): 965-971; R.L. Guerrant, M.D. DeBoer, S.R. Moore, R.J. Scharf, and A.A.M. Lima, "The Impoverished Gut: A Triple Burden of Diarrhoea, Stunting and Chronic Disease," *Nature Reviews Gastroenterology & Hepatology* 10 (2013): 220-229; W. Checkley, G. Buckley, R.H.Gilman, et al., "Multi-country Analysis of the Effects of Diarrhoea on Childhood Stunting," *International Journal of Epidemiology* 37, 4 (2008): 816-830.

33 J.A. Painter, R.M. Hoekstra, T. Ayers, R.V. Tauxe, C.R. Braden, F.J. Angulo, and P.M. Griffin, "Attribution of Foodborne Illnesses, Hospitalizations, and Deaths to Food Commodities by Using Outbreak Data, United States, 1998-2008," *Emerging Infectious Diseases* 19, 3 (2013): 407-415.

34 S. Hoffmann, B. Devleesschauwer, W. Aspinall, et al., "Attribution of Global Foodborne Disease to Specific Foods: Findings from a World Health Organization Structured Expert Elicitation," *PLoS ONE* 12, 9 (2017): e0183641.

35 J.N. Ssemanda, M.W. Reij, G. van Middendorp, et al., "Foodborne Pathogens and Their Risk Exposure Factors Associated with Farm Vegetables in Rwanda," *Food Control* 89 (2018): 86-96.

36 P. Gerber, H. Steinfeld, B. Henderson, et al., *Tackling Climate Change through Livestock - A Global Assessment of Emissions and Mitigation Opportunities* (Rome: FAO, 2013).

37 J. Poore and T. Nemecek, "Reducing Food's Environmental Impacts through Producers and Consumers," *Science* 360, 6392 (2018): 987-992.

38 A. Mottet, C. de Haan, A. Falcucci, G. Tempio, C. Opio, and P. Gerber, "Livestock: On Our Plates or Eating at Our Table? A New Analysis of the Feed/Food Debate," *Global Food Security* 14 (201): 1-8.

39 J. Heinke, M. Lannerstad, D. Gerten, et al., "Water Use in Global Livestock Production: Opportunities and Constraints for Increasing Water Productivity," *Water Resources Research* 56, 12 (2020): e2019WR026995.

40 J. Heinke, M. Lannerstad, D. Gerten, et al., "Water Use in Global Livestock Production: Opportunities and Constraints for Increasing Water Productivity," *Water Resources Research* 56, 12 (2020): e2019WR026995.

41 United Nations Educational, Scientific and Cultural Organization (UNESCO), *The United Nations World Water Development Report 2021: Valuing Water* (Paris: 2021); FAO and Intergovernmental Technical Panel on Soils (ITPS), *Status of the World's Soil Resources (SWSR): Main Report* (Rome: 2015).

42 Intergovernmental Science-Policy Platform on Biodiversity and Ecosystem Services (IPBES), *The Assessment on Pollinators, Pollination and Food Production: Summary for Policymakers* (Bonn: 2019).

43 T. Beal, C.D. Gardner, M. Herrero, L.L. Iannotti, L. Merbold, S. Nordhagen, and A. Mottet, "Friend or Foe? The Role of Animal-Source Foods in Healthy and Environmentally Sustainable Diets," *The Journal of Nutrition* 153, 2 (2023): 409-425.

44 J. Heinke, M. Lannerstad, D. Gerten, et al. "Water Use in Global Livestock Production: Opportunities and Constraints for Increasing Water Productivity," *Water Resources Research* 56, 12 (2020): e2019WR026995.

45 P. Gerber, H. Steinfeld, B. Henderson, et al., *Tackling Climate Change through Livestock - A Global Assessment of Emissions and Mitigation Opportunities* (Rome: FAO, 2013).

46 FAO and ITPS, *Status of the World's Soil Resources (SWSR): Main Report* (Rome: 2015); N. Ramankutty, Z. Mehrabi, K. Waha, L. Jarvis, C. Kremen, M. Herrero, and L.H. Rieseberg, "Trends in Global Agricultural Land Use: Implications for Environmental Health and Food Security," *Annual Review of Plant Biology* 69 (2018): 789-815.

47 T. Beal, C.D. Gardner, M. Herrero, L.L. Iannotti, L. Merbold, S. Nordhagen, and A. Mottet, "Friend or Foe? The Role of Animal-Source Foods in Healthy and Environmentally Sustainable Diets," *The Journal of Nutrition* 153, 2 (2023): 409-425.

48 FAO, International Fund for Agricultural Development (IFAD), UNICEF, World Food Programme (WFP), and WHO, *The State of Food Security and Nutrition in the World 2022* (Rome: FAO, 2022).

49 D.D. Headey and H.H. Alderman, "The Relative Caloric Prices of Healthy and Unhealthy Foods Differ Systematically across Income Levels and Continents," *The Journal of Nutrition* 149 (2019): 2020-2033.

50 K. Hirvonen, Y. Bai, D.D. Headey, and W.A. Masters, "Affordability of the EAT-Lancet Reference Diet: A Global Analysis," *Lancet Global Health* 8, 1 (2020): e59-e66.

51 J.L. Leroy, P. Gadsden, T. González de Cossío, and P. Gertler, "Cash and In-Kind Transfers Lead to Excess Weight Gain in a Population of Women with a High Prevalence of Overweight in Rural Mexico," *The Journal of Nutrition* 143, 3 (2013): 378-383; J.L. Leroy, P. Gadsden, S. Rodriguez-Ramirez, and T. Gonzalez De Cossio, "Cash and In-Kind Transfers in Poor Rural Communities in Mexico Increase Household Fruit, Vegetable, and Micronutrient Consumption but Also Lead to Excess Energy Consumption," *The Journal of Nutrition* 140, 3 (2010): 612-617.

52 C. Hawkes, M.T. Ruel, L. Salm, B. Sinclair, and F. Branca, "Double-Duty Actions: Seizing Programme and Policy Opportunities to Address Malnutrition in All Its Forms," *Lancet* 395, 10218 (2020): 142-155.

53 M. Herrero, D. Mason-D'Croz, P.K. Thornton, et al., "Livestock and Sustainable Food Systems: Status, Trends, and Priority Actions," in *Science and Innovations for Food Systems Transformation*, eds. J. von Braun, K. Afsana, L.O. Fresco, and M. Hag Ali Hassan, 375-399 (Cham, Switzerland: Springer International Publishing, 2023).

54 S.M. Pires and B. Devleesschauwer, "Estimates of Global Disease Burden Associated with Foodborne Pathogens," in *Foodborne Infections and Intoxications*, eds. J. Glenn Morris, Jr. and D.J. Vugia, 3-17 (London: Elsevier, 2021).

55 E. Blackmore, A. Guarín, S. Alonso, D. Grace, and B. Vorley, *Informal Milk Markets in Kenya, Tanzania and Assam (India): An Overview of Their Status, Policy Context, and Opportunities for Policy Innovation to Improve Health and Safety* (Nairobi: International Livestock Research Institute (ILRI), 2020); S. Henson, S. Jaffee, and S. Wang, *New Directions for Tackling Food Safety Risks in the Informal Sector of Developing Countries* (Nairobi: ILRI, 2023).

56 J. Poore and T. Nemecek, "Reducing Food's Environmental Impacts through Producers and Consumers," *Science* 360, 6392 (2018): 987-992.

57 C.J. Bryant, "Plant-Based Animal Product Alternatives Are Healthier and More Environmentally Sustainable than Animal Products," *Future Foods* 6 (2022): 100174.

58 A. Mukherji, C. Arndt, J. Arango, et al., Achieving *Agricultural Breakthrough: A Deep Dive into Seven Technological Areas* (Montpellier, France: CGIAR, 2023).

59 I.D. Brouwer and E. Talsma, "Solving Global Nutrition and Dietary Challenges: More than Proteins," in *Our Future Proteins: A Diversity of Perspectives*, eds. S. Pyett, W. Jenkins, B. van Mierlo, L.M. Trindade, D. Welch, and H. van Zanten, 468-482. (Amsterdam: VU University Press, 2023).

BOX 1

a T. Beal, C.D. Gardner, M. Herrero, L.L. Iannotti, L. Merbold, S. Nordhagen, and A. Mottet, "Friend or Foe? The Role of Animal-Source Foods in Healthy and Environmentally Sustainable Diets," *The Journal of Nutrition* 153, 2 (2023): 409-425.

b A. Mukherji, C. Arndt, J. Arango, et al., *Achieving Agricultural Breakthrough: A Deep Dive into Seven Technological Areas* (Montpellier, France: CGIAR, 2023).

c World Health Organization, *Red and Processed Meat in the Context of Health and the Environment: Many Shades of Red and Green*, Information Brief (Geneva: 2023).

BOX 2

a R.D. Semba, "The Rise and Fall of Protein Malnutrition in Global Health," *Annals of Nutrition and Metabolism* 69, 2 (2016): 79-88.

b R.D. Semba, "The Rise and Fall of Protein Malnutrition in Global Health," *Annals of Nutrition and Metabolism* 69, 2 (2016): 79-88; D.S. McLaren, "The Great Protein Fiasco," *Lancet* 304, 7872 (1974): 93-96; D.S. McLaren, "The Great Protein Fiasco Revisited," *Nutrition* 16, 6 (2000): 464-465.

c R.D. Semba, "The Rise and Fall of Protein Malnutrition in Global Health," *Annals of Nutrition and Metabolism* 69, 2 (2016): 79-88; D.S. McLaren, "The Great Protein Fiasco," *Lancet* 304, 7872 (1974): 93-96.

d R.D. Semba, M. Shardell, F.A. Sakr, et al., "Child Stunting is Associated with Low Circulating Essential Amino Acids," *EBioMedicine* 6 (2016): 246-252.

e J.E. Arsenault and K.H. Brown, "Dietary Protein Intake in Young Children in Selected Low-Income Countries Is Generally Adequate in Relation to Estimated Requirements for Healthy Children, Except When Complementary Food Intake Is Low," *The Journal of Nutrition* 147, 5 (2017): 932-939.

f J.E. Arsenault and K.H. Brown, "Effects of Protein or Amino Acid Supplementation on the Physical Growth of Young Children in Low Income Countries: Review of Published Intervention Trials," *Nutrition Reviews* 75, 9 (2017): 699-717.

g J.E. Arsenault and K.H. Brown, "Effects of Protein or Amino Acid Supplementation on the Physical Growth of Young Children in Low Income Countries: Review of Published Intervention Trials," *Nutrition Reviews* 75, 9 (2017): 699-717.

h M. Arimond, M. Zeilani, S. Jungjohann, K.H. Brown, P. Ashorn, L.H. Allen, and K.G. Dewey, "Considerations in Developing Lipid-Based Nutrient Supplements for Prevention of Undernutrition: Experience from the International Lipid-Based Nutrient Supplements (iLiNS) Project," *Maternal & Child Nutrition* 11, S4 (2015): 31-61; K.G. Dewey, "The Challenge of Meeting Nutrient Needs of Infants and Young Children during the Period of Complementary Feeding: An Evolutionary Perspective," *The Journal of Nutrition*143, 12 (2013): 2050-2054.

CHAPTER 8

1 J. Fanzo, L. Haddad, K.R. Schneider, et al., "Viewpoint: Rigorous Monitoring Is Necessary to Guide Food System Transformation in the Countdown to the 2030 Global Goals," *Food Policy* 104 (2021): 102163; K.R. Schneider, J. Fanzo, L. Haddad, et al., "The State of Food Systems Worldwide in the Countdown to 2030," *Nature Food* 4, 12 (2023): 1090-1110.

2 World Bank, *Taxes on Sugar-Sweetened Beverages: Summary of International Evidence and Experiences* (Washington, DC: 2020).

3 World Health Organization (WHO), "Existence of Price Subsidies for Healthy Foods," updated April 25, 2022. https://www.who.int/data/gho/data/indicators/indicator-details/GHO/existence-of-price-subsidies-for-healthy-foods

4 Evaluations of the program from select states indicate moderate success in increasing household expenditures on vegetables; M. Steele-Adjognon and D. Weatherspoon, "Double Up Food Bucks Program Effects on SNAP Recipients' Fruit and Vegetable Purchases," *BMC Public Health* 17, 946 (2017): 1-7.

5 H. Alderman, D. Gilligan, J. Leight, T. Mamo, M. Mulford, and H. Tambet, "Including Scalable Nutrition Interventions in a Graduation Model Program: Experimental Evidence from Ethiopia," IFPRI Discussion Paper 2208, IFPRI, Washington, DC, 2023; D.K. Olney, A. Gelli, N. Kumar, H. Alderman, A. Go, and A. Raza, "Social Assistance Programme Impacts on Women's and Children's Diets and Nutritional Status," *Maternal & Child Nutrition* 18, 4 (2022): e13378.

6 B.M. Popkin, S. Barquera, C. Corvalan, et al., "Toward Unified and Impactful Policies for Reducing Ultraprocessed Food Consumption and Promoting Healthier Eating Globally," *Lancet: Diabetes & Endocrinology* 9, 7 (2021): 462-470.

7 E.C. Keats, L.M. Neufeld, G.S. Garrett, M.N.N. Mbuya, and Z.A. Bhutta, "Improved Micronutrient Status and Health Outcomes in Low- and Middle-Income Countries Following Large-Scale Fortification: Evidence from a Systematic Review and Meta-Analysis," *The American Journal of Clinical Nutrition* 109, 6 (2019): 1696-1708.

8 J.K. Hanson and R. Sigman, "Leviathan's Latent Dimensions: Measuring State Capacity for Comparative Political Research," *Journal of Politics* 83, 4 (2021): 1495-1510.

9 P. Evans, *Embedded Autonomy: States and Industrial Transformation* (Princeton, NJ: Princeton University Press, 1995); A. Kohli, *State-Directed Development: Political Power and Industrialization in the Global Periphery* (New York: Cambridge University Press, 2004).

10 D. Pomeranz and J. Vila-Belda, "Taking State-Capacity Research to the Field: Insights from Collaborations with Tax Authorities," *Annual Review of Economics* 11, 1 (2019): 755-781; J. Weigel, "The Participation Dividend of Taxation: How Citizens in Congo Engage More with the State When It Tries to Tax Them," *Quarterly Journal of Economics* 134, 4 (2020): 1849-1903.

11 World Bank, *International Debt Report 2023* (Washington, DC: 2023).

12 J.R. Behrman and J. Hoddinott, "Programme Evaluation with Unobserved Heterogeneity and Selective Implementation: The Mexican PROGRESA Impact on Child Nutrition," *Oxford Bulletin of Economics and Statistics* 67, 4 (2005): 547-569.

13 A.U. Ahmed, J.F. Hoddinott, S. Roy, E. Sraboni, W.R. Quabili, and A. Margolies, *Which Kinds of Social Safety Net Transfers Work Best for the Ultra Poor in Bangladesh?* (Washington, DC, and Rome, Italy: IFPRI and World Food Program, 2016).

14 M.L. Niebylski, K.A. Redburn, T. Duhaney, and N.R. Campbell, "Healthy Food Subsidies and Unhealthy Food Taxation: A Systematic Review of the Evidence," *Nutrition* 31, 6 (2015): 787-795.

15 E.J. Gómez, "Government Response to Ultra-Processed and Sugar Beverages Industries in Developing Nations: The Need to Build Coalitions across Policy Sectors," in *The Political Economy of Food System Transformation*, eds. D. Resnick and J. Swinnen, 133-154. (Oxford, UK: Oxford University Press, 2023).

16 Food and Agriculture Organization of the United Nations (FAO), "Food and Agriculture Policy Decision Analysis Tool" https://fapda.apps.fao.org/fapda/#main.html; International Trade Administration (ITA), "Botswana-Country Commercial Guide" (Washington, DC: 2024).

17 *The Namibian*, "Botswana Fruit, Veg Ban Backfires," October 15, 2022; U.S. International Trade Administration, "Botswana-Country Commercial Guide" (Washington, DC: 2024).

18 United States Department of Agriculture (USDA), *Nigeria: Sugar Annual* (Washington, DC: 2023).

19 R. Moodie, E. Bennett, E.J.L. Kwong, T.M. Santos, L. Pratiwi, J. Williams, and P. Baker. "Ultra-Processed Profits: The Political Economy of Countering the Global Spread of Ultra-Processed Foods—A Synthesis Review on the Market and Political Practices of Transnational Food Corporations and Strategic Public Health Responses," *International Journal of Health Policy and Management* 10, 12 (2021): 968-982.

20 A.C. Holland and B.R. Schneider, "Easy and Hard Redistribution: The Political Economy of Welfare States in Latin America," *Perspectives on Politics* 15, 4 (2017): 988-1006.

21 WHO, *Global Report on the Use of Sugar-Sweetened Beverage Taxes, 2023* (Geneva: 2023).

22 G. Fretes, C. Corvalán, M. Reyes, L. Smith Taillie, C.D. Economos, N.L.W. Wilson, and S.B. Cash, "Changes in Children's and Adolescents' Dietary Intake after the Implementation of Chile's Law of Food Labeling, Advertising and Sales in Schools: A Longitudinal Study," *International Journal of Behavioral Nutrition and Physical Activity* 20, 1 (2023): 40.

23 S.J.M. Osendarp, H. Martinez, G.S. Garrett, L.M. Neufeld, L. Maria De-Regil, M. Vossenaar, and I. Darnton-Hill, "Large-Scale Food Fortification and Biofortification in Low- and Middle-Income Countries: A Review of Programs, Trends, Challenges, and Evidence Gaps," *Food and Nutrition Bulletin* 39, 2 (2018): 315-331.

24 Such policies encompassed measures to define national NCD targets and NCD action plans and efforts to reduce unhealthy diets (restrictions on marketing to children, saturated fatty acids and transfats policies, salt/sodium policies), harmful use of alcohol, and tobacco demand, as well as public education and awareness campaigns on physical activity; L.N. Allen, S. Wigley, H. Holmer, and P. Barlow, "Non-Communicable Disease Policy Implementation from 2014 to 2021: A Repeated Cross-Sectional Analysis of Global Policy Data for 194 Countries," *Lancet Global Health* 11, 4 (2023): e525-e533.

25 L.N. Allen, S. Wigley, H. Holmer, and P. Barlow, "Non-Communicable Disease Policy Implementation from 2014 to 2021: A Repeated Cross-Sectional Analysis of Global Policy Data for 194 Countries," *Lancet Global Health* 11, 4 (2023): e525-e533.

26 B.M. Popkin, C. Corvalan, and L.M. Grummer-Strawn, "Dynamics of the Double Burden of Malnutrition and the Changing Nutrition Reality," *Lancet* 395, 10217 (2020): 65-74.

27 S. Jaffee, S. Henson, L. Unnevehre, D. Grace, and E. Cassou, *The Safe Food Imperative: Accelerating Progress in Low- and Middle-Income Countries* (Washington, DC: World Bank, 2019).

28 See Bloomberg Philanthropies, "Partnership for Healthy Cities," accessed January 2023. https://www.bloomberg.org/public-health/building-public-health-coalitions/partnership-for-healthy-cities/

29 M. Nestle, *Food Politics: How the Food Industry Influences Nutrition and Health* (Berkeley: University of California Press, 2013); E. James, M. Lajous, and M.R. Reich, "The Politics of Taxes for Health: An Analysis of the Passage of the Sugar-Sweetened Beverage Tax in Mexico," *Health Systems & Reform* 6, 1 (2020): e1669122; P. Baker and S. Friel, "Food Systems Transformations, Ultra-Processed Food Markets and the Nutrition Transition in Asia," *Globalization and Health* 12, 1 (2016): 80; E.J. Gómez, "The Politics of Ultra-Processed Foods and Beverages

Regulatory Policy in Upper-Middle-Income Countries: Industry and Civil Society in Mexico and Brazil," *Global Public Health* 17, 9 (2022): 1883-1901.

30 M. Mialòn, B. Swinburn, and G. Sacks, "A Proposed Approach to Systematically Identify and Monitor the Corporate Political Activity of the Food Industry with Respect to Public Health Using Publicly Available Information," *Obesity Reviews* 16, 7 (2015): 519-530.

31 E. Bennett, S.M. Topp, and A.R. Moodie, "National Public Health Surveillance of Corporations in Key Unhealthy Commodity Industries–A Scoping Review and Framework Synthesis," *International Journal of Health Policy and Management* 12 (2023): 6876.

32 I. Torres, J.J. Villalba, D.F. López-Cevallos, and S. Galea, "Governmental Institutionalization of Corporate Influence on National Nutrition Policy and Health: A Case Study of Ecuador," *Lancet Regional Health: Americas* 29 (2024): 100645.

33 P. Wood and M. Tavan, "A Review of the Alternative Protein Industry," *Current Opinion in Food Science* 47 (2022): 100869.

34 J. Shen, Z. Zhu, M. Qaim, S. Fan, and X. Tian, eds., "E-Commerce Improves Dietary Quality of Rural Households in China," ZEF Discussion Papers on Development Policy No. 329, Center for Development Research, Bonn, Germany, 2023.

35 T. Reardon and R. Vos, "How Resilience Innovations in Food Supply Chains Are Revolutionizing Logistics, Wholesale Trade, and Farm Services in Developing Countries," *International Food and Agribusiness Management Review* 26, 3 (2023): 455-466.

36 Zero Hunger Coalition, *From Pledge to Action: Assessing Progress of the Zero Hunger Private Sector Pledge and Pledging Companies towards SDG2* (Zero Hunger Coalition, 2023).

37 T. Durotoye, I. Ilegbune, D. Schofield, V. Ajieroh, and O. Ezekannagha, "Industry Self-Regulation of Food Fortification Compliance: Piloting the Micronutrient Fortification Index in Nigeria," *Food and Nutrition Bulletin* 44, 1_ suppl (2023): S74-S84.

38 Feed the Truth and Corporate Accountability, "Food and Agriculture Corporate Transparency (FACT) Index," n.d. https://corporateaccountability.org/resources/fact-index/

39 L.N. Allen, S. Wigley, and H. Holmer, "Assessing the Association between Corporate Financial Influence and Implementation of Policies to Tackle Commercial Determinants of Non-communicable Diseases: A Cross-Sectional Analysis of 172 Countries," *Social Science & Medicine* 297 (2022): 114825.

40 L.N. Allen, S. Wigley, and H. Holmer, "Assessing the Association between Corporate Financial Influence and Implementation of Policies to Tackle Commercial Determinants of Non-communicable Diseases: A Cross-Sectional Analysis of 172 Countries," *Social Science & Medicine* 297 (2022): 114825.

41 J. Clapp, W.G. Moseley, B. Burlingame, and P. Termine, "Viewpoint: The Case for a Six-Dimensional Food Security Framework," *Food Policy* 106 (2022): 102164.

42 R. Patel, "What Does Food Sovereignty Look Like?" *Journal of Peasant Studies* 36, 3 (2009): 663-706.

43 F. Anderl and M. Hißen, "How Trust Is Lost: The Food Systems Summit 2021 and the Delegitimation of UN Food Governance," *European Journal of International Relations*, 30, 1 (2023): 151-175.

44 Office of the United Nations High Commissioner for Human Rights, *Fact Sheet No. 34: The Right to Adequate Food* (Geneva: 2010).

45 W.K. Taylor, "On the Social Construction of Legal Grievances: Evidence from Colombia and South Africa," *Comparative Political Studies* 53, 8 (2020): 1326-1356.

46 See FAO, "The Right to Food around the Globe," updated January 2021. https://www.fao.org/right-to-food-around-the-globe/en/. Explicit provisions clearly recognize the right to food or freedom from hunger while implicit ones emphasize rights to well-being or an adequate standard of living that indirectly affect one's right to food.

47 D. Resnick and J. Swinnen, "Introduction," in *The Political Economy of Food System Transformation: Pathways to Progress in a Polarized World*, 1-31 (Oxford, UK: Oxford University Press, 2023).

48 D. Resnick, "Food Systems Transformation and Local Governance," in *Global Hunger Index: Food Systems Transformation and Local Governance* (Bonn, Germany, and Dublin, Ireland: Welthungerhilfe and Concern Worldwide, 2022).

49 J. Thorpe, T. Sprenger, J. Guijt, and D. Stibbe, "Are Multi-Stakeholder Platforms Effective Approaches to Agri-Food Sustainability? Towards Better Assessment," *International Journal of Agricultural Sustainability* 20, 2 (2022): 168-183.

50 C. van Bers, A. Delaney, H. Eakin, et al., "Advancing the Research Agenda on Food Systems Governance and Transformation," *Current Opinion in Environmental Sustainability* 39 (2019): 94-102.

51 A. Moragues-Faus, "The Emergence of City Food Networks: Rescaling the Impact of Urban Food Policies," *Food Policy* 103 (2021): 102107.

52 S. Scott, Z. Si, T. Schumilas, and A. Chen, "Contradictions in State-and Civil Society-Driven Developments in China's Ecological Agriculture Sector," *Food Policy* 45 (2014): 158-166.

53 A. Buyse, "Squeezing Civic Space: Restrictions on Civil Society Organizations and the Linkages with Human Rights," *International Journal of Human Rights* 22, 8 (2018): 966-988; D. Resnick and S. Deshpande, "Illiberal Democracy and Nutrition Advocacy," *Development Policy Review* 41, 6 (2023): e12726.

54 A. Moragues-Faus, "The Emergence of City Food Networks: Rescaling the Impact of Urban Food Policies," *Food Policy* 103 (2021): 102107; T. Zerbian and E. De Luis Romero, "The Role of Cities in Good Governance for Food Security: Lessons from Madrid's Urban Food Strategy," *Territory, Politics, Governance* 11, 4 (2023): 794-812.

55 M.C. Herens, K.H. Pittore, and P.J.M. Oosterveer, "Transforming Food Systems: Multi-Stakeholder Platforms Driven by Consumer Concerns and Public Demands," *Global Food Security* 32 (2022): 100592.

56 K. Schneider, J. Fanzo, J. Haddad, et al., "The State of Food Systems Worldwide in the Countdown to 2030," *Nature Food* 4, 12 (2023): 1090-1110.

57 C. Zorbas, D. Resnick, E. Jones, et al., "From Promises to Action: Analyzing Global Commitments on Food Security and Diets since 2015," IFPRI Discussion Paper 2238, IFPRI, Washington, DC, 2024.

REGIONAL DEVELOPMENTS

AFRICA

1 W. Willett, J. Rockström, B. Loken, et al., "Food in the Anthropocene: The EAT-Lancet Commission on Healthy Diets from Sustainable Food Systems," *Lancet* 393, 10170 (2019): 447-492; Food and Agriculture Organization of the United Nations (FAO), International Fund for Agricultural Development (IFAD), UNICEF, World Food Program (WFP), and World Health Organization (WHO), *The State of Food Security and Nutrition in the World 2023: Urbanization, Agrifood Systems Transformation and Healthy Diets Across the Rural-Urban Continuum* (Rome: FAO, 2023); V. Abe-Inge and E. Miezah Kwofie, "Accounting for Environmental-Nutrition Trade-offs," in *AGRA Africa Agriculture Status Report 2023: African Food Systems in Empowering Africa's Food*

Systems for the Future*, eds. J.M. Ulimwengu, J. Njuguna, and S. Maina, Chapter 8, 143-162 (Nairobi: Alliance for a Green Revolution in Africa (AGRA), 2023).

2 FAO, African Union Commission (AUC), United Nations Economic Commission for Africa (ECA) and WFP, *Africa - Regional Overview of Food Security and Nutrition 2023: Statistics and Trends* (Accra: FAO, 2023).

3 G. Gatica-Domínguez, P.A.R. Neves, A.J.D. Barros, and C.G. Victora, "Complementary Feeding Practices in 80 Low- and Middle-Income Countries: Prevalence of and Socioeconomic Inequalities in Dietary Diversity, Meal Frequency, and Dietary Adequacy," *The Journal of Nutrition* 151, 7 (2021): 1956-1964.

4 E.O. Verger, A. Le Port, A. Borderon, et al., "Dietary Diversity Indicators and Their Associations with Dietary Adequacy and Health Outcomes: A Systematic Scoping Review," *Advances in Nutrition* 12, 5 (2021): 1659-1672; T. Ahmed, M. Hossain, and K.I. Sanin, "Global Burden of Maternal and Child Undernutrition and Micronutrient Deficiencies," *Annals of Nutrition and Metabolism* 61, Suppl. 1 (2012): 8-17; R.L. Bailey, K.P. West, and R.E. Black, "The Epidemiology of Global Micronutrient Deficiencies," *Annals of Nutrition and Metabolism* 66, Suppl. 2 (2015): 22-33; R.E. Black, C.G. Victora, S.P. Walker, et al., "Maternal and Child Undernutrition and Overweight in Low-Income and Middle-Income Countries," *Lancet* 382, 9890 (2013): 427-451; GBD 2017 Diet Collaborators, "Health Effects of Dietary Risks in 195 Countries, 1990-2017: A Systematic Analysis for the Global Burden of Disease Study 2017," *Lancet* 393, 10184 (2019): 1958-1972.

5 The 21 countries are Burkina Faso, Chad, Democratic Republic of Congo, Egypt, Eswatini, Ethiopia, Gambia, Ghana, Guinea Bissau, Kenya, Lesotho, Madagascar, Malawi, Mali, Mauritania, Mozambique, Niger, Rwanda, Sudan, Uganda and Zimbabwe; African Union, *The Cost of Hunger in Africa (COHA) Continental Report: Social and Economic Impact of Child Undernutrition* (Durban: 2022).

6 X. Han, S. Ding, J. Lu, and Y. Li, "Global, Regional, and National Burdens of Common Micronutrient Deficiencies from 1990 to 2019: A Secondary Trend Analysis Based on the Global Burden of Disease 2019 Study," *EClinicalMedicine* 12, 44 (2022): 101299.

7 FAO, AUC, ECA, and WFP, *Africa - Regional Overview of Food Security and Nutrition 2023: Statistics and Trends* (Accra: FAO, 2023).

8 T. Beal, F. Ortenzi, and J. Fanzo, "Estimated Micronutrient Shortfalls of the EAT-*Lancet* Planetary Health Diet," *Lancet Planetary Health* 7, 3 (2023): e233-237.

9 W. Marivoet and J.M. Ulimwengu, "Mapping the Nutrient Adequacy of Farm Production and Food Consumption to Target Policy in Uganda," *Development Policy Review* 40, 3 (2022): e12596; W. Marivoet, J.M. Ulimwengu, and L.M. Sall, *Policy Atlas on Food and Nutrition Security and Resilience: Kenya* (Washington, DC: IFPRI, 2020); W. Marivoet, J.M. Ulimwengu, and L.M. Sall, *Policy Atlas on Food and Nutrition Security and Resilience: Burkina Faso* (Washington, DC: IFPRI, 2020); W. Marivoet, J.M. Ulimwengu, and L.M. Sall, *Policy Atlas on Food and Nutrition Security: Rwanda* (Washington, DC: IFPRI, 2020); W. Marivoet, J.M. Ulimwengu, and L.M. Sall, *Policy Atlas on Food and Nutrition Security: Ghana* (Washington, DC: IFPRI, 2020).

10 I.K. Sharma, S. Di Prima, D. Essink, and J.E.W. Broerse, "Nutrition-Sensitive Agriculture: A Systematic Review of Impact Pathways to Nutrition Outcomes," *Advances in Nutrition* 12, 1 (2021): 251-275; M.T. Ruel, A.R. Quisumbing, and M. Balagamwala, "Nutrition-Sensitive Agriculture: What Have We Learned So Far?" *Global Food Security* 17 (2018): 128-153.

11 D.K. Olney, L. Bliznashka, A. Pedehombga, A. Dillon, M.T. Ruel, and J. Heckert, "A 2-Year Integrated Agriculture and Nutrition Program Targeted to Mothers of Young Children in Burkina Faso Reduces Underweight among Mothers and Increases Their Empowerment: A Cluster-Randomized Controlled Trial," *The Journal of Nutrition* 146 (2016): 1109-1117.

12 The program was implemented in Burkina Faso, Tanzania, Senegal, and Côte d'Ivoire from 2013 to 2016; S. Nordhagen, J. Nielsen, T. van Mourik, E. Smith, and R. Klemm, "Fostering CHANGE: Lessons from Implementing a Multi-country, Multi-sector Nutrition-Sensitive Agriculture Project," *Evaluation and Program Planning* 77 (2019): 101695.

13 A. Collishaw, S. Janzen, C. Mullally, and H. Camilli, "A Review of Livestock Development Interventions' Impacts on Household Welfare in Low- and Middle-Income Countries," *Global Food Security* 38 (2023): 100704.

14 R. Rawlins, S. Pimkina, C.B. Barrett, S. Pedersen, and B. Wydick, "Got Milk? The Impact of Heifer International's Livestock Donation Programs in Rwanda on Nutritional Outcomes," *Food Policy 44* (2014): 202-213; M. Jodlowski, A. Winter-Nelson, K. Baylis, and P.D. Goldsmith, "Milk in the Data: Food Security Impacts from a Livestock Field Experiment in Zambia," *World Development 77* (2016): 99-114.

15 A. Omer, D. Hailu, and S.J. Whiting, "Egg Consumption of Children under Two Years of Age through a Child-Owned Poultry and Nutrition Intervention in Rural Ethiopia: A Community-Based Randomized Controlled Trial," *Journal of Agriculture and Food Research* 9 (2022): 100354.

16 H. Alderman, D.O. Gilligan, J. Leight, M. Mulford, and H. Tambet, "The Role of Poultry Transfers in Diet Diversity: A Cluster Randomized Intent to Treat Analysis," *Food Policy* 107 (2022): 102212.

17 S. Passarelli, R. Ambikapathi, N.S. Gunaratna, et al., "A Chicken Production Intervention and Additional Nutrition Behavior Change Component Increased Child Growth in Ethiopia: A Cluster-Randomized Trial," *The Journal of Nutrition*, 150 (2020): 2806-2817.

18 H. Alderman, U. Gentilini, and R. Yemstov, *The 1.5 Billion People Question: Food, Vouchers, or Cash Transfers?* (Washington, DC: World Bank, 2017).

19 M.T. Ruel, H. Alderman, and the Maternal and Child Nutrition Study Group, "Nutrition-Sensitive Interventions and Programmes: How Can They Help to Accelerate Progress in Improving Maternal and Child Nutrition?" *Lancet* 382, 9891 (2013): 536-551.

20 D. Olney, A. Gelli, N. Kumar, et al., "Nutrition-Sensitive Social Protection Programs within Food Systems," IFPRI Discussion Paper 2044, IFPRI, Washington, DC, 2021.

21 J. Manley, Y. Balarajan, S. Malm, et al., "Cash Transfers and Child Nutritional Outcomes: A Systematic Review and Meta-Analysis," *BMJ Global Health* 5 (2020): 1-9; R. de Groot, T. Palermo, S. Handa, L.P. Ragno, and A. Peterman, "Cash Transfers and Child Nutrition: Pathways and Impacts," *Development Policy Review* 35, 5 (2017): 621-643.

22 World Bank, *The State of Social Safety Nets 2018* (Washington, DC: 2018).

23 WFP, *State of School Feeding Worldwide 2020* (Rome: 2020).

24 A. Gelli, E. Aurino, G. Folson, et al., "A School Meals Program Implemented at Scale in Ghana Increases Height-for-Age during Midchildhood in Girls and in Children from Poor Households: A Cluster Randomized Trial," *The Journal of Nutrition* 149, 8 (2019):1434-1442.

25 A. Gelli, "School Feeding and Girls' Enrollment: The Effects of Alternative Implementation Modalities in Low-Income Settings in Sub-Saharan Africa," *Frontiers in Public Health* 3 (2015): 76.

26 E. Aurino, A. Gelli, C. Adamba, I. Osei-Akoto, and H. Alderman, "Food for Thought? Experimental Evidence on the Learning Impacts of a

Large-Scale School Feeding Program," *The Journal of Human Resources* 58, 1 (2023): 74-111.

27 B. Barnabas B, S.A. Agyemang, E. Zhllima, and M. Bavorova, "Impact of Homegrown School Feeding Program on Smallholders' Farmer Household Food Security in Northeastern Nigeria," *Foods* 12, 12 (2023): 2408; H. Alderman, D. Bundy, and A. Gelli, "School Meals Are Evolving: Has the Evidence Kept Up?" *World Bank Research Observer* (2024): lkad012.

28 T.A. Desalegn, S. Gebremedhin, and B.J. Stoecker, "Successes and Challenges of the Home-Grown School Feeding Program in Sidama Region, Southern Ethiopia: A Qualitative Study," *Journal of Nutritional Sciences* 11 (2022): e87.

29 I.C. Ohanenye, C.U. Emenike, A. Mensi, et al., "Food Fortification Technologies: Influence on Iron, Zinc and Vitamin A Bioavailability and Potential Implications on Micronutrient Deficiency in Sub-Saharan Africa," *Scientific African* 11 (2021): e00667; A. Olanbiwoninu, A. Greppi, T. Awotundun, E.A. Adebayo, G. Spano, D. Mora, and P. Russo, "Microbial-Based Biofortification to Mitigate African Micronutrients Deficiency: A Focus on Plant-Based Fermentation as Source of B-group Vitamins," *Food Bioscience* 55 (2023): 102996.

30 A.C. Palmer, K. Healy, M.A. Barffour, et al., "Provitamin A Carotenoid-Biofortified Maize Consumption Increases Pupillary Responsiveness among Zambian Children in a Randomized Controlled Trial," *The Journal of Nutrition* 146, 12 (2016): 2551-2558; C. Hotz, C. Loechl, A. Lubowa, et al., "Introduction of B-carotene-rich Orange Sweet Potato in Rural Uganda Resulted in Increased Vitamin A Intakes among Children and Women and Improved Vitamin A Status among Children," *The Journal of Nutrition* 142, 10 (2012): 1871-1880; J.W. Low, M. Arimond, N. Osman, B. Cunguara, F. Zano, and D. Tschirley, "A Food-Based Approach Introducing Orange-Fleshed Sweet Potatoes Increased Vitamin A Intake and Serum Retinol Concentrations in Young Children in Rural Mozambique," *The Journal of Nutrition* 137, 5 (2007): 1320-1327; P.J. Van Jaarsveld, M. Faber, S.A. Tanumihardjo, P. Nestel, C.J. Lombard, and A.J.S. Benad'e, "B-carotene-Rich Orange-Fleshed Sweet Potato Improves the Vitamin A Status of Primary School Children Assessed with the Modified-Relative-Dose-Response Test," *The American Journal of Clinical Nutrition* 81, 5 (2005): 1080-1087.

31 E. Birol, D. Asare-Marfo, J. Fieldler, et al., *Cost-Effectiveness of Biofortification*, Progress Brief No. 25 (Washington, DC: HarvestPlus, 2015).

32 HarvestPlus, HarvestPlus Database of Biofortified Crops Released, accessed November 20, 2023. https://bcr.harvestplus.org/varieties_released/dashboard

33 The African countries where testing is ongoing with no releases yet are Benin, Chad, Central African Republic, Egypt, Eritrea, Eswatini, Gabon, Gambia, Guinea, Liberia, Morocco, Senegal, South Sudan, Togo, and Tunisia; HarvestPlus, *Biofortified Crops Around the World* (Washington, DC: 2020).

34 J.K. Foley, K.D. Michaux, B. Mudyahoto, et al., "Scaling Up Delivery of Biofortified Staple Food Crops Globally: Paths to Nourishing Millions," *Food and Nutrition Bulletin* 42, 1 (2021): 116-132.

35 E.C. Keats, L.M. Neufeld, G.S. Garrett, M.N.N. Mbuya, and Z.A. Bhutta, "Improved Micronutrient Status and Health Outcomes in Low- and Middle-Income Countries Following Large-Scale Fortification: Evidence from a Systematic Review and Meta-analysis," *The American Journal of Clinical Nutrition* 109, 6 (2019): 1696-1708.

36 R. Engle-Stone, M. Nankap, A.O. Ndjebayi, et al., "Iron, Zinc, Folate, and Vitamin B-12 Status Increased among Women and Children in Yaoundé and Douala, Cameroon, 1 Year after Introducing Fortified Wheat Flour," *The Journal of Nutrition* 147, 7 (2017): 1426-1436.

37 F. Rohner, M. Leyvraz, A.G. Konan, et al., "The Potential of Food Fortification to Add Micronutrients in Young Children and Women of Reproductive Age: Findings from a Cross-Sectional Survey in Abidjan, Côte d'Ivoire," *PLoS ONE* 11, 7 (2016): e0158552.

38 45 countries have legislation for mandatory salt fortification: 45 with iodine, 1 with iron, and 1 with fluoride.

39 30 countries have legislation for mandatory wheat flour fortification: 29 with folate and/or iron, 14-16 with vitamins B1, B2, B3, B12 and/or zinc, and 11 with vitamins A and/or B6.

40 12 countries have legislation for mandatory maize flour fortification: 12 with folate and iron, and 8-10 with vitamins A, B1, B2, B3, B6, B12 and/or zinc.

41 25 countries have legislation for mandatory oil fortification: 25 with vitamin A and 5 with vitamin D.

42 Global Fortification Data Exchange, Legislation Scope and Monitoring Protocols Database, accessed November 20, 2023. https://s3-us-west-2.amazonaws.com/gfdx-published-files/legislation_scope_and_monitoring_protocols.csv

43 M. Sablah, J. Klopp, D. Steinberg, Z. Touaoro, A. Laillou, and S. Baker, "Thriving Public-Private Partnership to Fortify Cooking Oil in the West African Economic and Monetary Union (UEMOA) to Control Vitamin A Deficiency: Faire Tache d'Huile en Afrique de l'Ouest," *Food and Nutrition Bulletin* 33, 4 Suppl (2012): S310-S320.

44 UNICEF and Economic Community of West African States (ECOWAS), *Regional Model Law for West and Central Africa Regulating the Marketing of Breastmilk Substitutes, Foods for Infants and Young Children and Related Feeding Utensils* (Dakar: UNICEF, 2022).

45 L. Casu, A.D. Diatta, I. Uzhova, et al., *Nutrition-Relevant Policy in West Africa: A Comprehensive Review* (Dakar: Transform Nutrition West Africa; Washington, DC: IFPRI, 2022).

46 S.V. Wrottesley, N. Stacey, G. Mukoma, K.J. Hofman, and S.A. Norris, "Assessing Sugar-Sweetened Beverage Intakes, Added Sugar Intakes and BMI Before and After the Implementation of a Sugar-Sweetened Beverage Tax in South Africa," *Public Health Nutrition* 24, 10 (2021): 2900-2910; N. Stacey, C. Mudara, S.W. Ng, C. van Walbeek, K. Hofman, and I. Edoka, "Sugar-Based Beverage Taxes and Beverage Prices: Evidence from South Africa's Health Promotion Levy," *Social Science & Medicine* 238 (2019): 112465.

47 L.E. Barry, F. Kee, J. Woodside, et al., "An Umbrella Review of the Effectiveness of Fiscal and Pricing Policies on Food and Non-alcoholic Beverages to Improve Health," *Obesity Reviews* 24, 7 (2023): e13570.

48 N. Nisbett, J. Harris, D.D. Headey, et al., "Stories of Change in Nutrition: Lessons from a New Generation of Studies from Africa, Asia and Europe," *Food Security* 15, 1 (2023): 133-149.

49 Scaling Up Nutrition, "SUN Countries," accessed November 15, 2023. https://scalingupnutrition.org/countries

50 These reporting frameworks are intended for all African countries, although not all countries have reported each year. Regarding the AATS for example, 51 of the total 55 countries reported data for the 2024 edition compared to 47 in the inaugural 2018 edition. The CNAS has data on all 55 countries.

51 African Union, *Continental Nutrition Accountability* Scorecard (Durban: 2019).

52 African Union, *Continental Nutrition Accountability* Scorecard (Durban: 2019); African Union, *3rd CAADP Biennial Review Report* (Durban: 2021).

MIDDLE EAST AND NORTH AFRICA

1 Food and Agricultural Organization of the United Nations (FAO), International Fund for Agricultural Development (IFAD), UNICEF, World Food Programme (WFP), World Health Organization (WHO), and United Nations Economic and Social Commission for Western Asia (UNESCWA), *Near East and North Africa: Regional Overview of Food Security and Nutrition 2022: Trade as an Enabler for Food Security and Nutrition* (Cairo: FAO, 2023).

2 FAO, IFAD, UNICEF, WFP, WHO, and UNESCWA, *Near East and North Africa - Regional Overview of Food Security and Nutrition: Statistics and Trends* (Cairo: FAO, 2023).

3 K.A. Abay, C. Breisinger, J. Glauber, S. Kurdi, D. Laborde, and K. Siddig, "The Russia-Ukraine War: Implications for Global and Regional Food Security and Potential Policy Responses," *Global Food Security* 36 (2023): 100675; C. Arndt, X. Diao, P. Dorosh, K. Pauw, and J. Thurlow, "The Ukraine War and Rising Commodity Prices: Implications for Developing Countries," *Global Food Security* 36 (2023): 100680.

4 Central Authority for Public Mobilization and Statistics (CAPMAS), accessed September 15, 2023. https://www.capmas.gov.eg/

5 FAO, IFAD, UNICEF, WFP, WHO, and UNESCWA, *Near East and North Africa - Regional Overview of Food Security and Nutrition: Statistics and Trends* (Cairo: FAO, 2023).

6 UNHCR, "Global Appeal 2024: Middle East and North Africa," accessed March 2024. https://reporting.unhcr.org/global-appeal-2024/regional-overviews/middle-east-and-north-africa

7 World Bank, *Beyond Scarcity: Water Security in the Middle East and North Africa*, MENA Development Report (Washington, DC: 2018).

8 R. Gatti, D. Lederman, N. Elmallakh, J. Torres, J. Silva, R. Lotfi, and I. Suvanov, *Balancing Act: Jobs and Wages in the Middle East and North Africa When Crises Hit*, MENA Economic Update, October 2023 (Washington, DC: World Bank, 2023).

9 G. Lopez-Acevedo, M.C. Nguyen, N. Mohammed, and J. Hoogeveen, "How Rising Inflation in MENA Impacts Poverty," *World Bank Blogs*, June 30, 2022.

10 D.D. Headey and H.H. Alderman, "The Relative Caloric Prices of Healthy and Unhealthy Foods Differ Systematically across Income Levels and Continents," *The Journal of Nutrition* 149, 11 (2019): 2020–2033; K. Hirvonen, Y. Bai, D.D. Headey, W.A. Masters, "Affordability of the EAT-Lancet Reference Diet: A Global Analysis," *Lancet Global Health* 8, 1 (2019): E59–E66.

11 K.A. Abay, N. Karachiwalla, S. Kurdi, and Y. Salama, "Food Price Shocks and Diets among Poor Households in Egypt," in *The Russia-Ukraine Conflict and Global Food Security*, eds. J. Glauber and D. Laborde, 129-134 (Washington, DC: IFPRI, 2023).

12 F. Belhaj, R. Gatti, D. Lederman, E.J. Sergenti, H. Assem, R. Lotfi, M.E. Mousa, *A New State of Mind: Greater Transparency and Accountability in the Middle East and North Africa*, MENA Economic Update (Washington, DC: World Bank, 2022).

13 C. Breisinger, Y. Kassim, S. Kurdi, J. Randriamamonjy, and J. Thurlow, "From Food Subsidies to Cash Transfers: Assessing Economy-wide Benefits and Trade-Offs in Egypt," *Journal of African Economies* 33, 2 (2024): 109–129.

14 K.A. Abay, L. Abdelfattah, M. Elkaramany, D. Elsabbagh, and S. Kurdi, "Nutrition-Sensitive Food Distribution amidst Inflationary Shock: Evidence from a Randomized Intervention in Egypt," IFPRI Discussion Paper 2218, IFPRI, Washington, DC, 2023.

15 Using an adjusted version of FAO's Household Dietary Diversity Score (HDDS), with a recall period of one week, reflecting consumption of 12 diverse food groups: (1) foods made from grains; (2) white roots and tubers; (3) 1egumes nuts and seeds; (4) milk and milk products; (5) meat and organ meat; (6) fish and seafood; (7) eggs; (8) vegetables; (9) fruits; (10) oils and fats; (11) spices condiments and beverages; and (12) sweets and sweetened beverages.

16 O. Ecker, P. Al-Riffai, C. Breisinger, and R. El-Batrawy, *Nutrition and Economic Development: Exploring Egypt's Exceptionalism and the Role of Food Subsidies* (Washington, DC: IFPRI, 2016); Egypt, Ministry of Health and Population, National Nutrition Institute, and UNICEF, *Nutrition Agenda for Action: A Policy Paper on Scaling Up Nutrition Interventions in Egypt* (Cairo: Ministry of Health and Population, 2017); K.A. Abay, H. Ibrahim, and C. Breisinger, "Food Policies and Obesity in Low- and Middle-Income Countries," *World Development* 151 (2022): 105775.

17 K.A. Abay, L. Abdelfattah, M. Elkaramany, D. Elsabbagh, and S. Kurdi, "Nutrition-Sensitive Food Distribution amidst Inflationary Shock: Evidence from a Randomized Intervention in Egypt," IFPRI Discussion Paper 2218, IFPRI, Washington, DC, 2023.

18 See, for example, O. Ecker, P. Al-Riffai, C. Breisinger, and R. El-Batrawy, *Nutrition and Economic Development: Exploring Egypt's Exceptionalism and the Role of Food Subsidies* (Washington, DC: IFPRI, 2016); Ministry of Health and Population, the National Nutrition Institute, and UNICEF, *Nutrition Agenda for Action: A Policy Paper on Scaling Up Nutrition Interventions in Egypt* (Cairo: 2017).

19 Measured using two outcomes developed by the Food and Agriculture Organization of the United Nations: (1) HDDS stands for Household Dietary Diversity Score, a qualitative measure of the household's consumption and food security, reflecting the economic ability of the household to access a variety of foods, ranging from 0 (consuming no food groups) to 12 (consuming twelve food groups). (2) FIES is the Food Insecurity Experience Score constructed based on eight questions on food-related behaviors and experiences associated with difficulties in accessing adequate food due to financial or other resource constraints, ranging from 0 (no insecurity at all) to 8 (maximum level of food insecurity). See FAO, "Household Dietary Diversity (HDDS)," accessed August 2023, https://www.fao.org/nutrition/assessment/tools/household-dietary-diversity/en/; FAO, *FIES Basics: The Food Insecurity Experience Scale: Measuring Food Insecurity through People's Experiences* (Rome: 2014).

CENTRAL ASIA

1 Food and Agriculture Organization of the United Nations (FAO), International Fund for Agricultural Development (IFAD), UNICEF, World Food Program (WFP), and World Health Organization (WHO), *The State of Food Security and Nutrition in the World 2023: Urbanization, Agrifood Systems Transformation and Healthy Diets across the Rural-Urban Continuum* (Rome: FAO, 2023).

2 Human Rights Watch, "Turkmenistan: Denial, Inaction Worsen Food Crisis," Sept. 23, 2020. https://www.hrw.org/news/2020/09/23/turkmenistan-denial-inaction-worsen-food-crisis#:~:text=Declining%20hydrocarbon%20income%20since%202014,the%20border%20closure%20with%20Iran

3 FAO, IFAD, UNICEF, WFP, and WHO, *The State of Food Security and Nutrition in the World 2023: Urbanization, Agrifood Systems Transformation and Healthy Diets across the Rural-Urban Continuum* (Rome: FAO, 2023).

4 FAO, "FAOSTAT: Suite of Food Security Indicators," accessed March 18, 2024. https://www.fao.org/faostat

5 UNICEF, "Malnutrition in Children," accessed March 18, 2024. https://data.unicef.org/topic/nutrition/malnutrition/

6 M. de Onis, E. Borghi, M. Arimond, et al., "Prevalence Thresholds for Wasting, Overweight and Stunting in Children under 5 Years," *Public Health Nutrition* 22, 1 (2019): 175-179 (2019).

7 WHO, "Global Health Observatory," accessed March 18, 2024. https://www.who.int/data/gho/data/indicators

8 C. Fang and M. Gurinović, eds., *Sustainable and Nutrition-Sensitive Food Systems for Healthy Diets and Prevention of Malnutrition in Europe and Central Asia* (Budapest: FAO, 2023).

9 WHO, "Global Health Observatory," accessed March 18, 2024. https://www.who.int/data/gho/data/indicators

10 R. Guthold, G. A. Stevens, L. M. Riley, F. C. Bull, "Worldwide Trends in Insufficient Physical Activity from 2001 to 2016: A Pooled Analysis of 358 Population-Based Surveys with 1.9 Million Participants," *Lancet Global Health* 6 (2018): e1077-e1086.

11 WHO, "Global Health Observatory," accessed March 18, 2024. https://www.who.int/data/gho/data/indicators

12 M. de Onis, E. Borghi, M. Arimond, et al., "Prevalence Thresholds for Wasting, Overweight and Stunting in Children under 5 Years," *Public Health Nutrition* 22, 1 (2019): 175-179.

13 FAO, IFAD, UNICEF, WFP, and WHO, *The State of Food Security and Nutrition in the World 2023: Urbanization, Agrifood Systems Transformation and Healthy Diets across the Rural-Urban Continuum* (Rome: FAO, 2023).

14 UNICEF, "Malnutrition in Children," accessed March 18, 2024. https://data.unicef.org/topic/nutrition/malnutrition/

15 S. Sousa, S. I. Lança de Morais, G. Albuquerque, et al., "Patterns of Street Food Purchase in Cities from Central Asia," *Frontiers in Nutrition* 9 (2022): 925771; G. Albuquerque, I. Lança de Morais, M. Gelormini, et al., "Availability and Nutritional Composition of Street Food in Urban Central Asia: Findings from Almaty, Kazakhstan," *International Journal of Public Health*, 67 (2022): 1604558.

16 J. Powles, S. Fahimi, R. Micha, et al., "Global, Regional and National Sodium Intakes in 1990 and 2010: A Systematic Analysis of 24 h Urinary Sodium Excretion and Dietary Surveys Worldwide," *BMJ Open* 3, 12 (2013): e003733.

17 Institute for Health Metrics and Evaluation (IHME), "GBD Compare," accessed March 18, 2024. http://vizhub.healthdata.org/gbd-compare

18 FAO, "FAOSTAT: Suite of Food Security Indicators," accessed March 18, 2024. https://www.fao.org/faostat

19 WHO, "Global Health Observatory," accessed March 18, 2024. https://www.who.int/data/gho/data/indicators

20 Global Diet Quality Project, accessed March 18, 2024. https://www.dietquality.org

21 Food Security Portal, "Vulnerability to Global Market Shocks V.2: Price Shocks to Major Staple Foods," accessed March 18, 2024. https://www.foodsecurityportal.org/node/2505 (2023).

22 Global Fortification Data Exchange, "Country Fortification Dashboard," accessed March 18, 2024. https://fortificationdata.org/

23 FAO, IFAD, UNICEF, WFP, and WHO, *The State of Food Security and Nutrition in the World 2023: Urbanization, Agrifood Systems Transformation and Healthy Diets across the Rural-Urban Continuum* (Rome: FAO, 2023).

24 FAO, IFAD, World Meteorological Organization (WMO), WHO, UNICEF, United Nations (UN), WFP, *Regional Overview of Food Security and Nutrition in Europe and Central Asia 2022: Repurposing Policies and Incentives to Make Healthy Diets More Affordable and Agrifood Systems More Environmentally Sustainable* (Budapest: FAO, 2023).

25 C. Fang and M. Gurinović, eds., *Sustainable and Nutrition-Sensitive Food Systems for Healthy Diets and Prevention of Malnutrition in Europe and Central Asia* (Budapest: FAO, 2023). https://doi.org/10.4060/cc3907en

26 World Bank, *Agrifood Trade and Food Security in Central Asia: Possible Implications of the War in Ukraine*, Washington, 2022.

27 K. McNamara and E. Wood, "Food Taboos, Health Beliefs, and Gender: Understanding Household Food Choice and Nutrition in Rural Tajikistan," *Journal of Health, Population and Nutrition* 38 (2019): 17.

28 U. Trübwasser, R. Verstraeten, L. Salm, et al., "Factors Influencing Obesogenic Behaviours of Adolescent Girls and Women in Low- and Middle-Income Countries: A Qualitative Evidence Synthesis," *Obesity Reviews* 22, 4 (2021): e13163.

29 K. McNamara and E. Wood, "Food Taboos, Health Beliefs, and Gender: Understanding Household Food Choice and Nutrition in Rural Tajikistan," *Journal of Health, Population and Nutrition* 38 (2019): 17.

30 R. Guthold, G. A. Stevens, L. M. Riley, and F. C. Bull, "Worldwide Trends in Insufficient Physical Activity from 2001 to 2016: A Pooled Analysis of 358 Population-Based Surveys with 1.9 Million Participants," *Lancet Global Health* 6 (2018): e1077-e1086.

31 For detailed discussion of policy issues related to responses to crises and trade openness and diversity see the Central Asia section of the *2023 Global Food Policy Report*, https://gfpr.ifpri.info/2023/04/11/regional-developments-central-asia-3/

32 K. Akramov and K. Chen, *High Value Crops Help Central Asia Revitalize Agriculture. Development Asia*, Policy Brief (Mandaluyong, Philippines: Asian Development Bank, 2020); K. Akramov, K. Chen, A. Park, J. Ilyasov, and S. Eltazarov, "Agricultural Development and Cooperation in Central Asia," in *Sino-Asia Agricultural Trade and Development Cooperation: Progress, Challenges and Outlook*, eds. K. Chen and R. Mao, Chapter 5, 115-162 (Montreal: Royal Collins Publishing Group Inc., 2023).

33 I. Lambrecht, S. Pechtl, K. Akramov, J. Aliev, and P. Khakimov, "A Changing Landscape? Plots, Crops, Infrastructure, and Livestock in the Khatlon Province," *IFPRI Blog*, March 29, 2024.

34 H. Takeshima, I. Lambrecht, K. Akramov, and T. Ergasheva, "Nutrition-Sensitive Agriculture Diversification and Dietary Diversity: Panel Data Evidence from Tajikistan" IFPRI Discussion Paper 2249, Washington, DC, 2024; K. Akramov and M. Malek, "Agricultural Diversity, Dietary Diversity and Nutritional Outcomes in Tajikistan," paper presented at the *2nd Global Food Security Conference*, Ithaca, New York, October 11-14, 2015; H. Takeshima, K. Akramov, A. Park, J. Ilyasov, and T. Ergasheva, "Agriculture-Nutrition Linkages with Heterogeneous, Unobserved Returns and Costs: Insights from Tajikistan," *Agricultural Economics* 51, 4 (2020): 553-565.

35 E. Bakhshinyan, L. Molinas, and H. Alderman, "Assessing Poverty Alleviation through Social Protection: School Meals and Family Benefits in a Middle-Income Country," *Global Food Security* 23 (2019): 205-2011.

36 G.M. Bui, "Strengthening Food Safety Systems in the Central Asian Regional Economic Cooperation Member Countries: Current Status, Framework, and Forward Strategies, " ADB Central and West Asia Working Paper Series No. 11, Asian Development Bank, 2022.

SOUTH ASIA

1 M. Sharma, A. Kishore, D. Roy, and K. Joshi, "A Comparison of the Indian Diet with the EAT-Lancet Reference Diet," *BMC Public Health* 20, 1 (2020): 1-13.

2 Global Diet Quality Project, 2024. www.dietquality.org/indicators

3 S.K.T. Baah, R.A.C. Aguilar, C. Diaz Bonilla, T. Fujs, C. Lakner, M.C. Nguyen, and M. Viveros, "September 2023 Global Poverty Update from the World Bank: New Data on Poverty during the Pandemic in Asia," *World Bank Blogs*, September 20, 2023.

4 Food and Agriculture Organization of the United Nations (FAO), International Fund for Agricultural Development (IFAD), UNICEF, World Food Programme (WFP), and World Health Organization (WHO), *The State of Food Security and Nutrition in the World 2023: Urbanization, Agrifood Systems Transformation and Healthy Diets across the Rural-Urban Continuum* (Rome: FAO, 2023).

5 K. Hirvonen, Y. Bai, D.D. Headey, and W.A. Masters, "Affordability of the EAT-Lancet Reference Diet: A Global Analysis," *Lancet Global Health* 8, 1 (2020): e59-e66.

6 A. Herforth, Y. Bai, A. Venkat, K. Mahrt, A. Ebel, and W.A. Masters, "Cost and Affordability of Healthy Diets across and within Countries: Background Paper for the State of Food Security and Nutrition in the World 2020," FAO Agricultural Development Economics Technical Study No. 9, FAO, Rome, 2020.

7 Y. Bai, R. Alemu, S.A. Block, D.D. Headey, and W.A. Masters, "Cost and Affordability of Nutritious Diets at Retail Prices: Evidence from 177 Countries," Food Policy 99 (2021): 101983; K. Raghunathan, D.D. Headey, and A. Herforth, "Affordability of Nutritious Diets in Rural India," Food Policy 99 (2021): 101982.

8 Y. Bai, R. Alemu, S.A. Block, D.D. Headey, and W.A. Masters, "Cost and Affordability of Nutritious Diets at Retail Prices: Evidence from 177 Countries," *Food Policy* 99 (2021): 101983.

9 D.D. Headey and H.H. Alderman, "The Relative Caloric Prices of Healthy and Unhealthy Foods Differ Systematically across Income Levels and Continents," *The Journal of Nutrition* 149, 11 (2019): 2020-2033.

10 Development Initiatives, *2018 Global Nutrition Report: Shining a Light to Spur Action on Nutrition* (Bristol, UK: 2018).

11 P. Pingali, B. Mittra, and A. Rahman, "The Bumpy Road from Food to Nutrition Security-Slow Evolution of India's Food Policy," *Global Food Security* 15 (2017): 77-84.

12 S. Desai and R. Vanneman, "Enhancing Nutrition Security via India's National Food Security Act: Using an Axe Instead of a Scalpel?" *India Policy Forum* 11 (2015): 67-113.

13 R. Khera, "India's Public Distribution System: Utilisation and Impact," *Journal of Development Studies* 47, 7 (2011): 1038-1060.

14 T. Kaul, "Household Responses to Food Subsidies: Evidence from India," *Economic Development and Cultural Change* 67, 1 (2018): 95-129.

15 A. Kishore, P.K. Joshi, and J.F. Hoddinott, "India's Right to Food Act: A Novel Approach to Food Security," *2013 Global Food Policy Report* (Washington, DC: IFPRI, 2014).

16 R. Khera, "Cash vs. In-Kind Transfers: Indian Data Meets Theory," *Food Policy* 46 (2014): 116-128.

17 R. Khera, "India's Public Distribution System: Utilisation and Impact," *Journal of Development Studies* 47, 7 (2011): 1038-1060; M. Pradhan, D. Roy, and V. Sonkar, "What Is the Effective Delivery Mechanism of Food Support in India?" *Economic and Political Weekly* 54, 42 (2019): 37.

18 R.L. Naylor, A. Kishore, U.R. Sumaila, et al., "Blue Food Demand across Geographic and Temporal Scales," *Nature Communications* 12, 1 (2021): 5413.

19 M. Sharma, A. Kishore, D. Roy, and K. Joshi, "A Comparison of the Indian Diet with the EAT-Lancet Reference Diet," *BMC Public Health* 20, 1 (2020): 1-13.

20 Calculated by authors using the Centre for Monitoring Indian Economy (CMIE) data 2015-2019. US dollar amount calculated using the 2019 currency exchange rate (1 US$ = 70.4 INR).

21 WHO, *The Growth of Ultra-Processed Foods in India: An Analysis of Trends, Issues and Policy Recommendations* (New Delhi: 2023).

22 P. Pingali, "Agricultural Policy and Nutrition Outcomes: Getting Beyond the Preoccupation with Staple Grains," *Food Security* 7 (2015): 583-591.

23 P.S. Birthal, D. Roy, and D.S. Negi, "Assessing the Impact of Crop Diversification on Farm Poverty in India," *World Development* 72 (2015): 70-92.

24 A. Kishore, P.K. Joshi, and J.F. Hoddinott, "India's Right to Food Act: A Novel Approach to Food Security," *2013 Global Food Policy Report* (Washington, DC: IFPRI, 2014).

25 A. Ahmed, J. Hoddinott, and S. Roy, "Food Transfers, Cash Transfers, Behavior Change Communication and Child Nutrition: Evidence from Bangladesh," IFPRI Discussion Paper 1868, IFPRI, Washington, DC, 2019.

26 C. Lane, "Meeting Health Challenges in Developing Asia with Corrective Taxes on Alcohol, Tobacco, and Unhealthy Foods," Working Paper No. 613, Center for Global Development, 2022; WHO, *The Growth of Ultra-Processed Foods in India: An Analysis of Trends, Issues and Policy Recommendations* (New Delhi: WHO, Country Office for India, 2023).

27 WHO, *The Growth of Ultra-Processed Foods in India: An Analysis of Trends, Issues and Policy Recommendations* (New Delhi: WHO, Country Office for India, 2023).

28 S. Bansal, "Food Warning Labels Are in the Deep Freeze," *Mint*, February 15, 2021.

29 M. Gupta, A. Kishore, D. Roy, and S. Saroj, "Post-Farmgate Food Businesses of India: The Enterprises, the Entrepreneurs, and the Employees," *Global Food Security* 36 (2023): 100665.

BOX 1

a S. Chakrabarti, A. Kishore, and D. Roy, "Effectiveness of Food Subsidies in Raising Healthy Food Consumption: Public Distribution of Pulses in India," *American Journal of Agricultural Economics* 100, 5 (2018): 1427-1449.

b P. Joshi, A. Kishore, and D. Roy, "Making Pulses Affordable Again: Policy Options from the Farm to Retail in India," *Economic and Political Weekly* 52, 1 (2017): 37-44.

EAST AND SOUTHEAST ASIA

1 A.-M. Thow, P. Farrell, M. Helble, and C.N. Rachmi, "Eating in Developing Asia: Trends, Consequences and Policies," Background paper for *Asian Development Outlook Update 2020* (Manila: Asian Development Bank, 2020).

2 B.M. Popkin, "The Nutrition Transition in Low-Income Countries: An Emerging Crisis," *Nutrition Reviews* 52, 9 (1994): 285-298.

3 GBD 2017 Diet Collaborators, "Health Effects of Dietary Risks in 195 Countries, 1990-2017: A Systematic Analysis for the Global Burden of Disease Study 2017," *Lancet* 393, 10184 (2019): 1958-1972.

4 Food and Agriculture Organization of the United Nations (FAO), "Food Security and Nutrition / Suite of Food Security Indicators," updated July 6, 2022. https://www.fao.org/faostat/en/#data/FS/metadata

5 Development Initiatives, *2021 Global Nutrition Report: The State of Global Nutrition* (Bristol, UK: 2021); W. Willett, J. Rockström, B. Loken, et al., "Food in the Anthropocene: The EAT-Lancet Commission on Healthy

Diets from Sustainable Food Systems," *Lancet* 393, 10170 (2019): 447-492.

6 M.S. Amarra and G.L. Khor (2015), "Sodium Consumption in Southeast Asia: An Updated Review of Intake Levels and Dietary Sources in Six Countries," in *Preventive Nutrition*, ed. A. Bendich (Cham, Switzerland: Springer, 2015).

7 Global Diet Quality Project, "Global Diet Quality Project," accessed November 2, 2023. https://www.dietquality.org/

8 World Food Programme (WFP), *Micronutrient Landscape in Southeast Asia. Status, Strategies & Future Directions* (Bangkok: 2022).

9 O. Huse, E. Reeve, P. Baker, D. Hunt, C. Bell, A. Peeters, and K. Backholer, "The Nutrition Transition, Food Retail Transformations, and Policy Responses to Overnutrition in the East Asia Region: A Descriptive Review," *Obesity Reviews* 23, 4 (2022): e13412; J. Harris, P.H. Nguyen, L.M. Tran, and P.N. Huynh, "Nutrition Transition in Vietnam: Changing Food Supply, Food Prices, Household Expenditure, Diet and Nutrition Outcomes," *Food Security* 12 (2020): 1141-1155; K. Sievert, M. Lawrence, A. Naika, and P. Baker, "Processed Foods and Nutrition Transition in the Pacific: Regional Trends, Patterns and Food System Drivers," *Nutrients* 11, 6 (2019): 1328; E.V. Goh, S. Azam-Ali, F. McCullough, and S.R. Mitra, "The Nutrition Transition in Malaysia; Key Drivers and Recommendations for Improved Health Outcomes," *BMC Nutrition* 6 (2020): 32.

10 World Health Organization (WHO), "Obesity and Overweight," updated June 9, 2021. https://www.who.int/news-room/fact-sheets/detail/obesity-and-overweight

11 NCD-RisC (NCD Risk Factor Collaboration), Country Risk Factor Data, accessed October 20, 2023. https://ncdrisc.org/data-downloads.html

12 FAO, UNICEF, WFP, and WHO, *Asia and the Pacific - Regional Overview of Food Security and Nutrition 2022: Urban Food Security and Nutrition* (Bangkok: FAO, 2023). https://doi.org/10.4060/cc3990e

13 A. Macfarlane, "Building Resilient, Equitable and Sustainable Food Systems in Asia," International Finance Corporation, September 26, 2022.

14 J. Harris, T. Hrynick, M.T.M. Thien, T. Huynh, P. Huynh, P. Nguyen, and A.-M. Thow, "Tensions and Coalitions: A New Trade Agreement Affects the Policy Space for Nutrition in Vietnam," *Food Security* 14 (2022): 1123-1141.

15 High Level Panel of Experts (HLPE), *Reducing Inequalities for Food Security and Nutrition* (Rome: FAO, 2023).

16 International Labour Organization (ILO), *Asia-Pacific Sectoral Labour Market Profile: Agriculture*, ILO Brief (Geneva: 2022).

17 Association of Southeast Asian Nations (ASEAN), *Regional Study on Informal Employment Statistics to Support Decent Work Promotion in ASEAN* (Jakarta: 2019).

18 B.M. Popkin, "The Nutrition Transition in Low-Income Countries: An Emerging Crisis," *Nutrition Reviews* 52, 9 (1994): 285-298.

19 S. Das and R. Paul, "Urbanization Trend of South, East, and Southeast Asian Countries: Influence of Economic Growth and Changing Trends in Employment Sectors," *Current Urban Studies* 9, 4 (2021): 694-719.

20 FAO, UNICEF, WFP, and WHO, *Asia and the Pacific - Regional Overview of Food Security and Nutrition 2022: Urban Food Security and Nutrition* (Bangkok: FAO, 2023).

21 P. Baker and S. Friel, "Food Systems Transformations, Ultra-Processed Food Markets and The Nutrition Transition in Asia," *Globalization and Health* 12, 1 (2016): 80.

22 P. Farrell, C.N. Rachmi, G. Mulcahy, M. Helble, and A.-M. Thow, "Food Environment Research Is Needed to Improve Nutrition and Well-Being in Asia and the Pacific," *Public Health Nutrition* 24, 14 (2021): 4706-4710.

23 FAO, *Climate Change, Biodiversity and Nutrition Nexus - Evidence and Emerging Policy and Programming Opportunities* (Rome: 2021).

24 W. David and D. Kofahl, *Food Culture of Southeast Asia: Perspective of Social Science and Food Science* (Kassel, Germany: Kassel University Press, 2017).

25 World Bank, Food Prices for Nutrition database, accessed October 20, 2023. https://databank.worldbank.org/source/food-prices-for-nutrition

26 Y. Bai, R. Alemu, S.A. Block, D.D. Headey, and W.A. Masters, "Cost and Affordability of Nutritious Diets at Retail Prices: Evidence from 177 Countries," *Food Policy* 99 (2021): 101983.

27 Asian Development Bank, *Key Indicators for Asia and the Pacific 2022*, 53rd ed (Manila: 2022).

28 WFP, *Food Security and Diets in Urban Asia: How Resilient Are Food Systems in Times of COVID-19?* (Bangkok: 2022).

29 Cargill, *Fixing Asia's Food System* (Singapore: 2018); M. Francois, B. Jesse, V. Lertkriangkraisorn, and S.M. Veranen, "How Grocers Could Use Sustainability to Transform Asian Food Systems," *McKinsey & Company Insights*, December. 13, 2022.

30 HLPE, *Reducing Inequalities for Food Security and Nutrition* (Rome: FAO, 2023).

31 HLPE, *Reducing Inequalities for Food Security and Nutrition* (Rome: FAO, 2023).

32 HLPE, *Reducing Inequalities for Food Security and Nutrition* (Rome: FAO, 2023).

33 ILO, *Asia-Pacific Sectoral Labour Market Profile: Agriculture*, ILO Brief (Geneva: 2022).

34 J.M. Dixon, J. Weerahewa, J. Hellin, et al. "Response and Resilience of Asian Agrifood Systems to COVID-19: An Assessment across Twenty-Five Countries and Four Regional Farming and Food Systems," *Agricultural Systems* 193 (2021): 103168.

35 J. Harris, T. Hrynick, M.T.M. Thien, T. Huynh, P. Huynh, P. Nguyen, and A.-M. Thow, "Tensions and Coalitions: A New Trade Agreement Affects the Policy Space for Nutrition in Vietnam," *Food Security* 14 (2022): 1123-1141.

36 O. Huse, E. Reeve, P. Baker, D. Hunt, C. Bell, A. Peeters, and K. Backholer, "The Nutrition Transition, Food Retail Transformations, and Policy Responses to Overnutrition in the East Asia Region: A Descriptive Review," *Obesity Reviews* 23, 4 (2022): e13412.

37 ASEAN, *ASEAN Food Safety Policy* (Jakarta: 2016).

38 O. Huse, E. Reeve, P. Baker, D. Hunt, C. Bell, A. Peeters, and K. Backholer, "The Nutrition Transition, Food Retail Transformations, and Policy Responses to Overnutrition in the East Asia Region: A Descriptive Review," *Obesity Reviews* 23, 4 (2022): e13412.

39 FAO, "Food-Based Dietary Guidelines: China" (Rome: 2022).

40 G. Acharya, E. Cassou, S. Jaffee, and E.K. Ludher, *RICH Food, Smart City. How Building Reliable, Inclusive, Competitive, and Healthy Food Systems Is Smart Policy for Urban Asia* (Washington, DC: World Bank, 2021).

41 G. Acharya, E. Cassou, S. Jaffee, and E.K. Ludher, *RICH Food, Smart City. How Building Reliable, Inclusive, Competitive, and Healthy Food Systems Is Smart Policy for Urban Asia* (Washington, DC: World Bank, 2021).

42 HLPE, *Reducing Inequalities for Food Security and Nutrition* (Rome: FAO, 2023).

43 B.A. Swinburn, V. I. Kraak, S. Allender, V.J. Atkins, P.I. Baker, J.R. Bogard, and W.H. Dietz, "The Global Syndemic of Obesity, Undernutrition, and Climate Change: The Lancet Commission Report," *Lancet*, 393 10173 (2019): 791-846.

44 HLPE, *Reducing Inequalities for Food Security and Nutrition* (Rome: FAO, 2023); GloPAN, *Food Systems and Diets: Facing the Challenges of the 21st Century* (London: 2016).

BOX 1

a Cambodia, National Institute of Statistics, *Report of Cambodia Socio-Economic Survey 2021* (Phnom Penh: Ministry of Planning, National Institute of Statistics, 2022).

b Development Initiatives, *2021 Global Nutrition Report: The State of Global Nutrition* (Bristol, UK: 2021).

c National Institute of Statistics, *Report of Cambodia Socio-Economic Survey 2021* (Phnom Penh: Ministry of Planning, National Institute of Statistics, 2022).

d Development Initiatives, *2021 Global Nutrition Report: The State of Global Nutrition* (Bristol, UK: 2021); Cambodia, National Institute of Statistics, Report of Cambodia Socio-Economic Survey 2021 (Phnom Penh: Ministry of Planning, National Institute of Statistics, 2022).

e Global Panel on Agriculture and Food Systems for Nutrition (GloPAN), *Food Systems and Diets: Facing the Challenges of the 21st Century* (London: 2016).

f Academy of Global Food Economics and Policy (AGFEP), *2022 China and Global Food Policy Report* (Beijing: 2022); AGFEP, *2023 China and Global Food Policy Report* (Beijing: 2023).

g Chinese Center for Disease Control and Prevention, *Report on Nutrition and Chronic Disease Status of Chinese Residents-2020* (Beijing: People's Medical Publishing House, 2021).

h M. Springmann, L. Spajic, M.A. Clark, et al., "The Healthiness and Sustainability of National and Global Food Based Dietary Guidelines: Modelling Study," *BMJ* 370 (2020): m2322.

i GloPAN, *Food Systems and Diets: Facing the Challenges of the 21st Century* (London: 2016).

j GloPAN, *Food Systems and Diets: Facing the Challenges of the 21st Century* (London: 2016).

k Cambodia, National Institute of Statistics, *Report of Cambodia Socio-Economic Survey 2021* (Phnom Penh: Ministry of Planning, National Institute of Statistics, 2022).

l *WFP, Food Security and Diets in Urban Asia: How Resilient Are Food Systems in Times of COVID-19?* (Bangkok: 2022).

LATIN AMERICA AND THE CARIBBEAN

1 E. Díaz-Bonilla, *What Is Food and Nutrition Security and How to Measure It?* (San José, Costa Rica: IICA, 2023) analyzes these and other indicators related to food security and nutrition.

2 Food and Agriculture Organization of the United Nations (FAO), International Fund for Agricultural Development (IFAD), UNICEF, World Food Program (WFP), and World Health Organization (WHO), *The State of Food Security and Nutrition in the World 2023. Urbanization, Agrifood Systems Transformation and Healthy Diets across the Rural-Urban Continuum* (Rome: FAO, 2023).

3 E. Díaz-Bonilla, "Haiti and Its Multiple Tragedies: Much More Needs to Be Done," LAC Working Paper 26, International Food Policy Research Institute (IFPRI), Washington, DC, 2022. https://doi.org/10.2499/p15738coll2.135035

4 FAO, FAOSTAT database, accessed January 2024, http://faostat.fao.org

5 See a more detailed discussion of these indicators by countries in E. Díaz-Bonilla, *What Is Food and Nutrition Security and How to Measure It?* (San José, Costa Rica: IICA, 2023).

6 E. Díaz-Bonilla, "Reflexiones sobre El Desarrollo Agropecuario, Rural y de Los Sistemas Agro-alimentarios en América Latina y El Caribe," *Revista Pensamiento Iberoamericano*, 80-84 (Madrid: Secretaría General Iberoamericana, 2023).

7 C. Hawkes, M.T. Ruel, L. Salm, B. Sinclair, and F. Branca, "Double-Duty Actions: Seizing Programme and Policy Opportunities to Address Malnutrition in All Its Forms," *Lancet* 395 (1028): 142-155.

8 United Nations Economic Commission for Latin America and the Caribbean (CEPAL), *Institucionalidad Social en América Latina y El Caribe: Eje Central para Avanzar Hacia un Desarrollo Social Inclusivo* (Santiago: 2023).

9 WFP and UNICEF, *All the Right Tracks: Delivering Shock-Responsive Social Protection in the Sahel–Learnings from the COVID-19 Response* (Rome: WFP, 2023).

10 E. Diaz-Bonilla, V. Piñeiro, and D. Laborde, "Latin America and the Caribbean: Food Systems in Times of the Pandemic," in *Advances in Food Security and Sustainability*, ed. M.J. Cohen, vol. 6, 263-288 (Cambridge, MA: Elsevier, 2021).

11 C.P.D Silva, A.C. Bento, and E. Guaraldo, "The Impact of Front-of-the-Packaging Nutrition Labelling Warnings on Consumer Habits: A Scoping Review Exploring the Case of the Chilean Food Law," *British Food Journal* 124, 13 (2022): 66-80.

12 World Bank, *Taxes on Sugar-Sweetened Beverages: Summary of International Evidence and Experiences* (Washington, DC: 2020).

13 L. Lefebvre, B. McNamara, and V. Piñeiro, "Realizing the Potential of Neglected Crops in Latin America," *IFPRI Blog*, July 5, 2023.

14 FAO, IFAD, Pan American Health Organization, UNICEF, and WFP, *Regional Overview of Food Security and Nutrition–Latin America and the Caribbean 2022: Towards Improving Affordability of Healthy Diets* (Santiago: FAO, 2023).

15 R. Remans, S.A. Wood, N. Saha, T.L. Anderman, and R.S. DeFries, "Measuring Nutritional Diversity of National Food Supplies," *Global Food Security* 3, 3-4 (2014): 174-182.

16 J. Dithmer, A. Abdulai, "Does Trade Openness Contribute to Food Security? A Dynamic Panel Analysis, *Food Policy* 69 (2017): 218-230.

17 FAO and IFPRI, *La Seguridad Alimentaria y El Comercio Agroalimentario en América Latina y El Caribe* (Santiago: 2023).

Made in United States
North Haven, CT
05 November 2026

21763083R00082